Remission towards Curing: Alzheimer's, Parkinson's and Multiple Sclerosis
Nutritional Integrative Therapies

James C. Tibbetts, STL, MBA
Anne Marie Tibbetts, MS, RD

Disclaimer Notice: You have the constitutional right to prescribe for yourself and to determine your own diet and detoxification methods but the writers and publisher assume no responsibility. If you use the information in this book without the approval of a health professional, you prescribe for yourself, which remains your constitutional right. The authors and publisher do not intend to diagnose or prescribe. Nutritionists and other health experts in the field of health and nutrition hold widely varying views.

The Scripture citations are taken in part or whole from various bibles including: *The New American Bible* (Thomas Nelson Publisher, 1970); *The Jerusalem Bible* (Doubleday & Co., 1966); *Revised Standard Version, King James Version* (Zondervan Bible Publishers, 1978); *The Holy Bible Douay-Rheims Version*, (Tan Books and Pub., 1971); *Holy Bible from the Ancient Eastern Text*, translation from the *Aramaic of the Peshitta* by George M. Lamsa, (Harper SanFrancisco,1961); *Aramaic English New Testament Peshitta English Aramaic critical Edition* translation by Andrew Michael Roth (Netzari Press, 2008); *Jewish New Testament* trans. by David H. Stern (Jewish New Testament Publications, Inc., 1989).

Published By
Jim Tibbetts
Living Foods Technology, LLC
P.O. Box 2533
Glenville, New York 12325

www.jimtibbetts.com

This book is dedicated to:

Pope John Paul II
& those seeking the Culture of Life

Pope John Paul II had Parkinson's disease, and even with this disease he gave his life fully to preaching the Gospel. The Vatican confirmed the diagnosis in 2003, after keeping it quiet for about 12 years. Sister Marie Simon-Pierre had Parkinson's disease in June 2005. She prayed to Jesus and to the late John Paul II (1920-2005). One morning after getting up, her Parkinson's had vanished, a mystery confirmed by a local medical team. She recounted her story to Vatican officials. ... (See section on prayer)

Jesus Christ is there for those who seek Him. Pray for you're healing in the spirit, and work towards your healing through nature with nutrition and fasting. A person need to choose daily, "the culture of Life" or "the culture of Death."

"For us too, Moses' invitation rings out loud and clear: 'See, I have set before you this day life and prosperity, death and disaster' (Deut 30:15 JB) . . . 'This invitation is very appropriate for us who are called day by day to the "daily duty" of choosing between the "culture of life" and the "culture of death".'" "The Gospel of Life is at the heart of Jesus' message." "Jesus says: 'I came that they may have life, and have it abundantly' (Jn 10:10)."
          Blessed Pope John Paul II - March 25, 1995,
          His Encyclical: *Gospel of Life*, versus 28, 1.

Table of Contents

Part III - The Nutritional Therapy Used

Introduction

This book is about the body going into remission and curing through a nutritional therapy approach! This book presents real people, some cured and some not, about clinical experience, journal studies, nutritional understandings and testimonials.

Remission implies that the disease is stopped but still exists and is dormant. Curing implies the person is self-healing. The strict plant-based diet is putting the disease into remission and over time the human system is heading to curing the disease. But if the person leaves the strict raw diet and goes back to the standard American meat-based diet, the disease could come back. In other words a person can remain free of the disease as long as they remain on a plant-based Live-food type of nutritional approach.

Throughout this book we have focused on plant-based nutrition and it will be called Live or Living or raw Plant-based Nutrition, this will help to distinguish it from the standard American vegetarian diet which is usually cooked and full of grains and healthy junk foods found in health food stores. There are other methods like fasting and exercise which are also needed to achieve optimum nutrition and curing of the disease.

Pharmaceutical drug usage is not the subject of this book but obviously they are not curing these diseases. Drug companies want to keep a disease in remission so that the person would need to keep taking pharmaceutical drugs for the rest of their lives. In this book, the disease is put into remission through a nutritional therapy approach and is able to get off drugs or most of them. They can live out their lives, in a normal and healthy way.

There is a psychological and spiritual dimension, which is also motivational. By using scriptures this book is both a moral teaching and a systematic teaching on the Jewish people and the early Christians who choose a plant-based diet. This was, for them, a moral choice for the Culture of Life over the Culture of Death, in relation to food and fasting. This dimension is usually needed to succeed.

This book is about the Culture of Life over the Culture of Death! All the chapters close with a spiritual section because without a conversion of heart and mind, the scientific center section could do them little good, since they may not move forward and follow the Live-Food Nutrition approach. Spirituality helps to open the heart. An open heart leads to an open mind and emotions, which leads to open hands, to do the work needed.

A nutritional approach to cure a chronic disease requires a lot of work to do the food preparation. If a person is not willing to put the time in and do the work of food prep; then they will probably not be put into remission or cured.

This book is years in the making. James Tibbetts is the primary author and wrote the first draft of this book, and Anne Marie Tibbetts gave her nutrition expertise and many corrections in the revisions.

We hope and pray that this book is beneficial to you in bringing you greater health, peace of mind and healing of PD, AD, and MS, and related diseases. When you are cured of your disease, to some degree, let us know; write us, we love to collect testimonials!

"My dear friend, I hope you are in good health and may you thrive in all other ways as you do in the spirit." 3 John 2

To your good health and thriving in the spirit,
James Tibbetts
Anne Marie Tibbetts

Part I – Medical, Nutritional Paradigms

Chapter 1
The Culture of Life

The famous 5th century monk <u>Dionysius the Areopagite</u> says, "Purified souls, being raised up to the heights of contemplation, participate in the Divine, 'Thus do we learn that it is the Cause and Origin and Being and Life of all creation. (Gen 1) It is a Principle of Illumination to them that are being enlightened; a Principle of Perfection to them that are being perfected; a principle of Deity to them that are being deified; and of Simplicity to them that are being brought into simplicity.'[a]"[1]

The Father of Medicine - Hippocrates (460-377 BC) stated, "Let your food be your medicine and let your medicine be your food."

a. A Seven-fold Therapy Methodology

The approach used here is primarily Evidence-Based Nutrition, but also taken into account are the journal studies and experience from Evidence-Based Medicine, whose focus is primarily pharmaceutical drugs. This book will describe the seven-part methodology of curing major degenerative diseases, like Parkinson's (PD), Alzheimer's (AD) and Multiple Sclerosis (MS). The major focus is primarily a nutritional and fasting approach. The other approaches are added in because they are also important in relation to nutrition. The seven categories are:

---

[a] Illumination: as in Purgation, Illumination and Union. Perfection: technical usage as in 1 Cor. 2:6; Phil. 3:15. Deity: as St. Bernard bluntly says: "To experience this state is to be deified." Simplicity: soul turns from complex world to having one desire - for God, in a simple and unified state, Mat 6:22.

1. Living Plant-based Nutrition
2. Juice and/or Water Fasting
3. Supplementation
4. Curative Exercises
5. Purification advanced methods (as needed)
6. Counseling or coaching
7. Prayer and Meditation

Healing occurs on three levels: physiological, psychological and spiritual. The roots of illness can start in the body and move into the soul, if the illness is rooted out of the body but not the soul, the roots of illness may grow back into the body. Or the roots of illness could start in the soul (mind, emotions and will) or the human spirit and grow from there. In the long run the body, soul and spirit need to be purified of this illness. Purification is a key concept.

1. Living Plant-based Nutrition
Plant-based nutrition is either vegetarian, vegan, raw vegan or Live-food nutrition. The problem with the plant-based diet approach today is that there are too many healthy-junk foods in the health food stores. For some people, eating French fries and potato chips are plant-based nutrition. To make the distinction for a healing plant-based nutrition diet, the term Live or Living is used. Actually the Latin term *"vegetus"* used for vegetarian means living or alive or dynamic. This is the type of food used in the healing process of chronic diseases. All raw plant-based foods like vegetables and fruits are "living foods" and are usually in their optimum state.

2. Juice and/or Water Fasting
Anyone can do a seven to ten day juice fast on their own; this is noted by most every book on fasting. If a person is going to fast longer than ten days, then a professional is helpful since a person is entering into the therapeutic fasting stage. A seven day fast is general housecleaning for the

body, but a fourteen day fast or longer involves more therapeutic healing for the body.

3. Supplementation

Most people want to see some scientific journal studies on the benefits of vitamins. Studies on vitamins have been out for a long time. *Geriatric Nutrition: The Health Professional's Handbook* (2006) states: "Nutrition-related risk factors may include inadequacy of essential nutrients, particularly vitamin B12, B6, folate, and the antioxidants vitamin C, vitamin E, and Beta-carotene. Recent studies suggest that individuals with cognitive impairment are at risk for nutrition-related problems.[2] [3] Several studies indicate that elderly people who live alone or in institutions have dietary intakes of vitamins and minerals below recommended levels."[4] [5] Many doctors usually don't want to waste their time with vitamins and minerals; they figure that's a job for a Registered Dietitian.

4. Curative Exercise

Sports like football, baseball, hockey, golf, tennis and the like are not curative exercise even though there might be some psychological benefit to them. Exercise routines like yoga and Pilates are curative exercises, this is what they were originally designed for and they accomplish healing. A Pilates' teacher noted that she has a lot of clients who play golf and tennis who have muscle problems because they only swing on one side of their body and she has to give them exercises to help them balance their muscles out.

5. Purification: Advanced Methods

This topic is a bit controversial but it is a method that is not fasting or supplementation, even though these can be purification methods. It involves complex methodologies such as neutralizing the chemical of a disease, or using homeopathy, or other energy methodologies.

Throughout this book we focus on two main ways of putting into remission or curing these diseases: juice fasting

3

and Live-Food nutrition. Curing through an 'antidote' can be neutralizing the chemical, pesticide, or poison that is the primary antagonist causing the disease.[b] Homeopathic medicine by itself could heal a disease, or advanced work by a chemist could develop an antidote for the poison that is behind the disease. But paying a chemist is expensive and not financially practical for most people. Actually both fasting and live-food nutrition purifies the body of chemicals, pesticides, or other poisons and could cure the disease.

6. Counseling

Counseling is oftentimes needed to keep the patient's feelings from getting in the way of the healing process. In the counseling chapter, an example is given of a person who was being cured of MS and following the diet perfectly but she became angry and that stopped the process of healing. She needed counseling to deal with her anger before the healing process could continue. Compliance is the biggest problem. Most people don't follow through with the plant-based diet, but eat what they want to. They need counseling to create behavior change.

7. Prayer and Meditation

Prayer is a spiritual activity. This is something that is partly outside our control since the person is entering into the supernatural realm, the realm of the Divine. Prayer can and will help in all circumstances of people who have PD and MS. But expecting a complete cure of PD and MS through prayer alone is rare in the literature. An example of a religious sister healed of Parkinson's through prayer is given in the discussion on prayer. Meditation is a process of slowly healing the psyche and bringing the person deeper into the spiritual life. Meditation is different from prayer, it is an activity of the soul, and prayer comes out of the human spirit.

---

[b] Neutralizing the chemical causing the disease, see section f, the daughter of Rebecca Carley, MD

b. People in Remission towards Curing

Are there any people with PD, AD or MS that have been cured? Yes, in the research done for this book, there are people around the country that have been cured. All of these were cured through a Live Plant-based diet with juicing and/or fasting.

Real names are given of some of those who have been cured, but those still struggling with PD or MS have been given fictional names and are not listed here. The reasons people are not cured can provide useful information. In this book the actual names of people who conquered Parkinson's, Alzheimer's and Multiple Sclerosis, and the people that helped put these people into remission or cured them are:

- Monica B. cured of Parkinson's by Dr. Shelton
- Parkinson's Patient of Tosca Haag, MD
- Parkinson's Patient of Dr. Ray Kent
- Parkinson's Patient of Fred Bisci, PhD
- Two Parkinson's Clients of Bill Irwin, MS, MSW
- Two Parkinson's Clients of Anne Wigmore's Institutes on the West Coast
- Parkinson's patient Andrea Proudfoot, Gerson Therapy hospital and Halleluiah Diet
- Parkinson's Patient in Alaska of Dr. Schulze
- MS Cure of Matt Goodman
- Dr. Graham's testimonial Jim's cure of MS
- Ms. W.O., an MS client of Dr. Shelton
- Fr. F.J., an MS client of Dr. Shelton
- Eddie in Brisbane, Australia, cured of MS
- Judi Hurst in Florida, cured of MS
- Pastor Bob East, cured of MS
- Lani of Central Point, OR, cured of MS
- Donna cured of MS
- Dale K. of Tennessee, cured of MS
- Pastor Michael Sustar of Phoenix, AZ, cured of MS

- Alan Greer cured of MS through diet
- Carol cured of MS through diet
- Darlene cured of MS through diet
- Robert Trincellito from New York, cured of MS
- Judy Livingstone cured of MS
- Ann Boroch, a naturopath practitioner, cured of MS
- Dr. F.J., Optometrist, cured of MS by Dr. Shelton
- Pam's mother with Alzheimer's by Dr. Graham
- A woman with Alzheimer's by Dr. Schultz
- Alzheimer's client by Dr. Scott's
- Dr. Roy Swank's patients in his studies
- Dr. John McDougall's patients in his study

Several Important Studies on MS noted are:

The low-fat diet treatment of MS was developed by Roy Swank, MD, who treated more than 5000 people over the past 50 years. The results were remarkable. Dr. Swank has four major journal studies that disucss data on curing MS through a low fat semi-vegetarian diet. (*Lancet*, 1990; *Nutrition*, 1991; *Am J Clin Nutr.*, 1988; *Arch Neurol,* 1970)

John McDougall, MD was mentored by Roy Swank, MD. Dr. McDougalls's Research and Education Foundation has funded a study with the Neurology Department in the School of Medicine, of Oregon Health and Science University in Portland, on the dietary treatment of Multiple Sclerosis (MS) with a low-fat vegan diet. This study with over 20 people that finished up in 2013, was very successful and the results will be published soon.

MS is close to Parkinson's and Alzheimer's in many of the disease parameters and medical issues. The testimonials and case studies presented here indicate not only MS, but also PD and AD, are curable. But PD and AD need a stricter diet than what Dr. Swank or Dr. McDougall are using to treat MS.

It is sad, but some people cured of MS and PD through this approach do not want to share their healings with others. One owner of an institute said they can't give out names or information because of legal and confidentiality agreements that their patients sign. The author knows from other sources that they have cured a lot of MS clients through this approach, basically using the Anne Wigmore (Hippocrates) diet.

Several foundations have been contacted and given a copy of an earlier version this book in the past including: The Michael J. Fox Foundation; Tom Hartman Foundation; and the Muhammad Ali Foundation. The author visited Fr. Tom Hartman in person and the staff at the Muhammad Ali Center.

c. Numbers and Stages of PD, AD and MS

Today, there are about 1.8 to 2 million Americans with Parkinson's disease (in 2002 about 1.4 million)[c] and about 50,000 - 60,000 new cases are diagnosed every year. Most people with Parkinson's are older but about four percent are under 50 years of age. Men are about one and a half times more likely to have Parkinson's than women. There are over 10 million people worldwide who have Parkinson's.

In 2002, the estimates differed from 1.2, 1.4 to 1.5 million.[6] PD was rare among the young but now Parkinson's is occurring in people under 60 at an estimated rate of 5 to 10%, and in some as early as in their twenties. Both the rate of PD and the incidence of younger people with PD are on the rise.

Alzheimer disease (AD) is the most common form of dementia and is classified as a neurodegenerative disorder.

---

[c] If we assume, as the pharmaceutical companies do, that 70% of people with PD are on the drug, *Sinemet*, then there are about 1,400,000 people with PD, (in a population of 270,000,000 in 2002 it is more now).

Short term memory loss is one of the first signs of AD. As the disease advances, symptoms can include confusion, irritability, and aggression, trouble with language, mood swings and long-term memory loss.[7]

In 2006, there were about 26.6 million, and in 2013 there were over 44.4 million people worldwide with Alzheimer's. One prediction is that it will affect 1 in 85 globally by 2050.[8] The World Health Organization estimated that in 2005, 0.379% of the people worldwide had dementia, and that the prevalence would increase to 0.441% in 2015 and to 0.556% in 2030.[9] The incidence of Alzheimer's has been shown to increase with age. Every five years, after the age of 65, the risk of acquiring the disease approximately doubles, increasing from 3 to as much as 69 per thousand person per year.[10] [11]

"In 1979, according to official statistics of the Centers for Disease Control, 653 people died of Alzheimer's Disease in the United States. In 1991, that figure leapt to 13,768. In addition, by 2002, over 58,785 people died of Alzheimer's disease in the United States. In other words, in a period of twenty-four years there has been an 8,902 percent increase in the deaths from Alzheimer's disease in the United States. Clearly we have a huge epidemic on our hands."[12] "The situation is similar in the United Kingdom."[13] A recent study (3/2014) at Rush University found the death toll was 503,400 rather than 83,000 because the death certificates did not list AD as a cause of death on many certificates.

There are over 5.2 million Americans of all ages with Alzheimer's disease in 2013. Alzheimer's is the 6th leading cause of death in the U.S. overall and 5th leading cause of death over age 65. Throughout the coming decades, the baby boom generation is going to add about 10 million to the total number of people in the U.S. with AD. Worldwide dementia is estimated to be at 75.6 million by 2030. These diseases are growing fastest in the developed countries (62%).

Alzheimer's places a great burden on caregivers (social, psychological, physical and economic) in developed countries[14] [15] and in developed countries it is one of the most costly diseases to society.[16] [17] A 1998 study estimated that the cost of Alzheimer's disease in the United States may be $100 billion each year.[18] Costs increase with dementia severity and the presence of behavioral disturbances.[19] Therefore any treatment that slows cognitive decline, delays institutionalization or reduces caregivers' hours will have economic benefits.[20] In 2013, the direct costs of caring for those with Alzheimer's to American society will total an estimated $203 billion. (Alzheimer's Association - web) In a 2007 study, the annual cost per Parkinson's patient was around $10,000 per year in the U.S.[21] An article from *Internal Medicine News* (3/2013) "The total cost of dementia to the U.S. economy ranged from $159 billion to $215 billion in 2010." The New York Times (4/2013) stated that dementia care cost is projected to double by 2040.

The total estimated worldwide cost of dementia was $604 billion (US dollars) in 2010. About 70% of the costs occured in Western Europe and North America. If dementia care was a country, it would be the world's 18th largest economy, and if it was a business it would exceed Walmart ($414 billion) and Exxon Mobil ($311 billion).[22]

What about people with MS? Most people are diagnosed between ages of 20 and 50. There are about 500,000 people who have MS in the US, and worldwide there are around 3 million (in 2010). There are four defined categories of MS:
- 85% have 'Relapsing-Remitting' who have flare-ups and relapses with acute worsening of neurologic function.
- 10% have 'Primary-Progressive' which is a slow continuous worsening of the disease.
- 50% of the 'Relapsing-Remitting' MS people develop 'Secondary-Progressive' MS which is continuously degenerating.

- 5% have 'Progressive-Relapsing' also a progressive degeneration but have acute relapses and attacks during partial recovery. All four are said to be incurable.[23]

As of 2008, globally MS is about two times more common in women than in men.[24] While in people over fifty, MS affects males and females almost equally.[25]

There are traditionally five stages in Parkinson's and the same could be said for MS. It is a continual degeneration of the neurological function. MS, AD and PD are similar in some ways neurologically.

Whereas in stage one and two it is possible to reverse PD and MS in under a year, for stage three and four it will probably take two years. This means that work on the person's part to bring it into remission is needed, which involves a strict vegetarian or raw vegan diet, with juicing, green powders and nutrients (supplements). Within six months, a person will notice a tremendous difference in their health and a reduction in symptoms. Within eight months, they should see a reduction of about 50% of the symptoms and 50% of the dependence on drugs to reduce symptoms. Within 12 to 16 months, they should be about 90-97% cured of Parkinson's. Everyone is different and more research is needed, but starving a disease like Parkinson's and MS to death is a long slow process.

Within nine months to a year a person should physiologically have reached the first stage of remission which is "neuro-plasticity." Parkinson's disease progression will have slowed to a crawl and this could be shown through an L-dopa PET brain scan. In the long run, the goal is to get off most pharmaceutical drugs. Drugs are poisons which usually interfere with the body's ability to put the disease into remission, because they affect the liver and other organs that are involved in detox and the curative process.

The 4 stages of Alzheimer's are usually termed: pre-dementia, early, moderate and advanced.[26] [27] Advanced Alzheimer's patients are usually confined to a bed or a chair. It is probably too late to cure the AD with the Living plant-based nutritional approach as discussed in this book. People with Pre-dementia and early stage Alzheimer's can definitely be treated with this approach, and within a year or two the AD should be put into remission. People with moderate stage AD would probably take at least two to three years to put it into remission. This is not just using the Living plant-based nutrition therapy but involves several long fasts per year, with two of the fasts being a 21-28 day juice fast.

One way to describe the severity of Parkinson's disease is using the Hoehn and Yahr scale, developed by Margaret Hoehn and Melvin Yahr in the 1960s. This scale describes five 'stages' of Parkinson's disease. The scale reflects the worsening of the disease but is not a linear indicator of the disease progression.[28]

- Stage I: Unilateral features of Parkinson's disease, including the major features of tremor, rigidity, or bradykinesia.
- Stage II: Bilateral features mentioned above, along with possible speech abnormalities, decreased posture, and abnormal gait.
- Stage III: Worsening bilateral features of Parkinson's disease, along with balance difficulties. Patients are still able to function independently.
- Stage IV: Patients are unable to live alone or independently.
- Stage V: Patients need wheelchair assistance, and/or are unable to get out of bed.

Disease corresponding to the stages IV and V was found in 37% and 42% of patients, with disease duration of 10 and 15 years, respectively. However, Hoehn and Yahr also found considerable variability; 34% of patients with a disease duration of 10 years or longer were still in stages I or II, reflecting heterogeneity of the disease.[29]

In 2008, the published literature, investigators statements and public presentations show that there are about 136 studies on MS research, while in 2009 there are about 129 studies. These studies are progressing through the drug development pipeline. Some of the highlights of this group in 2008 are:
• 11 large-scale studies involving more than 1000 people with MS – up from 3 in 2002
• 37 oral drugs under study for treating MS or its symptoms; 5 are in larger, phase 3 trials
• Novel strategies for progressive disease, including cannabis extract for neuroprotection, and results of a study on low-dose naltrexone.[30]

Alzheimer's disease is not well understood by Allopathic medicine and their current treatment is drugs that help with the symptoms of the disease and mask these symptoms. As of 2012, there have been over 1,000 clinical trials that have been or are in progress on AD.[31]

There are few studies that are dealing with plant-based nutrition with fasting as a therapy for MS, possibly a few for AD and none for PD (in our review of the literature). The influence of nutrition on drug therapy is probably involved in some of these other drug studies. Remember there are billions of dollars in pharmaceutical drugs for MS, AD or PD, but the pharmaceutical companies don't make money on selling fruits and vegetables used in nutrition therapies. Furthermore, doctors know how to give out drugs in 10 minutes or less, but nutritional therapies can take an hour or more to explain and longer to train a client in a nutritional approach and get them motivated to try it. Insurance companies do not pay for this time to train patients.

The efforts of an optimal nutritional approach, such as a Live Plant-based approach, can be used to protect and repair the brain and spinal cord. Nutritional studies fall under the category of novel strategies for progressive disease, but sadly no there are few to no studies discussing this.

d. Possible Causes of PD, AD and MS

We approach the causes of PD, AD, and MS from an alternative perspective; reviewing books and articles citing journal studies; "While scientists know Alzheimer's disease involves progressive brain cell failure, the reason cells fail isn't clear."[32]

Parkinson's and Alzheimer's diseases are very closely related and people with PD sometimes end up with AD and vice versa. Journal articles often use data from the two together in their studies. In terms of pathophysiology, PD usually has Lewy bodies in the brain as does AD in a different form.[33] The clinical and pathological data often overlap and the most typical symptom of Alzheimer's disease, dementia, occurs in advanced stages of PD, while it is also common to find neurofibrillary tangles in brains affected by PD.[34]

There is no evidence for a genetic cause for Alzheimer's but in 1% to 5% of the cases there are some genetic similarities that have been identified.[35] Other hypotheses exist in trying to explain the cause of the disease. There are various hypotheses on AD including: the cholinergic hypothesis[36] which proposes that AD is caused by reduced synthesis of the neurotransmitter acetylcholine, but medication treatment for acetylcholine deficiency has not been very effective. Other cholinergic effects have also been proposed, for example, initiation of large-scale aggregation of amyloid,[37] leading to generalized neuroinflammation.[38]

The amyloid hypothesis postulated that extracellular beta-amloid deposits are the fundamental cause of the disease.[39] The Tau Hypothesis is the idea that tau protein abnormalities initiate the disease cascade.[40] The Oxidative stress and dys-homeostasis of biometal (biology) metabolism may be significant in the formation of the pathology.[41] [42]

Another hypothesis asserts that the disease may be caused by age-related myelin breakdown in the brain.[43] Iron released during myelin breakdown is hypothesized to cause further damage. Homeostatic myelin repair processes contribute to the development of proteinaceous deposits such as beta-amyloid and tau.[44] Some have hypothesized that dietary copper may play a causal role, where there is a copper excess and a zinc deficiency.[45] Studies have shown an increased risk of developing AD with environmental factors such as the intake of metals, particularly aluminum.[46]

In the role of protein aggregation in mitochondrial dysfunction and neurodegeneration in Alzheimer's and Parkinson's Diseases, these have been identified as a protein mis-folding disease (proteopathy), caused by plaque accumulation of abnormally folded beta amyloid and tau amyloid proteins in the brain.[47] Exactly how disturbances of production and aggregation of the beta-amyloid peptide gives rise to the pathology of AD is not known.[48]

In the pathology of Alzheimer's disease inflammation processes also seems to have a role since inflammation is a general marker of tissue damage in any disease, and may be either secondary to tissue damage in AD or a marker of an immunological response.[49]

Is the current treatment of Parkinson's obsolete? In the *Better Brain Book*, David Perlmutter, MD, an expert in brain disease and its treatment, writes about Parkinson's, "The current mode of treatment is sorely inadequate and obsolete. The sad truth is that the standard drug treatment for Parkinson's merely masks the symptoms and does nothing to stop the progression of the disease. In some ways it may actually make it worse. When discussing risk factors for neurological diseases I noted that people who have been exposed to particular toxins, such as insecticides used in farming or gardening or other chemicals on the job, are prime candidates for Parkinson's disease. This makes perfect sense, because toxins increase the production of free radicals in the body, particularly in the brain. It's true, however, that not everyone who is exposed to these toxins will eventually develop Parkinson's disease. Why are some people more vulnerable to the damaging effects of toxin-generated free radicals than others? Interestingly, the answer may have more to do with the liver than the brain. The liver is the body's main detoxifying organ. Its primary job is to render chemicals harmless before they can enter the bloodstream and circulate throughout the body's tissues and cells. Many Parkinson's patients have weaker-than-normal liver function and therefore have a flawed detoxification system."[50]

In the book *The Brain Gate*, Robert Hatherill, PhD, an expert in this field, explains: "Researchers have struggled for more than a century to figure out what causes Parkinson's disease. Until about twenty years ago, our understanding of its causes remained murky; there were few clear clues: no single entity – infection, stress, genetics, or age – seemed to account for the tremors and gradual paralysis of Parkinson's that afflict over 1.2 million in the United States alone. Then, in 1982, a series of bizarre events occurred. Since the disease usually occurs in older people in the sixth decade of life, doctors found it strange that young drug users started turning up at hospitals showing signs of Parkinson's disease. Scientists found a toxic contaminant present in the synthetic street heroin being used that caused this strange outbreak of Parkinson's and solved the mystery. 'Foreign' chemicals such as pesticides were actually causing Parkinson's disease. An alarming study published in the *Journal of the American Medical Association* claimed that environmental chemicals cause the majority of Parkinson's disease. Other published studies indicated the same troubling connection. While most scientists don't accept it, Parkinson's disease has become the first documented brain ailment of the industrial revolution. Pollutants that taint our food supply may foster new generations of brain illnesses."[51]

Experts estimate that at least twenty-five percent of the American population is likely to suffer from heavy metal poisoning. These heavy metals include cadmium, aluminum, lead, and mercury, all of which are increasingly being linked to brain disease."[52]   In all or most all, of the cases of Parkinson's and Alzheimer's, one or more of these heavy metals can often be found in the brain. It is known that heavy metals, mostly lead, are found in the brain of almost all Parkinson's patients. Aluminum is found in most, if not all, Alzheimer's patients. Mercury is found in most, if not all, Autism patients. These heavy metals also cause inflammation, which is also found in these different brain diseases. All of these can be detoxified from the body through a raw vegan diet with juicing and/or fasting.

In doing a review of the literature, there are about fourteen possible causes that stand out. Most likely these people with AD, PD and MS could be cured, or their disease could be put into remission, through fasting and a raw vegan nutrition therapy. These are the possible causes of Alzheimer's, Parkinson's and MS diseases and/or things that reinforce and feed the disease. The chances are that it is more than one of these or several together:

1. Heavy metal toxicity
2. Pesticides
3. Pharmaceutical or street drugs
4. Vaccines or chemical poisons
5. Excitotoxins and other chemical additives
6. Fungi, mold, yeast
7. Bacteria and pathogenic microorganisms
8. Toxic (denatured) Animal Proteins
9. Internal Cellular Toxins (i.e. parasites)
10. External Environmental Toxins
11. NeuroInflammation in brain and CNS
12. pH &/or sodium-potassium levels are off
13. Allergy to meat and gluten
14. Food additives and/or colors (i.e. glutamate)

Most of these possible causes will cause neuroinflammation. The definition of and studies done on neuroinflammation are found in the articles of the *Journal of Neuroinflammation* publication online, established by

Professor W. Sue T. Griffin of Univ. of Arkansas Medical Sciences and Prof. Robert E. Mrak at the University of Toledo. The inflammation is part of the pathways and cycle of these neuro-diseases like PD, MS, ALS and Alzheimer's and the mental disorders like Schizophrenia. The inflammatory mechanisms have been known and discussed for decades but neurodegeneration has met with vigorous criticism. Perhaps this is why living plant-based foods are so effective, because they reduce and eliminate the neuro-inflammation and thus the disease!

In MS, apart from demyelination, the other sign of the disease is inflammation. One explanation is that the inflammatory process is caused by T cells, a kind of lymphocyte that plays an important role in the body's defenses. The attack of myelin starts the inflammatory processes, which triggers other immune cells and the release of soluble factors like cytokines and antibodies and other destructive proteins.[53]

What is important is to find a cure that works for the majority of the people and a Live-food plant-based nutrition therapy with juice fasting does work for the majority of the people.

Animal-based proteins (see chapter 11 on meat) are possibly causing the Lewy Bodies and other deformed proteins in the brain. That's a reason why the journal studies have shown that a strict vegan nutritional approach slows down the disease progression, or stops it completely. Abram Hoffer, MD discusses "a chronic schizophrenic woman who was unable to come to my office because she was rigid and catatonic." He fasted her for 30 days and she got well but her conditions came back when she started eating again. He tested her for food allergies. "She was allergic to all meats: as soon as she ate meat her major symptoms recurred. She then went on a vegetarian diet and remained well. Since then I have fasted at least 200 schizophrenic patients. More than 60 percent were well after the fast."[54]

Abram Hoffer, MDin his book *Healing Schizophrenia*, writes of a study he did, "During our study with fasting, over a four-month period 60 patients (schizophrenic) went through a fast, usually at home. … Forty were well at the end of the fast and have remained well since. They do not need any medication but must avoid the foods which they are allergic. The other 20 did not improve whatsoever. The 40 who recovered have remained well since, but thirty were allergic to dairy foods. Two were also allergic to beef. One was allergic to smoking, one to aspirin, and the rest to sugar and other foods. Other orthomolecular physicians have found similar recoveries."[55] This could be more appropriately called an intolerance, as a true allergy would cause them to break out in a rash or have trouble breathing.

Another possibility which is seldom discussed because it is rather scary is BSE. Bovine spongiform encephalopathy (BSE, also known as mad cow disease) has surfaced (in the 1970's) in Great Britain, France, Switzerland, Canada, Spain, Germany, Japan, Russia, and in 1988, there was a confirmed death from JD in Manchester, NH.[56] Health authorities consider it to be the most likely cause of a new variant of Creutzfeldt-Jakob disease (vCJD), a fatal brain disease that, as of May 2003, has affected 139 people worldwide. Bovine spongiform encephalopathy is a fatal central nervous system disease first identified in the UK in 1986. This disease distorts normal proteins in human brain and nerve cells; a similar thing occurs in Alzheimer's. There is a history of connections between AD and BSE.[57] Another source says, it affects less than 200,000 people in the US.[58]

Laura Manuelidis is a top neurodegenerative disease scientist at Yale University. In 1989, she published the results of a study that examined the post mortem brains of forty-six Alzheimer-disease patients and found six cases, or 13 percent of the patients had died of CJD.[59] Thus they were mis-diagnosed. A second study by the University of Pittsburgh in the journal of Neurology in 1989, examined the brains of fifty-four presumed Alzheimer patients and found three cases of CJD, or 5.5 percent.[60] Thus the Pittsburgh and Yale studies suggest that somewhere between 5.5 percent and 13 percent of Alzheimer's diagnoses are really CJD (mad cow disease). That means that out of 5.2 million people with Alzheimer's in the U.S. in 2013, 5.5 to 13 percent of them (286,000 to 676,000) actually have /or had mad cow's disease. What this suggests is that it comes from animals eating other animal parts, which is done at farms to save money!

e. The Silver Bullet

The mindset coming out of the medical community and the pharmaceutical industry is looking for this magical "silver bullet" to kill Parkinson's and MS. It is based on the Germ Theory, in which the medical community wants to kill the germ or condition (some now call it gene expression) with a drug, and the silver bullet is the magical drug. Yet, as we know, the real problem is not one of a germ, but primarily one of the internal biological environments, the Biological Terrain! That is why a plant-based nutrition system works.

When a scholar does a serious review of the literature, the problem of dopamine is only one of several of the problems with Parkinson's. A second problem is mitochondrial damaged cells, a third are Lewy Bodies, a fourth is the Electron Transfer Chain Dysfunction and a fifth is heavy metal toxicity. Scientists need to find several different bullets (or drugs) and not just one, for example:

- a silver bullet, for dopamine
- a gold bullet, for mitochondrial damage cells
- a bronze bullet, for Lewy Bodies/amyloid plaques
- an aluminum bullet, for heavy metal toxicity
- a lead bullet, for Electron Transfer Chain Dysfunction
- a steel bullet, for neuro-inflammation.

They could need at least five to six drugs to cure Parkinson's, AD or MS, as one drug is not going to solve all these issues.

There is an urgent need for integrative medical management. The allopathic model, based on the Germ Theory that currently dominates Parkinson's management, is obsolete. A scientist in this field, Parris Kidd, PhD points out, "that the major adverse side effects of the various drugs currently in use for the disease, combined with the limitations for the dopamine replacement strategy, dictate the need for alternatives."[61] Studies show that after five years these drugs no longer work but actually increase the Parkinson's downward spiral.

The pharmaceutical drugs are creating an illusion of success which is only masking the conditions, and the killing off of the dopamine cells in the brain continues, month by month, year by year. Not only does this create an illusion of "quality of life," but it weakens the motivation to use natural means like plant-based foods, especially Live-Plant-based Food nutrition therapy.

The medical institutions and foundations are guiding the thinking about Parkinson's and MS. They are looking for a "silver bullet," a pharmaceutical drug. So everyone is frantically searching for this pharmaceutical drug, this silver bullet.

f. A Medical Antidote for PD, AD & MS

Most people assume that there is no medical cure for PD, AD and MS. On the other hand, yes, there does seem to be a medical cure for PD, AD and MS, and other related brain disorders, but the chemical cure, which is an antidote is not allowed.

If there is a cure, what is the cure and why is it not allowed? It fairly clear that there is a lot of evidence that pesticides, industrial and household poisons, pharmaceutical drugs and vaccinations all have a high probability of being the primary cause of Parkinson's and also MS. All of these chemicals can have antidotes to neutralize the chemicals. For instance if you have a strong acid, a strong base could be added to neutralize the acid. The same can be done with any chemical, an antidote can be developed to neutralize the harmful effects of that chemical.

Today we have the technology through laboratory work involving blood and urine, hair and skin cell analysis, and other sophisticated forms of medical analysis to determine exactly what foreign chemicals are lodged in the body. Then through testing like CT scans, ultrasounds and other scanning and laboratory techniques it can be determined where in the body this foreign chemical is found. The science today is advanced enough to go right down to the molecular level; they do it all the time in laboratories. Once the type of chemical and where it is lodged is determined, a chemical antidote can be made up and administered to neutralize the foreign chemical, that is probably causing or part of the Parkinson's and MS.

Rebecca Carley, MD developed an antidotes to these drugs doing this for her daughter. Dr. Carley is from Long Island and successfully pioneered a treatment to reverse the injuries from vaccines such as autism and autism spectrum disorders. But she was threatened to lose her medical license by the NY state department of health, for speaking out.[62] For reasons like this most medical doctors do not want to speak out or devise an antidote method to reverse these diseases. Besides Dr. Carley was successful because she had a chemistry background.

Dr. Carley proposed that through vaccinations it affects the Allergy-Immune Diseases then through the auto-antibodies to Myelin that affects the Nervous system. Then through the nervous system the central (Encephalitis) it affects and perhaps causes things like Autism, Multiple Sclerosis, Parkinson's, Lou Gehrig's Disease and others. Rebecca Carley, MD states, "The research I have done over the past 11 years PROVES that vaccines cause a corruption in the immune system that leads to all autoimmune disease, non-traumatic seizures and cancer, in people and in pets. The fact that I have developed a protocol which reverses all vaccine-induced diseases using natural therapies was the true reason for the NYS medical board's attack against me, since I never had a complaint against me by any patient, even when I was a surgeon, before my only child was brain damaged from vaccines, and I learned how to reverse it."[63] And she successfully reversed her child's brain damage using this method.

Perhaps she can be called a Wild Duck. She is a Wild Duck, someone starting a cultural revolution! But the medical industry stopped her cultural revolution and silenced her as a Wild Duck quacking about the Truth!

This medical doctor, Rebecca Carley, MD brings out the question that perhaps these neurological diseases did not really exist, except in minor cases, until modern technology and medicines came about, and then they increased greatly when people started to become vaccinated. Perhaps, the more vaccinations a person receives, the more they will cause diseses and strengthen the disease to continue.

Two other doctors possibly using this method are Sherry Rogers, MD an environmental doctor in NY, who is an expert and author in this field, she has completely healed several Parkinson's patients. And also a holistic medical doctor, Gabriel Cousens, MD MD(H) who healed two clients with MS. One MS client Dr. Cousens had a pesticide removed or neutralized, that was found to be in their body, and another MS client had a chemical (possible vaccination) neutralized that they had been given as a child. Once these were removed, the MS went away and these people live normal lives today.   Dr. Cousens is a holistic and a homeopathic doctor with his own natural pharmacy so he is not the usual doctor just using allopathic methods of drugs.

g. Masking the Symptoms with Drugs
and other common questions

In the *Better Brain Book*, David Perlmutter, MD, an expert in brain disease and its treatment, writes about Parkinson's, "The current mode of treatment is sorely inadequate and obsolete. The sad truth is that the standard drug treatment for Parkinson's merely masks the symptoms and does nothing to stop the progression of the disease."

Another major problem is that studies are showing that drugs are limited and usually only help alleviate symptoms for about five years. Then the use of drugs starts to cause the Parkinson's to progress faster.

These drugs are only masking the symptoms, a smoke screen, the disease continues to get worse. The drugs are not slowing down or stopping the progress. Studies show that after several years, some studies say five years; the drugs actually do no good and make the disease progress faster. So the longer you stay on drugs, the less your chances are to succeed in defeating Parkinson's. The drugs are building up toxicity I the body, weakening it.

Non-drug therapies are highly beneficial in Parkinson's disease, but seldom prescribed. Today, nearly 2 million Americans, mostly men, face the agony of Parkinson's disease in later years. Experts who provide physical, occupational, speech and nutritional therapy tell why their services should be utilized for Parkinson's patients in a managed care environment.[64]

A very long term, (*Neurology*, 2008) three decade study of nearly 9,000 people begun in the early 1960's and showed that obesity increased the risk of Alzheimer's by about 293%. This means obesity nearly triples the risk of having Alzheimer's.[65] Similar results would probably be found for both Parkinson's and MS.

Some turn to drugs to help reduce the shaking in Parkinson's. Actually the shaking is part of the physiological response to the condition, the body wants to get rid of the poison or toxin and shaking can help to dislodge it and get it into the bloodstream to get rid of it. Thus shaking can be a good thing and on a Living Plant-based diet with lots of juices (liquids) and fasting the poison or toxin could be flushed out of the body.

Are people ever misdiagnosed because of heavy metal toxicity? Yes, heavy metal toxicity mimics Parkinson's. A lot of patients today are misdiagnosed when it comes to heavy metal toxicity. The only way a doctor can be totally convinced that a patient has Parkinson's is to do a PET brain scan, otherwise that person could be misdiagnosed just by looking at the symptoms or other clinical evidence. A brain scan is very expensive and usually not covered by insurance. A brain scan can show the deterioration in the brain neurons of someone that has Parkinson's disease.

There are journal studies that indicate nutrition is a factor and can help PD, AD and MS. The nutritional signposts give a sense of direction away from meat-based diets towards plant-based diets.

People who eat a Mediterranean diet have a lower risk of AD,[66] [67] and it may improve outcomes in those with the disease.[68] Those who eat a diet high in saturated fats and simple carbohydrates have a higher risk.[69] The Mediterranean diet is heading in the right direction but it is not putting AD or PD into remission, a person has to go next major step to a raw vegan diet to do that.

The risk of dying from Alzheimer's disease is twenty-six percent higher among the non-Hispanic white population than among the non-Hispanic black population whereas the Hispanic population has a thirty percent lower risk than the non-Hispanic white population.[70] This is a very important statistic since the non-Hispanic white population diet is the standard American diet which is one of the worst in the world.

The three things that have been found helpful for AD are mental stimulation, exercise, and a balanced diet. These have been found to delay cognitive symptoms but not the brain pathology.[71]

Whereas there is evidence that a vegan diet does slow the progression of these diseases and a raw vegan and Living foods diet actually stops these diseases. But if a person goes back to the standard American meat-based diet for more than a month the disease does come back.

h. Live-Food Zone Nutrition

Live plant-based nutrition therapy and fasting is the first known cure of Parkinson's (1943), as will be noted later, through a raw vegan diet and fasting. The research in this book has found in the treatment of the diseases of MS, AD and PD a consistent pattern: avoid dairy, avoid most grains and avoid meats; eat mostly raw fruits and vegetables with periods of fasting. Nearly all the books and studies and testimonials say the same thing.

Lawrence C. Katz, PhD, professor of Neurobiology, explains that, "A long series of investigations by Dr. Michael Merzenich at the University of California, San Francisco, has shown the adaptability of connections in the adult brains. Recent findings by Dr. Jon Kaas at Vanderbilt University and Dr. Charles Gilbert at Rockefeller University have shown directly that neurons in the adult brain can actually grow new 'wires' to connect one another. The beneficial effects of neurotrophins have been documented in hundreds of experiments at leading universities throughout the world. The first neurotrophin was discovered almost 50 years ago as a substance that not only kept certain types of nerve cells alive but also caused them to sprout many new branches. Later it was named Nerve Growth Factor or NGF, which is found throughout the body but was scarce in the cerebral cortex."[72]

"In the early 1980's, Yves Barde at the Max Planck Institute in Munich, Germany, finally succeeded in purifying a molecule from the brain that behaved just like NGF. Named Brain-Derived Neurotrophic Factor, or BDNF, it was found almost everywhere in the brain, including the cerebral cortex. Research by Bai Lu at the National Institutes of Health, Erin Schumann at Cal Tech, and Tobias Bonhoeffer at the Max Planck Institute in Munich, has shown that neurotrophins help increase the strength of connections in the hippocampus, a part of the brain that is critical for learning and memory."[73] Now both NGF and BDNF are built on superior nutrition and eating Live Plant-based Foods in the Live-Food Zone! If a person goes back to eating the Standard American Diet, the disease could and probably will come back. This has been the experience of others with the disease of MS.

The basic benefits of plant-based nutrition for Parkinson's, Alzheimer's and other brain diseases are:

- Anti-Oxidant
- Anti-Neuro Inflammatory
- Anti-Protein aggregation
- Anti-Excitotoxicity
- Mitochondria Protectors
- Balanced pH and sodium-potassium cellular levels
- Reduced pathogenic microorganisms and fungi levels
- Mitochondria Protectors
- Supports starving the disease to death

- Supports Brain homeostasis
- Neuroprotection leading to neuroplasticity
- Neuroplasticity leading to neuro-regeneration

'Supports starving the disease to death' needs a little explanation. Parkinson's, Alzheimer's and MS are like scavenger diseases which feed on dead and dying material. Living Foods starve the disease (bacterial, viral, or whatever). For instance, Journal studies indicate that the vegan diet is the only successful diet to treat Parkinson's. Live Plant-based Food diets have cured AD, PD and MS. Using MRI's the brain scar tissue also has been shown to clear up in both MS and in Parkinson's patients' brains.

The first known account of being cured by this method is from Dr. Herbert Shelton in 1943. He was one of the great medical practitioners back in the 40's, 50's and 60's, using Living Plant-based Foods and fasting in his practice. Monica B., age 39, had been diagnosed with Parkinson's disease; she had previously suffered with Parkinsonism for six years. She fasted three times under the supervision of Dr. Shelton: 30 days, 14 days and later another 14 days. Monica was at the health school for nine months which served a Living Foods diet. After she had fasted thirty days, the tremor immediately reoccurred, but not as severely as before the fast. After the second fast, the tremors were less and after the third fast, the tremors were gone. For more than ten years, Dr. Shelton remained in contact with Monica and she had no recurrence of her tremors and she lived a healthy, normal life."[74]

A Living Plant-Foods or raw vegan diet does the same thing to Parkinson's, Alzheimer's, and MS: it starves the disease to death. It is known that the long-term survivors are mostly vegans and those in remission are mostly raw vegans or eating Live-Foods.

As the famous Greek physician Hippocrates said, "The body heals itself. The patient is only Nature's assistant." The key insight is: germs don't cause disease, they develop in a diseased environment. This inner environment is the zone, the place within the body that Live-Food nutrition is needed.

i. The Sevenfold Path of Purification

Christianity began with the Aramaic phrase: "Purify thyself and believe the Good News." (Mk 1:15)

There are actually seven levels of purification that a person needs to practice.
The Sevenfold Purification includes:
1. Purification of the Body
   Mt 16:24; Lk 9:23; 1 Cor 9:27; 2 Cor 7:1; 3 John 2
2. Purification of the Soul (mind, emotions, will)
   Rom 12:2; Heb 4:12; Lk 1:46
3. Purification of the Spirit
   Matthew 5:3-10
4. Purification of Family Relationships
   Matthew 5:17-48
5. Purification of Social Relationships
   Matthew 6:1-7:12
6. Purification of the Relationship with
   The Living Planet
   Deut 20.19-20; Ps 24:1; Ps 145:9
7. Purification of the Relationship with
   The Communion of Saints
   Heb 11:10; 12:1, 13, 14; 2 Cor 3:18; Eph 4:1-6

We are involved in all seven levels to some degree and need purification on all seven levels as a way of life to become happy, health and holy.

Part II

Evidence for MS, PD and AD
Remissiona to Cures

Jesus was a Physician - Jesus may have been brought up
as a carpenter, but the evidence suggests that he later became
versed in the healing arts and became a well-known
physician. Jesus knew the Essenes and the Therapeutae
Jewish communities, who are strong in the healing arts.
Origen, an early Church Father asserts that Jesus was not a
carpenter as he grew up, '. . . that in none of the Gospels
current in the Churches is Jesus Himself ever described as
being a carpenter.' The oldest translation of Mark 6 states,
"Jesus son of Joseph the carpenter," later translations write,
Jesus the carpenter, son of Joseph. Twice Jesus referred to
himself as a physician: Lk 4:23, Mk 2:15-17 which are
confirmed in parallel text Mk 2.17 and Lk 5:32. Jesus spent
about a third or more of his time healing people in the
Gospels. Finally, some of the early Church Fathers called
Jesus the Divine physician.[d]

a. Optimum Evidence through Case Studies
and Testimonials

There is evidence that Parkinson's, Alzheimer's and
Multiple Sclerosis have been cured through nutritional
means. The following are case histories and testimonials.
True it is not a lot of evidence but a few here, dozen there,
and some more along the way adds up and shows a
significant nutritional evidence of a direction that works to a
great degree! The approach in this book takes into account
the psychological and the spiritual dimensions of healing
which nearly all journal studies avoid.

---

[d] Jim Tibbetts, *Jesus and Mary were Kosher Vegetarian*, (2013).

In the next three chapters will be a short review of the literature on some of the cures for PD, AD and MS. Journal studies are important but simple testimonials are also just as important as nutritional signposts pointing the direction to go.

Scientific studies with statistics are considered the best type of studies and for some things that is true but in a way nutrition case studies are the best type of study because everyone 1. biochemically, 2. physiologically and 3. anatomically is a little different. All these little bits add up to a larger amount and when 4. psychological and 5. cultural differences are added in, it makes a large amount of error. A historical case study works with every single person as an individual who is unique and different which gives a better overall physical (above 1, 2, 3, 4 ,5) historical understanding and proof of healing or remission.

In addition to that it's not just the math or statistics that are the problem. The major problem is the people who do the study and their agenda's. These agenda's usually bring them money, job security and fame. Scientific evidence is a new kid on the block in the last 100-200 years. Medicine, case studies and testimonials have been around for over 3,000 years and only in the last 150 years or so has scientific evidence with statistics and proofs have become something of importance.

By using testimonials and case studies we are using real people and not statistics. These real people are relating their stories with all the various influences in their lives. "Not all human life can be reduced to a unit of data in a RCT: indeed, the bias in the positivist paradigm itself reproduces a narrow scientism."[75] (*Achieving Evidence-Based Practice*)

In the book, *Science in the Private Interest, has the Lure of Profits Corrupted Biomedical Research?* by Seldon Krimsky (2004)[76] gives an excellent overview of this issue of bias in the journal literature. 'Funding bias,' in other words, private funding can bias the outcome of studies toward the interests of the sponsor.[77] [78] Also association between funding source and study outcome *New England Journal of Medicine,*[79] "Marcia Angel, former editor of The *New England Journal of Medicine*, commented that it was her impression 'papers submitted by authors with financial conflicts of interest were far more likely to be biased in both design and interpretation.'[80]

A work on *Achieving Evidence-Based Practice* notes; "There are pressures upon researchers to publish in more prestigious, high-impact journals: 'As long as journals continue to pursue their current editorial policies then we are restricting our view of a broader scientific picture. More worrying, though, if statistical significance increases the chance of a researcher's work being published, might not he or she be tempted to tamper a little with data? After all, a career might depend on it.'"[81] "The process of peer review by professional journals is itself acknowledged as biased, with questions of method and name bias, publication bias and differing value ascribed to differing traditions of enquiry (Wilkie 1997)."[82] Another problem is magnifying trivial differences through risk factor statistics can be used.[83]

For a deeper explanation of this problem of journal studies see Jim Tibbetts book; *The Bioethics of Drug Intervention and Plant-based Nutrition Therapy.*

Using case studies is a superior method when various case studies and testimonials can be combined as has been done in this book. In fact most scientific studies get started with a case study showing results. Hopefully this book will become the basis for journal studies.

Chapter 2
Evidence of MS Remissions to Cures

St. Anthony the Great (d. 350) says, "And those who are monks, and are zealous to achieve the full measure of sanctity and purity, should take particular care always to keep themselves such that they can say with the Apostle, 'I keep under my body, and bring it into subjection.' (1 Cor 9.27) Striving to attain perfect purity, it is needful to bear the labors of repentance; both in the soul and body, harmoniously and in equal measure.'"[84]

a. Studies and Case Histories

Many health professionals do not like the idea that multiple sclerosis (MS), a degenerative disease of the nervous system, might be linked to diet. One of the main factors of the link with diet appears to be the strongest contact we have with our environment: our daily food intake. Although wealthy countries generally have higher rates of MS and less affluent countries have lower ones, there is one exception: Japan. Even though the Japanese live in a modern, industrialized country with all the stress, pollution, and smoking habits common to other industrialized nations, their rice-based diet is more characteristic of the foods consumed in poorer nations where MS is less common. The Japanese case provides strong evidence that a diet heavy in animal foods, not other 'modern' scourges, may lay the foundation for MS.

One theory (*American Journal Medicine*) holds that the MS attacks are caused by a decreased supply of blood to the sensitive brain tissues[85] [86] Of course, all aspects of a diet filled with rich foods can cause problems, but animal fats—especially those from dairy products—have been the most closely linked to the development of MS.[87] Another theory suggests that feeding cow's milk to infants lays the foundation for nervous system injury later in life. Cow's milk has only one-fifth as much linoleic acid (an essential fatty acid) as human breast milk. Linoleic acid makes up the building blocks for nervous tissues. It may be that children raised on a high animal-fat diet deficient in linoleic acid (as most children are in our society) develop a weaker nervous system that is susceptible to problems as they age. Analysis of brain tissues has shown that people with MS have a higher saturated fat content in their brains than people without the disease.[88] What precipitates the attacks of MS is unknown, but the suspected culprits include viruses, allergic reactions, and disturbances of the flow of blood to the brain. Most likely, the offender is connected to the circulatory system in the brain or spinal cord, because the lesions and scarring characteristic of MS are centered in nerve cells near blood vessels.

Two studies published in the *British Medical Journal* set the ball rolling on Fats and MS. In 1973, a study testing sunflower seed oil, showed that the frequency, severity, and duration of attacks were reduced in the group who took the sunflower seed oil.[89] Later, in 1978, a trial was conducted by Professor David Bates and co-workers at Newcastle University with 116 patients with MS. The Newcastle study shows that someone with MS can be helped with evening primrose oil. It showed the effectiveness of polyunsaturates for MS.[90]

These results may mean that patients who stick closely to the low saturated/high PUFA diet have less demyelination and therefore less damage. This would fit with other findings that patients on the diet seem to have shorter and less severe relapses. Professor Michael Crawford believes that the diet may work as a remission agent.[91]

b. Swank and McDougall Low fat Diet for MS

Roy Swank, M.D., former head of University of Oregon's neurology department and was a practicing physician at Oregon Health Sciences University, observed that MS patients improved on a forced low-fat diet. In the 1950s, Swank began treating his own patients with such a diet. He got excellent results, so for the next 35 years he treated thousands of MS patients in this way. By any medical standard, his results have been remarkable: patients' conditions improved by as much as 95 percent.[92] Patients fared better if they had detected the disease early and had, had few attacks, but even long-time MS sufferers experienced a slowdown of the disease's progression. Originally Swank was most concerned with limiting saturated fat, but over the years he had become more attuned to the dangers of all kinds of fat. His MS diet was about 20 percent fat by calories, but not necessarily vegetarian. Swank's results are unchallenged by other studies. Three important findings emerged from Swank's research:

1. The earlier an MS patient adopted a low-fat diet, the better the chance of avoiding deterioration and death from the disease.
2. Patients who limited their saturated fat intake to less than 20 grams a day no longer showed the expected deterioration from the disease.
3. Among patients whose saturated fat intake was 17 grams or less daily, the death rate over a 35-year period was 31 percent—close to normal. The death rate was 21 percent for the patients who kept to that low level of fat consumption and who started the diet within three years of diagnosis of the disease. On the other hand, patients consuming more than 25 grams of saturated fat daily had a death rate of 79 percent over the period of the study; nearly half of those deaths were directly due to MS.[93]

But instead of advocating a low-fat vegetarian diet for MS patients, many doctors either ignore Swank's work or dismiss it because they think the diet would be too difficult to follow.

Roy Swank, MD, was the mentor for John A. McDougall, MD, on the subject of Multiple Sclerosis. Dr. McDougall points out that, "Dr. Swank developed a low fat diet for treating MS patients. He recommended not more than 40 to 50 grams of total fat per day (compared to 150 to 175 grams in the American/ Canadian diet) and 0 to 15 grams of saturated fat per day (compared to 140 to 165 grams). There was no limit on the amount of carbohydrate from starches, vegetables, and fruits. Polyunsaturated fats were increased a little from 15 to 25 to 20 to 35 grams per day. His research soon showed that with adherence to the diet, relapses decreased by about 70 percent in the first year of treatment (from 1 relapse per year to 0.2 per year). Then after the first year, there was continued improvements, about 5% fewer relapses per year for the next 2 years. For the first 16 years of treatment with a low fat diet, the rate of exacerbation (new attacks and/or decline) was decreased by 95%. Dr. Swank learned that early cases of people with MS did especially well on the diet. As the years with the disease accumulate then the response to diet was expected to be less dramatic."[94] [95] [96] [97]

(*Lancet*, 1990; *Nutrition*, 1991; *Am J Clin Nutr.*, 1988; *Arch Neurol*, 1970)

The low-fat diet treatment of MS was developed by Roy Swank, MD who treated more than 5000 people over the past 50 years and the results are remarkable.

The Swank Diet focuses on drastically reducing saturated fats, but includes a small amount of low fat dairy foods, egg whites, and skinned white-meat chicken and white fish. The McDougall Diet is a vegetarian diet, avoiding animal products. Dr. McDougall points out that, "The McDougall diet is very low in saturated fats. As an internist

35

concerned about all aspects of a patient's health, I prescribe a stricter and, I believe, a much more effective (and tastier) diet. Even low fat dairy and meat products are a health hazard causing infectious diseases, allergic reactions, as well as delivering high loads of animal protein (causing osteoporosis, kidney stones, liver, and kidney damage) and some meats contain hormones and environmental chemicals. These animal foods are completely deficient in dietary fiber and meat contains no carbohydrates. Although lower in fat and cholesterol, low fat meats and dairy products can still contain substantial amounts of both harmful ingredients. The dairy proteins are of particular concern to me because they are the leading cause of autoimmune diseases."[98]

Dr. McDougall gives an insightful dialogue with his mentor Dr. Swank. "More than 20 years ago, during one of my many visits with Dr. Swank at his Oregon medical school office, I asked him, "Why is it that when MS patients ask their doctors about changing their diet, they are told this is quackery? And why does the MS Society offer a similar message? You have published in the world's most respected scientific journals." He leaned back in his chair, took a moment for thought, and then explained, "You know, most people in this country expect to be cured by a pill, and to have a cure that is almost instantaneous. With the low fat diet, the people actually have to work to get better, and have to cure themselves. And as far as the MS Society is concerned, John, they don't mention it because they didn't discover it. It wasn't their research dollars that found this treatment. So they're not going to tell anybody. I discovered it in my small office here, in the basement of the University of Oregon Medical School." So it is not just money that keeps people from highly effective dietary cures, egos are also involved—the well-known business doctrine, 'Not Invented Here,' is working to keep you and your family sick. Self-centered people think, 'If I didn't invent it, then there is no real reason for me to promote it, especially when there is no fame or fortune in it for me.'"[99]

c. McDougall MS Study

John McDougall, MD is a board certified internist, who has been caring for people with diet and lifestyle medicine and is the co-author with his wife of 8 books. He has the McDougall program in Santa Rosa, California and lectures widely on plant-based diets. As noted above he took on the data of Dr. Swank about MS and did his own vegan study on MS as noted below.

Taken from his website; "The McDougall Research and Education Foundation has funded a study on the dietary treatment of Multiple Sclerosis (MS) with the Oregon Health and Science University in Portland. The Neurology Department of the School of Medicine, headed by Dennis Bourdette, MD and under the supervision of Vijayshree Yadav, MD, enrolled patients in the McDougall Program for intervention with a low-fat vegan diet. This is a single-blind, controlled trial using the latest MRI technologies and Neurologic evaluations." This study finished up in 2013 and Dr. McDougall gave a talk showing some data on it at Neal Barnard, MD, conference on Nutrition and the Brain, 2013. It is very successful from this talk. Dr. McDougall's study on MS is in the process of being publishing in a journal. At this time no data is available but the point is his study on over 20 MS clients on a lot-fat vegan diet is very successful.

d. Hallelujah Acres Testimonials of Remission, Cure

These previous studies show that a low fat diet helped but didn't always cure MS. The subjects in the studies were not following a raw vegan nutrition approach. There is a book on MS written by Ann Boroch, a naturopath practitioner, who cured her MS from reading other books on this topic and made the appropriate plant-based dietary changes.

Here are several testimonials mostly from The Hallelujah Diet website. These people have used a raw vegan diet with juicing approach to cure MS. The diet is very similar to and in some places identical to the Alleluia Diet, discussed in these talks, which Jim Tibbetts emphasizes in this work.

In 1976, George Malkmus, a Baptist minister, was cured of colon cancer through the Gerson diet. The Gerson diet created by Dr. Max Gerson and the Gerson Institute in San Diego, CA., became famous for curing cancer with this diet (80/20 raw diet with 6 8oz. glasses carrot and 6 glasses green drink plus a supplement regime; green drinks are a variety of greens, cucumber, kale spinach and other greens juiced.). Rev. Malkmus named the Hallelujah Diet as an expression of gratitude after his healing, which was basically using the Gerson diet. Rev. Malkmus changed it by using barley grass powder instead of making 6 fresh green drinks but he still emphasizes 6-12 8oz. glasses of carrot juice daily. Later he made other small adaptations, such as moving away from promoting 100% raw to promoting 85% raw, and adding a supplement line.

Let us read through the following testimonials to show that there is a pattern with the Hallelujah diet. Some people start to feel better in a few weeks, but it takes at least 3 to 4 months to start seeing serious results and it takes about 9 to 12 months to get off all or most all the medications and to be 90% or completely cured. In the following talk on the Olympic Live-Food awards, Judy Livingstone was cured of MS by a Hallelujah Acres health minister, Bill Irwin, a psychologist, who modified the diet and who also believes counseling is needed to cure these types of diseases. Rev. Malkmus disagreed with Bill Irwin on this point, that counseling is needed to be completely healed.

These testimonials are not case studies, but give good examples of a few of the many people that have been helped or cured through a raw vegan nutrition approach:

2001 testimonial: I learned of the healing properties of raw vegetable & fruit juices after I was diagnosed with multiple sclerosis in 1991. I went on a cleansing diet first and then took in only raw vegetable juices for the better part of a year . . . . The only solid food I ate was in the form of salads and/or fruit. As of this date (9/14/94), I have not had any symptoms of multiple sclerosis. I praise God for showing me how to become healed.

June of 1997: Judi Hurst in Florida started having problems. She started losing her balance, her left side became numb. Her eyes became weak, making it difficult to read or even think. The first doctor said it was stress; another thought it was a stroke, which turned out to be false. She became fatigued, her smile disappeared and her speech became slurred, even though she was a vocal major in college and directed a large 100-person church choir. She could no longer sing or play the piano as she lost orientation on the keyboard. She started using a cane as her legs became weak and her eyes swollen. She had pain from an elbow surgery earlier which continued. Finally, her doctor diagnosed her with Multiple Sclerosis.

In May 1998, she began the Hallelujah Diet, a raw vegan diet. She began being a steward of the body God had entrusted to her. She was overweight and lost 75 pounds on the diet, dropping from a size 22 to a size 12! Her strength came back and she could sing and play the piano. The healing of the Multiple Sclerosis was a process and took time; eventually she could walk without a cane, her pain in her elbow also went away and she achieved a full recovery.[100]

Pastor Bob East, was crippled by Multiple Sclerosis in the prime of his life. He changed his diet to the Halleluiah diet (before 1994) and went on to become a middle-aged mountain climber. Pastor Bob, now in his mid-60s, no longer experiences any symptoms of MS, which medical doctors consider to be an incurable disease that gets progressively worse.[101]

Debi's testimonial: "After doing a moderate amount of study, my husband (who is very supportive) and I adopted The Hallelujah Diet, and almost immediately set about weaning myself off all the medications the doctors had me on. It took 2 months, but eventually I was even able to discontinue the morphine patches. On The Hallelujah Diet, I gradually got better and better. We stayed strictly on the diet for 6 months. Then, a little at a time, I started going back to my old SAD, [Standard American Diet] until I was completely off The Hallelujah Diet and back on the meat, sugar, and cooked food diet again. On the SAD, my symptoms soon returned, and it was back to the doctors for my 'health care.' First it was one drug, then two and then more and more until finally I was on 6 different drugs. Finally, I said 'NO MORE' to the neurologists. This gave me a very bad reputation for being a difficult patient, and this went into my medical records. Each time a doctor wanted to add another drug I refused until I ferociously dreaded any future doctor appointment and was willing to do almost anything to put an end to this endless drug regimen the doctors insisted I be on. While on The Hallelujah Diet I was able to eliminate all my drugs and my MS exacerbations almost totally went away. How long will it take us to realize that our health is our choice?"[102]

Steve's testimonial: "The truth is I am not sure if my deliverance from MS symptoms is from a direct healing from the Lord due to prayer or as a result of following the Hallelujah Diet ideas. I give the Lord praise as either one is from him. I use to bend over with tremendous shocking feelings going through my left arm and up through my neck. I use to hit my arm against the wall to try to make it stop and told my parents I thought I was having a heart attack. I couldn't even explain all the terrible symptoms I was having. It was like every nerve in my arm was being shocked all at once. I finally went to the neurologist and after many tests the diagnosis was MS. Now after following the advice in your book and others like it, I have been symptom free for two years now and also work out with weights and jog. Keep up the great research and praise the Lord."[103]

Anonymous submission: "In January 2001, pain struck my body with searing force and my muscles began to ache continuously. I lacked energy and I eventually became as weak as a child. I did not have the strength to hold a coffee cup to my mouth and chores that once were undertaken with gusto, became impossible to perform. Signs of depression were also setting in. I no longer could perform my roles as homemaker, wife and mother. During the months of my illness, I had been too many doctors, specialists and naturopaths. I was diagnosed first of all with Fibromyalgia and then with Rheumatoid Arthritis and Multiple Sclerosis. Drugs or hundreds of vitamins and other additives were the only answer for me. I avoided the drugs as I had seen the results of years of drug-taking in the aged fold for whom I had cared for. I was swallowing 64 different vitamin and supplement tablets a day as well as 30 drops of other concoctions. I was a walking Health-food shop, with no money left in the bank. My cousin was visiting Queensland from New South Wales, and he told me about the Hallelujah Diet. I decided it was worth a try because my future didn't look good. Only the day before my cousin's visit, I'd been to a specialist in Brisbane, who'd told me I'd be in a wheelchair within two years."

"I began juicing and eating a mainly raw food diet on the 8th of May, 2002. I will never forget the first five days as the toxins began to be released from my body. I had almost every reaction one could get. I was vomiting, had diarrhea, was shivering cold, and had a constant migraine for four days and my face broke out in a severe rash. On the sixth day, as soon as I awoke, even before I moved a muscle, I knew something was different. On that beautiful morning of the 13th of May, I was able to swing my legs over the side of the bed and walk to the bathroom. Tears flowed as I was overcome with emotion. Since then, I have been improving daily. I am now able to walk, ride my pushbike, entertain and live a relatively normal life. My friends and family are amazed at the dramatic results that are irrefutable evidence for all to see. I have never felt so well. On saying that, I must admit that during the last three years I have sometimes lapsed back into careless eating habits, only to find that within weeks I'm lacking energy, not sleeping well and generally not feeling well. Does this not prove that what we eat is who we are?"

"I give thanks to my Lord and the many people who have been praying for me. I believe my health is my responsibility. This was specially so in my case as there was nothing the doctors and other health professionals could do. I don't think about being on a diet. It's more a lifestyle change. We all make choices daily, what we wear, where we go and what we feed our bodies. Since I've been feeding my body living, healthy food, it has responded positively and begun to heal itself."[104]

Charlie (husband) and I (no name) explain: "During the year 1999, I started experiencing numerous physical problems that resulted in a diagnosis of Multiple Sclerosis in the year 2000. I had lost most of the feeling in my hands, arms, legs and feet, and on most days, even walking was a chore. Then about every 3-months, I would experience a relapse, and the doctor would place me on high doses of steroids. I was also on 9 daily medications . . . In June 2005, I started on The Hallelujah Diet. Almost immediately after making the diet change, my headaches were gone, and it wasn't long before I was able to eliminate most of my medications. My doctor was shocked at my improvement. It has now been almost 2-years since I adopted The Hallelujah Diet and I have my life back! I have lost 28 pounds; I am once again able to work in my garden, wash my car, and my energy has been restored. I thank God for showing me these great truths regarding diet and how diet affects the body. Now I am singing praises to God for this miraculous healing in my life. Hallelujah!"[105]

Phyllis Heacock, Alexandria, VA.: "It has been the difference between excellent health and a wheelchair for me. . . . After reading it, I began The Hallelujah Diet and Lifestyle with fabulous results. I feel better today than ever, and have had no prescription drugs since I began the diet. Today, no one would ever suspect that I have MS. I have had no new exacerbations. I have been and remain over 90% symptom free -- only a few nuisance reoccurrences when I allow myself to get under too much stress."[106]

Linda L.: "I was diagnosed with MS in June 2001(although, of course, I knew something was wrong since 1996). I had already tried the conventional methods of treatment for MS. I was not getting better, just slowly getting worse. I had to rest almost all day so I would be able to have enough energy to cook dinner and do the dishes in the evening. I had developed muscle weakness in my left arm and left leg. It was difficult to walk most days and definitely painful and difficult to walk or even move until about noon each day. Most of the time, I couldn't walk up the stairs, in fact most nights I would crawl up the stairs and sit and rest about every 4 or 5 steps. In the mornings, I couldn't even hold a cup of coffee in my left hand. I was unsteady and off balance. I couldn't mentally function without assistance."

"By January, I had read enough information that I decided to try the Hallelujah diet. I had nothing to lose. My neurologist wasn't very thrilled with me and said what you eat has nothing to do with anything. But, never-the-less, I told him I was going to try it for 6 months. Well, I started the Hallelujah Diet in January 2002. I was on the diet for about 3 months before I noticed any difference in my MS symptoms. However, my irritable bowel syndrome that I had had for about 7 years, was gone after 3 days on the diet. My digestive problems (which I've had since I was a teenager,) were gone after about 1 week, and my chronic sinusitis that the doctor had told me I would always have was gone right away too. After 3 months, I realized that I wasn't having to take naps anymore. Then that my balance was better, and I didn't have numbness and tingling and aching in my torso anymore, and then in my arms and legs, etc."

"I have now been on the diet for only 9 months, and everyone around me (including myself) are amazed at how well I am doing. I feel better than I have felt in 5 years and I keep getting better. Almost all of my MS symptoms are gone. And I am off all my MS medicines. The only thing I am taking now is one injection per month of B12 for pernicious anemia (a condition caused when your body quits producing an enzyme that allows your body to absorb B12). I haven't even had a headache since I began this diet. Last month, my husband had to go on a business trip, so I went with him. I walked all over the city. Less than 1 year ago I could hardly walk from one room to the next without being totally worn out. Praise God for bring such a simple answer which has allowed me to live again! I feel great!"[107]

Dave & Sherry Orcutt, Plant City, Florida: "In December 2001 Dave went to the Emergency Room because of an accident and then eight weeks later; Dave's doctor confirmed he had MS and that he was to start taking the A, B or C drug for the rest of his life. But he refused all the toxic choices and told the doctor he was going to look for an alternative. . . As I prayed and contemplated this change, I was working as a Financial Controller at our church. A pastor brought a young lady into my office and suggested I listen to her testimony. One year previously she had MS so severely she was in a wheelchair, her body riddled with pain daily and she had refused all drug therapy. She had 12 lesions (11 in her brain and 1 in her spine. Dave only had 1 in his spine). She went on this (Hallelujah) diet and in six months her lesions were one-half the size. After one year, her MS was gone and today she teaches aerobics. . . . We started the

(Hallelujah) diet immediately [about March]. In July 2002, we decided to go to the Health Minister training in Shelby. . . Our ministry called, 'Back to Eden Health Ministry' was born in September 2002 and we have touched over 400 lives since its beginning."

"Following are the health improvements we have experienced on the diet: Dave (husband) threw his walker away -- most days his MS symptoms are non-existent. Gone are: severe arthritis pain (he used to take 800 mg of Ibuprofen twice a day for the pain), facial cancers, 44 pounds, body odor, toe fungus, acid reflux, headaches, snoring, an undiagnosed chest lump, severe joint pain, bad breath, and he is now growing hair back on his head -- on a bald spot he has had for twenty plus years."

"Sherry (wife) -- is now off blood pressure and thyroid medicine (taken for 10 years before making the diet change), facial wrinkles have lessened and now have healthier hair. Healed and gone are: allergies, 50 pounds, three Years of bronchitis/pneumonia (and has not returned), athlete's foot, bladder incontinence, acid reflux, body odor, bad breath, dandruff, bleeding gums, large bunion (almost gone), shoulder pain from previous injuries, hand, facial skin smoother, black moles disappearing, and for 32 years I was anemic and now give blood regularly."[108]

"Amberlee (our daughter) -- At 15, no one would expect that she would be experiencing many health problems, but we noticed several of her health problems had disappeared. She lost 41 pounds and found self-esteem and joy. Acne and bleeding gums are gone, achy joints, knee lock ups, headaches, PMS and menstrual pain, dandruff, acid reflux are gone, and stretch marks have disappeared, and the constant cough she had for two years disappeared. Today, Amberlee, at age 18, is a beautiful, young, healthy, woman!"[109]

Kathleen & John G. of Wayne County, GA.: "John was diagnosed with relapsing and remitting MS in April 2001. Friends of ours had told us about the H-acres diet after having lifesaving results with cancer. We resisted for a year, then we started it May 2002. We were considering a cane or other helpful walking instrument for John at this time. In July 2002, we had almost successfully been on the transitional diet for 6 weeks. It was a big change from our usual Cajun to the core diet. It's October 2002, and John has not had a relapse since we started the diet. Sometimes he thinks something is starting but it never manifests. We are pleased with the results and have chosen to continue at a slow pace. Many people have asked how we lost our weight. We tell them, 'We chose to get healthy.'"

Kathy: "I've been a vegetarian since I was 15, but still ate cheese, sugar and processed foods. A friend sent me a link to this site, and I was immediately intrigued. I studied nutrition in college and wasn't buying the SAD (standard American Diet) as healthful. I was diagnosed with MS in 1989. I started the Hallelujah Diet about 6 months ago, and I am off all medications. I was never able to exercise because it aggravated the symptoms. I can now go for 30 minutes on the Nordic Track with no problem! I can sleep! I'm hoping for reversal of nerve damage in my hands. Don't give up hope people!"[110]

Susan G.: "I was diagnosed with MS in 9/99, with some very devastating symptoms. After the doctors told me there was no cure, and sent me home with a load of drugs, I began researching diet, and searching for folks who had been cured through nutrition. I have been on the HD (Halleluiah diet) after reading 'God's Way,' and then went 100% raw since 2/01. The results are astounding. Through a few months of raw, I have experienced a complete remission and a gradual reversal of my symptoms. At this time, I have regained bowel/bladder control, no more numbness, no fatigue at all (as a matter of fact, increased mental alertness and clarity), I no longer use a cane to walk, and added strength to both legs. At this time, I walk with a limp due to weakness in my left leg, but even that will disappear with time and proper raw nutrition. I fully support the HD in curing the incurables and look forward to being able to live the rest of my life disease- free."[111]

Lani of Central Point, OR - "I have been on a quest for health ever since being diagnosed with multiple sclerosis (MS) many years ago. My journey has been a long but steady one. My diet has been an evolution over the decades based on a tremendous amount of reading, experimenting, and finding what worked and didn't work for me. I have gone from the SAD diet, to the Macrobiotic diet, to a vegetarian diet, to a raw vegan diet, and finally to The Hallelujah Diet. My MS has been in complete remission for many years, and I am now an energetic person, teach yoga 3 days a week, along with raw food preparation classes. I feel The Hallelujah Diet is so appropriate for those seeking better health. Eating 85% raw and 15% cooked allows people not to feel deprived, and it's an easy diet to follow once you have learned the basics."[112]

Eddie (7/5/2006) - "My name is Peter and I live in Brisbane, Australia. I'm writing regarding my friend Eddie, who has had Multiple Sclerosis for approximately 15 years. He has been in a wheelchair for the past 6 years and was losing muscle strength, vision, and memory. He also had bladder infections and continuous constipation problems. He had to be helped to transfer from the wheelchair at all times and was ill with whatever flu or cold going around. The doctor's diagnosis was an ongoing decline in all body functions and eventually death! Eddie's response was that God was in charge, and he started to follow The Hallelujah Diet. That was 3 years ago. The results: Now transferring from wheelchair by himself, No bladder infections for 2 years, No flu's or colds for 2 years, No more memory loss at all, No constipation at all, Vision improved -- Had to get weaker glasses, Now standing unaided on walking frame for

5 minutes, Now believes he will walk again, Hair re-growing and has to shave every day now, Increased motor co-ordination, All blood tests normal, Robust Life." [113]

Donna – "I was diagnosed with Multiple Sclerosis (MS) 15-years ago. For the first 5-years, while my children were young, I was very sick. Then about 10-years ago, after returning from a clinic in Reno where I had gone looking for help with my MS, I came upon your book, "God's Way To Ultimate Health," in a book store. I read the book, immediately knew it was God's answer to my physical problems, and started the Hallelujah Diet. After just a few weeks on the diet, my MS symptoms started going away. Prior to the diet change, I was wiped out by noon and had no energy to do anything the rest of the day, but now my energy was returning. It has been 10-years since that day I started on The Hallelujah Diet, and I am thrilled to report that I am totally well, and haven't seen a doctor for my MS since then. I don't even say that I have MS anymore, because all symptoms are totally gone." (7/10/2007, first written) [114]

Dale K. of Tennessee – "About 5-years ago, while painting our house, I became extremely fatigued and started slurring my words. I went to the hospital and an MRI showed lesions on my brain. My hearing was damaged and my vision impaired to the extent I couldn't see very well. Then I started having balance problems, tremors in my feet and lower legs, and I started dragging my right foot. About three months after the first attack, I was diagnosed with Multiple Sclerosis. I was completely devastated. The symptoms I was experiencing and the diagnosis devastated me. I prayed fervently for God to heal me, or show me what to do. That is when someone gave me a copy of George Malkmus' tapes on 'How to Eliminate Sickness.' Immediately after listening to the tape, I went on The Hallelujah Diet, and within a week started feeling better. Soon thereafter my whole body began to improve and my energy returned. The tremors and shakes that were so uncomfortable went away, my balance improved, and the dizziness disappeared. My eyesight, according to my eye doctor is continuing to improve, and I have not had another attack, nor do I expect to. It is wonderful to feel normal again and to know I am going to continue to feel great every day, just as long as I remain on The Hallelujah Diet." [115]

   C. B., Maricopa, Arizona; "I am a 51 year old married woman who in January 2005, at age 47, was diagnosed with Multiple Sclerosis. Between January 2005 until I began The Hallelujah Diet in July 2008, I suffered an exacerbations every six months that would last anywhere from two weeks to one month. My last relapse was in May 2008 and was the worst ever. My brother-in-law told me about The Hallelujah Diet in July 2008 and suggested it might help my condition. He showed me a testimony of a woman who had her Multiple Sclerosis go into remission after adopting The Hallelujah Diet. That testimony inspired me enough to start the journey. It has been almost a year now since I adopted the diet and since making the diet change I have not experienced even one relapse. In fact, I feel great. I bicycle six miles three times a week, walk miles twice a week, and swim once a week. I have lost 14 pounds and many inches. I have no other option than to continue eating food that is in its original state, just as God told us we should eat in Genesis 1:29. I will never go back to the old way of eating because my health depends on my choices, and I know that with God's strength, truth, and promises, I can continue making healthy choices for myself. I am blessed to have a husband who desires to be healthy also, and so we continue on this journey together, standing strong against those who would challenge us to forsake The Hallelujah Diet. My daughter and her boyfriend have recently joined us on the diet." Maricopa, AZ *(Population 1040)*

   Pastor Michael Sustar of Phoenix, AZ – "Two years ago I was diagnosed with Multiple Sclerosis, and the symptoms continued to worsen, until I could barely shuffle along or climb even a few stairs. My eyesight was also deteriorating rapidly . . . I adopted The Hallelujah Diet and within just eleven weeks, I was able to walk normally, bound up stairs, and my eyesight had improved tremendously. My wife Monica, who had thyroid problems, has also seen considerable improvement since the diet change."[116]

These are a few of the many testimonials cited on their website and in their literature for MS. On contacting Olin Idol, a leader in the H.A. movement about Parkinson's, he said they only have about 5 people who were helped and claim being cured to some degree, that he was aware of.

Even though the few people just mentioned were not in any official study, they really had MS and were really cured of MS. This is extremely important. A medical doctor with Parkinson's once told me, "Many medical doctors lack common sense!" There is some truth in that statement, sometimes medical doctors and researchers tend to lack common sense because they don't want to accept these simple testimonials. Like most people they want to see hundreds of cures in a study that lasts 10 years or longer. If they don't see this happen, then they throw the baby out with the bathwater and discard the preliminary evidence. What was just presented are a few short testimonials of people being healed of MS related to this organization and its Living Plant-based nutrition diet. Praise-God!

e. Alan Greer the Remission, Cure

One of the best known and most publicized people with MS whose lives have changed as a result of identifying their food sensitivities are Alan Greer.[117] "The other well-publicized exclusion diet with a successful outcome is the Rita Greer diet. Rita Greer began experimenting with foods for her husband Alan when he was severely disabled and doctors had written him off as a hopeless case. Her first breakthrough was when she accidentally discovered that Alan felt better on a diet that totally excluded meat - something she was forced to do through sheer poverty. From that, it was a short step to discover that he reacted badly to eggs and cheese and all saturated fat. Rita also decided to follow the principles of the gluten-free diet and cut out everything made with wheat, barley, oats, and rye."

"With much trial and error, hard work, study of nutrition, and the creativity that goes with being a gifted artist, Rita eventually came up with a diet that suited Alan's body perfectly. She kept him on this basically vegan diet for about four years, during which time he made gigantic improvements to the point where the wheelchair and walking aids were banished with the bedpans to the lumber room. His regeneration was so startling that some doctors were doubtful that he had ever had MS at all, as his improved condition did not tally with his medical notes. There is no doubt, however, that Alan Greer did and does have MS. It is just that he no longer eats the foods that were having a toxic effect on him."[118]

This just shows that persistence pays off, especially when dealing with nutrition. The following testimonials of Carol and Darlene are case studies of complete recovery of advanced MS. (Which are described in the book: *The MS Recovery Diet.*[119])

f. Carol the Remission, Cure

Carol was diagnosed with MS at thirty-two and later read about the Dr. Swank diet and other nutritional approaches which she tried. "Carol's serene countenance gives an impression of a young woman in her thirties, not a fifty-one-year-old. Adding to this, several years of yoga show in her good posture and easy movements. Certainly, this is not the picture of a woman who has MS."

"She then related that over the last almost twenty years, she had given information about her MS diet – the Swank diet – to about a hundred people. "Of course, I haven't been able to follow up on everyone, but the three people I know who followed the diet are now essentially symptom-free. All those folks that I know of who decided it was too extreme or that they couldn't give up some foods are now quite progressed in their disease," Carol said. "I don't understand. When my MS was bad, I was so depressed and desperate to do anything. If the way out of MS was to only eat gruel, then I would have done just that."[120]

"As the years went by and Carol lived free of symptoms, she became more lax about her diet, eating a lot of things she hadn't before. She even dared to eat foods with high fat, including Mexican food. In the fall of 1989, Carol's MS returned with a vengeance. Both of her legs felt like trunks, and she shuffled like a surgery patient. She was horrified. 'This is it!' she told herself, 'I'm not going downhill.'"

"Carol returned to strictly following the diet and three weeks later she was again symptom-free. Carol has rarely strayed since. Laughing at herself, Carol explained how she weaned herself from her favorite chocolate ambrosia pie. 'Every time I looked at the pie, I'd superimpose an image of myself in a wheelchair on it.' That killed her craving."[121]

So she's in a state of permanent remission and, as long as she stays on her strict diet, including lots of fruits and vegetables, she can live a normal lifestyle. It a strict diet or is it a normal, healthy diet, it's the rest of the world that is off-base eating the standard American diet. The important thing is that when she returned to the strict Living plant-based diet she became symptom-free. The following story of Darlene is even more dramatic.

g. Darlene the Remission, Cure

This testimony of complete recovery of advanced MS is dramatic and shows the power of living nutrition when a person perseveres week after week, month after month, year after year as Darlene did.[122] This is really a story of the Ann Wigmore diet combined with other diets since Darlene took wheat grass juice, which was promoted by Ann Wigmore back in the 1970's.

In 1974, Darlene's whole being was ravaged by her rapidly progressing multiple sclerosis. The overwhelming, paralyzing fatigue had robbed her of all vitality. "I was tired, I didn't care about anything." Darlene recalled her arms and legs were lost in numbness, preventing her from doing any activity. Even worse, she was often beset with intermittent spasms, in which her muscles would tremor, and cramps, in which her muscles would tighten in excruciating pain.

"MS also affected her vision, making the world a blurry place, taking away any possibility of reading or doing handwork. Darlene's cognitive abilities, such as thinking and reasoning, were lost in an MS fog. She became increasingly emaciated because, after eating, she experienced punishing pain in her chest and around her heart. Darlene added another reason she go so thin was that often she was just too tired to chew and swallow. Finally, Darlene experienced difficulty swallowing and breathing, the last-stage symptoms. Her days were spent sleeping or just lying down because she had neither the ability nor energy to do anything else."[123]

"The symptoms initially began a few years before 1970, but she dated the start of her progressive MS to 1970. During this time, she visited doctors and took their advice and prescriptions. But nothing helped, and the medications only gave bad side effects and reactions. She continued to worsen and by 1974 the MS was full blown. She and her husband started looking elsewhere and discovered Sr. Bridgette MacDougall, who was one of the early pioneers in the diet/nutrition approach to multiple sclerosis. She gave up gluten, limited fat intake and sugar.

"Careful as she was about following the diet, after six months, Darlene was discouraged because she felt that she hadn't registered any progress. Then, while praying, she realized that the pain in her chest and around her heart after she ate was gone. That one bit of progress was enough. She redoubled her efforts." [124]

Darlene explained that she always tried to "remember the depths, from which she had climbed," rather than look at all she still couldn't do. "That helps" she said, "as well as being aware of the little things. Recovery from MS is all about almost imperceptible steps forward." After a while, more confident, she began to vary her foods a little. "I noticed that some things on MacDougall's list [to avoid] didn't bother me." Darlene said. "And some of the things he said were OK did bother me." She kept a food diary, being especially careful to track new foods, which she introduced at a rate of one a week. For her, reactions to foods came quickly in the form of indigestion or echoes of past symptoms.

"In minute steps, Darlene kept getting better. 'After I could walk without help, and it was hardly good walking, it took another two to three years before I could do stairs,' she told me. Fortunately, her cognitive skills and ability to think and remember were among the first things to clear up. Her vision was another symptom that improved early on. This allowed her to read labels and to do her own research on MS and nutrition."

"Through the healing years, mindful that the anemia could return, Darlene had her trusted family physician monitor her. A good and compassionate man, he was supportive of her diet and was impressed by her results. Upon his request, she wrote up her experience, giving the details of what she did. Her doctor passed the essay on to some of his other patients with MS. None of them followed through, with one person going so far as to say that it was 'too much work.' Darlene noted that the same holds true now. She shook her head over all the unnecessary pain and suffering because of people's ignorance and unwillingness to take charge of their MS."[125]

h. Joseph Malfara the Remission, Cure

Joseph Malfara of Toronto, Ontario, Canada is 58 (1913) and for 18 years (in 2013) he had multiple sclerosis (MS). Through some raw fooders he found out about raw foods and was told about the Hippocrates Health Institute (HHI). "It took me a year to make up my mind, and I first visited Hippocrates for my MS condition … After three weeks, I did not see any results. I may have improved some, but I didn't notice anything. As it turns out, I had actually spent the three weeks detoxing. So I booked for one more week, and what a week! Slowly my legs were getting stronger. I could walk with a stride, and lots of good things happened in week four. I went home with confidence that I was on the right path. I continued eating raw food for about eight more months. But I was losing so much weight that I panicked and started re-introducing cooked foods, including chicken and other meat." "Over the next year and a half, my health started to decline from my poor food choices. My walking got worse. I would get sick with colds, sometimes even pneumonia." Joseph took a trip to Brazil and then Bulgaria for this MS but it did not help but only got worst.

Finally, my sister Rene and my sweetie Laura said, "You got better at Hippocrates, what are you doing wasting your time and money traveling all over the world? You tried this before and got better!" So I thought about it for a few weeks, and booked another trip to HHI. For the next three weeks Joe did a number of different therapies for his MS and also for Lyme disease that he did not know he had. He continued eating the raw foods and drinking wheat grass juice and he wrote, "I am slowly getting better. My head is much clearer, and Laura has noticed a big improvement in my ability to communicate. My thinking, speaking and writing are so much better. I have started going to the gym every day – something I had not done in three years. My upper body is getting stronger, and after six weeks I have started resistance training to strengthen my legs. I learned that I have to work on my legs in the evening, to prevent fatigue with my walking during the day. To date, I have also

55

lost 25 pounds without even trying, just by eating great living and energetic food." Towards the end of his 12 week stay Joe started walking on his own for short distances. "It took a long time to get this way, and it will not go away in 9 or 12 weeks. If only there was a magic bullet!" He ends the article saying, "Yours, now in better health, and continuing to get better on this life learning journey, Joe Malfara."[126]

i. Olympic Plant-based Cure Zone

People struggling with major degenerative diseases like Parkinson's and MS need to move into the Plant-based Cure Zone in an Olympic way. They need to imagine that they are trying out for the Olympics'. It is hard work for months in order to start to see results when training for the Olympics. It is usually 9 to 18 months to see full results in being cured from a degenerative disease. Whether a person is training for the Olympic Games or for an Olympic Cure of their degenerative disease, they need support, coaching and proper nutrition. When a person has to battle cancer, Parkinson's, MS or other major degenerative diseases, this battle embodies the Olympic Spirit!

In the 2012 Olympics, one athlete said, 'I haven't had a dessert in 2 years.' Sometimes it is individual work and other times its team work as in the 2014 winter Olympics several teams swept the metals such as America in skiing and Russia in the 50 meter cross country. Another Olympian said, 'I haven't watched TV since last summer.' Training is what makes athletes Olympians, it's an investment to be the best, and for a degenerative disease you are trying to optimize your body to overcome the disease. The person needs to try to be their best. Olympic athletes have time constraints, like the rest of us, but they have learned to utilize their time to maximize their training. People with degenerative diseases also have to learn to utilize their time in preparing the Live-Foods, fasting and juicing to maximize their bodies' ability to cure the disease, or at least to put it in remission. These people need to make a long-term commitment to live in the Plant-based Cure Zone to maintain their optimal health and healing.

An Olympic champion is the culmination of a lot of hard work, blood, sweat and tears. It involves a legacy of excellence, a fire-brand of possibilities, and striving towards perfection. The discipline that is required to overcome a major degenerative disease requires similar aspirations, but work in the area of nutrition and fasting. Upon conquering the disease, the person can say, 'Wow! Did I really do that?' They will have achieved a tremendous joy and peace.

In the 2012 summer Olympics, 85 countries won at least 1 medal and 7 countries won a medal for the 1st time. Yet it helps to be your own country, Russia in its country in 2014 won 33 medals and 13 gold, the most of any country in 2014 (America won 28 medals, 9 gold). The 'Olympic Plant-based Cure Achievement Awards' is not about countries but about degenerative disease categories. A total of 98 events in 15 winter sport disciplines were held at Sochi, Russia (2014), there are at least 98 degenerative diseases that can be cured with a Living Plant-based nutrition therapy with about 15 different disciplines involved in this type of therapy.

Winning is not a competition between individuals, but a competition to beat the disease or diseases they struggle with. Every two (or four) years there should be a contest and it will have examples of cures through Live-Foods or plant-based foods. The cures will be analyzed and in each major disease category a Gold, a Silver and a Bronze Achievement award will be given. The contestants will be people who have conquered the degenerative disease and are models of Olympic champions who overcame the many barriers to win freedom from the bondage of the disease. They will continue to live in the Plant-based Cure Zone which keeps the disease at a distance and their health optimal.

The 2014 Olympic Plant-based Cure Awards has given a Bronze award to Robert Trincellito, a Silver award to Matt Goodman and a Gold award to Judy Livingstone for their Live-Food Cures of MS. During the years 2008 and 2014, their case histories were studied and were deemed a model for others to follow in their fight to overcome MS. Following are their stories."

j. Robert Trincellito the Remission, Cure

The person who received the Bronze Award, Robert Trincellito from New York (age 43 in 2008). He was officially diagnosed with MS on 1/7/08. Based on his MRI and his history, he had had MS for between 5 to 8 years. He had psoriasis, crippling migraines and volatile moods accompanied with depression, due to severe hormonal imbalances. He also had a large patch of de-myelinization in the brain. Some of his symptoms included double vision, massive mood swings, confusion and loss of sight in his left eye (optical neuritis: treated with steroids, cleared up in a couple of weeks, Christmas 2007). The doctor put him on several drugs. One drug made him suicidal and he was taken off of it.

Robert comments: "I do believe the meds were actually counterproductive during this time because, since being 100% off of them, I do feel finally, totally free and at peace. I was told that this one drug was a synthetic peptide, along with amino acids, so it didn't seem to be chemically invasive. It was, for me, totally mentally invasive. I honestly believe that the meds made my burgeoning body sluggish."

Robert found a nutritionist, and even though he followed the regimens of supplements prescribed, he experienced minimal progress, with noticeable side effects such as hypersensitivity and insomnia. Shortly afterwards, it was a friend, Jennifer, who introduced him to a lifestyle of a raw diet, good food combinations, and detoxification through colon hydrotherapy. The results were immediate. His moods began to stabilize and his psoriasis quickly disappeared. His energy levels were heightened, his focus sharpened, his migraines ceased to exist and he lost 50 pounds, presently weighing a healthy 166 pounds which is normal for his height and build.

Robert joined an MS support group and he e-mailed me this comment in the midst of my questions about his MS: "James, I am so proud of what I've done. After attending a few MS group sessions soon after being diagnosed back in Feb or March of '08, and listening to hopeless, groaning about medications and Doctors, I vowed that this would not be my fate. I could not believe that this is what was in store for me. I was more scared of people with MS than I was of having MS myself.

So, on Feb 9, 2008, one day after my 42nd birthday, I CHOSE to begin my path to wellness. I made mistakes but have continued to move on and grow. It was also on this day that I wrote my mantra, 'I choose to live presently, in retrospect of my own future that will be without regret. James, if I'm in a wheelchair 20 years from today, I will have no regrets because I am accountable to, and respectful of, my future self. Getting MS hasn't been a tragedy for me. It hasn't ruined my life, it has saved it."

Robert relates a regression that happened in May 2009: "Back in May, I felt some numbness in my lower right leg and sensitivity to cold. I was extremely stressed due to a very personal matter and had completely abandoned all my hard work and efforts concerning diet, juicing, and exercise. I made a rare visit to my neurologist. He called it a 'sensory exacerbation.' He also said that it didn't mean my MS was getting worse, he said it seemed that it was just poking its head out to take a look around. He prescribed steroids which I did not take and a MRI which I refused to get. I immediately fasted for the next 3 days and did colonics. The symptoms quickly went away and I've never looked back." This is an important event because it shows that after 6 months he was in remission, as long as he continued on the raw diet and detoxification regime.

In September of 2008, Robert started eating raw foods (80/20 raw) and was not a vegetarian before that time. In October 2008, he started doing colonics once a week for a month and since then, twice a month. He also did juicing, smoothies and juice fasting on a weekly basis. Robert has been drinking juice almost daily since September 2008. On some days he just drank juice without ever thinking about it. Starting in February 2009, he would juice fast for one day a week and in April, he started fasting 2 to 3 days once a month. He would usually use green juices on a fast: "Some fast days might be a fruit smoothie for breakfast and killer green juices the rest of the day. In fact, that is pretty much my average daily regimen."

On asking the question, did the juice fasting seem to help the MS? Robert replied, "I do believe so. I feel so well and healthy just fasting that my body continues to thank me for all my efforts. The pure fact that my psoriasis is gone, which existed like gloves on my hands, is a testament that my immune system is correcting itself."

On asking another question, did you find doing colonics helped the MS symptoms or recovery? Robert replied, "Absolutely! I believe in colonics so much in treating my MS that I've become a licensed colonic therapist! I have been self-treating for the better part of 6 months. The benefits are so noticeable and absolutely invaluable to all, but more so and especially MS-ers!! My overall wellness response was incredible." (Before November 2008 Robert never did an enema.)

Robert continued: "As I've stated in the past, my approach to my MS is simple, treat my overall wellness and immune system, which in turn will correct the 'errors' that have unwittingly occurred in my body."

On asking: What do others think of your being healed of MS? Robert replied: "Citizens love what I've done, MS-ers not as much."

Within a month after starting a raw food diet, Robert noticed that his new diet approach helped with the symptoms of MS and his entire well-being. Physically, he noticed that his MS symptoms started going away within the first two months. Cognitively, in his thinking processes, it was more gradual in that the symptoms faded away within four months. He recognizes the change in his life and well-being and states: "All I can say is that no one, including myself, recognizes that man I am now from who I used to be. I have been reborn. My mission from day one was to get my immune system to STOP attacking my nervous system. With all the changes I've experienced, I believe: mission accomplished."[e]

Two things can be noticed about Robert's testimonial that was influential in putting his MS into complete remission. First, is that he moved into a raw foods orientation, of approximately 80% raw, 20% cooked, which is a standard raw vegan diet. The second thing is he did detoxification methods along with his new raw foods diet. He did colonics, juicing and juice fasting to detoxify. Thus, it was both his raw vegan diet and detoxification methods that changed his biochemistry enough to put the MS into complete remission for several years (September 2008 to September 2010). It takes the body years to rebuild in its quest for healing, and in the meantime, he can live a perfectly normal, healthy lifestyle with his Living Foods diet, juicing, and juice fasting program! This is an excellent witness of nature's power to heal!

k. Matt Goodman the Remission, Cure

-----

[e] E-mails confirming status of MS: August 2009, September 2010; Robert's website is: www.fifthstreetwellness.com

Matt is a very pragmatic person and states clearly that "I manage it, and don't believe in a cure." This is what this book is all about putting MS into remission and managing it. But in the plant-based nutrition world it could be considered cured. By staying on a strict raw vegan therapeutic nutritional approach as pointed out in this book the MS stays in remission, but some just say, they're cured!

The person who received the Silver Award is Matt Goodman. In November 1997 Matt Goodman was diagnosed with Multiple Sclerosis by a neurologists before his 26th birthday. He was in good shape as a personal trainer. Eventually he could walk but not exercise or run and was on various pharmaceutical drugs. He got a video by George Malkmus of Hallelujah Acres. He took action and made the transition to 100% raw foods. He experienced a strong detox period of about three to four weeks. After just six months on a 100% raw food diet, Matt was running at full speed. In nine months Matt was leaping over boulders and running in the Adirondack Mountains. He also does yoga and meditation. June 2003, Matt and his dog started hiking the Appalachian Trail and traveled over 2,600 miles on rugged terrain, with a 65 pound backpack, from Maine to Tennessee! Today Matt is medication free and has not worked with a medical doctor since 1998. He wrote a book on his healing journey called, *To the Brink.*

Matt said "I had a real bad flare-up (in 1999), and I stopped eating cooked foods," he said. "I felt that starting to eat raw food was the beginning of the self-healing (process). It took about six months before I started to feel a lot stronger." Now Matt feels better than when he was diagnosed. Matt and his wife, Sandy, stick to their raw foods lifestyle. He explained, "I eat mostly raw, juice fast as often as often as I can, but Sandy does not, nor should she live as strict as I do.[127]

In an email interview he gave a deeper understanding of his remission. In 1997 Matt saw three neurologists, 2 were renowned at Jefferson and Univ. Penn. First he tried Solumedrol/ Prednisone, but only for an unsuccessful healing of optic neuritis and weakened legs, but after a sleepless - 5 days, "I was done with drugs until 5 months later I succumbed to Interferon injections (Avonex) for another 5 months until I got off it." An MRI showed lesions on the brain in 1997.

Over the next year he did well without drugs until one week he had a major flare-up. "I immediately opened to raw in desperation, then fasting a year and a half later. Lived strict like a monk: raw, fasting, yoga, for 3+ years, then walked from Maine to Tennessee, 1600 miles, at a ridiculous fast clip passing most people. All of this was almost 6 years after my diagnosis."

"When I got home I did tree-work for 2.5 years, and today still work more than full-time today in retail management and live on a 4th gen heirloom cranberry farm with wife and pets. However, by no means am I running up any mountains. I am more than 10 years older, autoimmune conditions take their toll, but there is dignity and strength dealing with all levels of disability and the aging process. This is somebody speaking with pretty incredible discipline, so there is no shame in struggle. I say this with a twinkle in my eye of course, knowing what happens when I allow the miraculous tools to do their magic. Dealing with any serious illness takes incredible strength. I am thankful that I am privy to the tools that wait for us to plunge."[128]

In asking for examples of his MS symptoms he had, he replied. "I've had every common symptom that I've heard and usually manage them all too varying degrees. Numb arms, legs, skipping/ double vision, blindness, weak bladder/ prostate, vertigo." On asking, have you had any recurring symptoms since you hiked the Adirondack Mountains? "I've hiked many mountains in the Adirondacks, but not since before I hiked the Appalachian Trail. Like I said, I manage all symptoms, and quite well I must say."

What was it like the first three months of being raw with MS? "Felt good after a 3-week cleanse, but nerves take a lot of patience to heal. Six months of very strict healthy regimen and I was running fast again!" What was it like from nine months to a year with MS? "MS can be debilitating very quick depending on a number of factors. Even at my strongest, I could put myself in a wheelchair in a matter of hours with a few bad choices piled on top of one another."

What was it like from a year into raw: to the second year of being raw with/without MS? "Unbelievable, especially when I started a diligent juiced fasting schedule: 1 day a week, 3-4 days in a row 1/month. Then 10 days, generally with the change of seasons. With yoga, properly combined and portioned raw and juice fasting, I don't believe in limits. Without these tools, MS is a nightmare."

Asking if yoga or other exercised helped? "Absolutely. I still do a full body self-massage, roll on balls, and at least some yoga almost every day. Most other exercise is retail management and yard-work." He uses green foods as one of his supplements.

Did you ever leave the raw food diet or pull back on raw foods and find the symptoms came back? "Sure. I've been mostly raw since 1999, but I've never been conventional. Nature is my teacher, not just humans with agenda. We'd eat all kinds of stuff foraging. My wife's a gourmet cook and dang straight I taste ☺

What Matt is describing here is typical in others with MS, they do great on a raw food diet until they leave it for a length of time, like a month, then the MS comes back with a vengeance as Darlene said in her interview. There is a biochemical threshold that an MS person needs to stay above.

Judy Livingstone (below) has worked hard to have several glasses of carrot juice every day and eat a raw diet and has had little to no symptoms. She also climbs mountains and does many other sports in Maine.

So you have any advice for those with MS?
MATT: "I definitely think virtually all illness can be managed if not overcome, with the implementation of some personally tailored, universal tools. At the same time, there is no shame in not being able to do it and taking medication. Slow down, ask for and receive help, and wear the warrior badge of dealing with health issues with dignity. Number one: don't feel guilty if you can't control it. Focus on the fundamentals – work to slow and halt the progression of symptoms. Be patient and be in the moment. Have belief in yourself and commit to follow through with your health goals."[129] His website: www.rawpower.info

The next case history is more of a case study of the whole experience and history of being cured of MS through Live-Food Nutrition. All of the testimonials given earlier could turn into a case-history like Matt's or Robert's or a case study like Judy's, but this is a lot of work. Jim personally travelled to visit Judy several times (once with Anne Marie) to write this case-history.

l. Judy Livingstone the Remission, Cure - A Case Study
Olympic Live-Food Cure - Winner of the Gold

This Case History on Judy Livingstone is a powerful story of Multiple Sclerosis being cured. It was written by Jim and Anne Marie's interviews and reviewed by her.
Judy Livingstone - MS Testimonial March 2010

The MS Diagnosis
"In 1989, Judy was a 40 year old female living in the Florida Keys with her husband and two children, and working at a hospital as a phlebotomist (a person who draws blood). She took a new job as a cashier in a busy

supermarket and noticed that she began to lose part of her visual acuity. Some of the keys on the keyboard were disappearing. She was referred to a neurologist at Miami-Dade hospital. After testing, and an MRI, four lesions were found on her brain and they determined she had Multiple Sclerosis (MS). These lesions appeared as 'white matter' on the MRI and indicated a deterioration of the myelin sheaths on the nerves.

"At that point, she was on the Standard American Diet (SAD). She started to feel really sick from the disease and had problems with her legs; she was beginning to get wobbly and unsteady at times as her motor skills were deteriorating.

"Her marriage began to fall apart and she got a divorce and moved back to Maine with her two sons, where she had three jobs. She was diagnosed with Multiple Sclerosis a second time from a doctor in Portland. When she moved to outside of Bangor, she was again diagnosed with MS by a neurologist in Bangor. She had three medical doctors who all gave her the MS diagnosis.

"After coming back to Maine, she started attending a Pentecostal Church. After a few years, she met a man, Ernie, who she dated. Ernie accepted her disease and they fell in love and got married. They bought a large parcel of land deep in the woods and built their house, in which they still live.

"The MS started getting worse. She started getting electrical shocks from her nervous system, and some drugs helped to deal with these issues, but the shocks were increasingly uncomfortable and it made her skin sensitive to touch. Her body would jump, like someone sticking her with pins. It didn't stay localized; it started in her face and back of head, and moved down her arm, and her skin would become very tender. These symptoms could last up to seven days, and then they might subside for a while, and then come back again. She didn't get much REM sleep as a result.

"At this point, she accepted medications for her MS. But the medications didn't help her much because the more she took them, the less mobile she became. The medication seemed to affect her mobility and didn't abate the progression of her disease.

"These shocks from her nervous system would come and go. The symptoms might last only three days; there seemed to be no pattern to it. She learned that MS runs its own course as there is no dependable pattern for its progression. It produces surprises and is different every day.

"Other symptoms of the disease are cluster headaches and photophobia; Judy couldn't find relief at all. The cluster headaches affected her eyes and being in the dark would make her more comfortable. She was prescribed oxygen to use on a regular basis. By breathing in about 8 liters of oxygen for 12 minutes it would take the headache away.

"Ptosis of the eyelids was another symptom that lasted a week or two, and was always connected with the cluster headaches. Then the eye would recover.

"Her gait started deteriorating after two years and her legs started being affected. She started using a cane and later, had to use a walker for adequate support while being mobile. She was prescribed an AFO lift-brace for one foot because she was beginning to drag it due to a primary foot drop. Her balance was not good and she wasn't able to walk easily without a walker. At first, it happened occasionally, but about 1 to 2 years later, she had to use the walker or have human assistance all the time. For the next fifteen years, it was almost constant.

"She was taking lots of medications including: Tegretol, Amitriptyline, Prozac, Xanax and Methotrexate, to name a few. The side effects of these drugs would make her almost helpless and her husband would have to take care of her. Ernie would often have to help her shower and dress.

"In 2002, her neurologist ordered another MRI. The scan showed 9 lesions on her brain. So the disease had progressed. She started to feel desperate and was willing to go anywhere, even out of the country, to find a cure. She knew that her disease was steadily progressing.

"A devastating symptom was memory loss. She couldn't do her checkbook anymore, because she couldn't think clearly; it was like being medicated. She couldn't do a task, because it was confusing and it was too difficult to do. She would forget the simplest things. She was not able to run the household anymore. Oftentimes, at home, she would usually just sit and watch television to pass the day.

"She started getting frustrated, having to use the walker all the time. She gradually lost her independence and became dependent on everyone around her. She was homebound, and when she fell, Ernie would bring her to the emergency room. The doctor thought she was depressed but Judy insisted that she was not depressed but frustrated. She told the doctors, "Wouldn't you be frustrated if you couldn't be independent anymore?" But the doctors put her on anti-depressant medications anyway. She says "My medicine cabinet was filled with bottles of pills, but I was getting worse by the day." She reflected, "My emotions got into all this, because I couldn't think about how to get better."

"She could not really say that the medication helped her symptoms, but they did help to make her sleep at times. But, on the other hand, she notes that the drugs didn't work well for sleeping either. She took the medications because the doctors said the drugs would work. Sometimes the drugs would increase some symptoms for a while. They would help a little on the balance in the beginning, but afterwards they did not really help anymore.

"Judy related that the doctors would suggest a drug saying, 'I don't know if it is going to work, it's worked in the past for other patients, so let's try this. If it doesn't work, we'll try this other drug. If you are lucky and this drug works, then it will be good for that symptom.' So Judy would try the drug, but it was like a guessing game. The only thing that actually worked for Judy was the oxygen for headaches. What made her the angriest was when the doctors would say something like: 'I am only here to listen to your symptoms; we don't have a cure for it.' Judy became very disillusioned with all the drugs she was taking.

The Turning Point

"There was a turning point in Judy's struggle, something that stopped the downhill progression of the disease and started a process of healing to take place.

"In 2003, Judy had been part of a local church for 11 years; she was on the worship team. It was a Pentecostal church and oftentimes the members would come over and pray over her when she was struggling with the disease. The prayers did not stop the disease but would help her emotions, and sometimes the symptoms for that day; the prayers gave her hope and gave her a lift in life.

"She was a confirmed Catholic, and at age 21, she changed and became Pentecostal. She has been slain in the spirit and was at the altar when she first prayed in tongues. She prays in tongues in her private life and believes it protects and relaxes her. Her husband was also Catholic and became Pentecostal and prays in tongues as well. She and Ernie have a strong prayer life together.

"When she was asked, 'Did you feel let down if people prayed over you and nothing happened?' she replied 'No, I have never blamed God for my MS. We have control over how we behave. I just feel everything happens for a reason, the body, soul and spirit are connected.'

"When asked, 'When at home, and had symptoms, would you pray?' She replied, 'Yes, I would feel better emotionally, but the symptoms wouldn't go away, I felt better because I released it and God's in control of my life. You have to stay in the WORD and feed your spiritual body.'

"One Sunday, a blind man, Bill Irwin, MSW with a seeing-eye dog came to their church. He heard her shuffling along the church corridor after the service and asked his wife to ask her what was wrong with her. His wife asked Ernie and he said, 'she has Multiple Sclerosis, and it is progressing rapidly. She is sort of in the latter stages of the disease and will soon be wheelchair bound.'

"'The next week, Bill told Ernie that I didn't need to be sick anymore and that he thought he could help me. So we got together and Bill said, 'If you really listen to me, and you really understand what I'm trying to tell you, you can get better, and maybe even well.' Bill has a 30 plus year background in Clinical Chemistry. He is a Christian Family and Marriage Counselor, a Health Minister, a Life Coach, and a nationally known professional Motivational Speaker. He has hiked the entire Appalachian Trail, with his Seeing-Eye Dog, Orient, and wrote a book about his journey. The book is called *Blind Courage*.

"Bill then explained what he wanted her to do. He suggested baby steps at first, which included juicing carrots and drinking a green powder drink made from barley, called *Barley Max*. He warned her that it didn't taste too good, but suggested she drink six glasses of it a day.

"Judy's first reaction to Bill was, 'What do I have to lose? I have tried everything else, and nothing worked. I've tried medicines and psychologists. So why not give this a try?' She told Bill that she was on lots of medications, 14 of them and that she needed the medications in order to stay better. Bill said, 'Take things as they come.'

"In the beginning, she just drank the carrot juice and Barley Max and started to feel a little more energy. After a while, Bill suggested that instead of continuing with baby steps that she go to the next level and fully change her lifestyle. Bill asked her if she was willing to do this and Judy told him that she was willing. Then he told her that she had to get all of the dairy and meat products out of her life. He said she should not consume any animal based products: anything that originated from a father and a mother. Next, he said she needed to get rid of caffeinated coffee, white flour and all processed or fried foods. In addition, Bill told them they needed to consume very little cooked foods and to arrange the meals so that 85% of everything they ate was raw. He also suggested that she begin to walk as rapidly as she could for a half hour a day and increase her speed until she could walk a mile in 15 minutes and then increase the time to an hour five times a week. 'Rigorous exercise is an absolute must for one to become optimally well and stay that way. It enhances all body functions and supports the immune system and takes away negative emotions such as depression, anxiety etc.,' he admonished her.

"An interesting part of Judy's new diet was that she did not take any supplements except for the green barley powder. She did take B12 for a while, but not diligently. And today she still takes no vitamins, which means the diet and juicing carrots gave her all the nutrients she needed to recover. She did turn slightly orange or brown color on her skin from all the carrot juice every day. It looked like a good tan.

"Ernie was very supportive and willing to do the lifestyle with Judy. So their home became a raw vegan one, whereas before they served the standard American diet. They arranged their meals to be 100% vegan and about 85% raw foods, having a little cooked food at dinner time. When she first started the diet, she gave up everything and went right to it. In the morning she ate only fruit, in afternoon only salad and at suppertime she ate some cooked food. She followed an 85/15 raw vegan diet which means about 85% of the food

71

is raw and only about 15 % is cooked, and zero animal products are allowed; it is a vegan diet.

"Exactly 4 months after beginning to follow diet, she got up about 5:30 am one morning and felt like she had energy. Ernie asked her was wrong. She said, 'I feel good!' He replied, 'What do you mean you feel good?' 'I can't explain it, but I just feel good, I have energy.' She replied.

"'Wow, what do you want to do?' her husband asked. She replied, 'Maybe later on today we can take a little walk. I haven't been for a walk outside in a long time. So let's take a walk.'

"Later that day, she and Ernie went for a walk but the AFO support the doctors had prescribed to stabilize her foot, didn't feel comfortable, so she took it off. It was then she noticed that her foot wasn't dropped; it was not hanging anymore. Walking further, she said to Ernie, 'I feel better without it.' She put the AFO support away in the closet that day and hasn't needed it since.

"About a week later, she said to Ernie, 'You know, I'm not having those visual symptoms or those awful cluster headaches.' He said, 'Yeah, I've noticed that.' So she stopped the deliveries of oxygen because the cluster headaches were gone. Two major symptoms of the disease were gone within about 4 months.

"Another early symptom that stopped was her legs jumping around in bed. She stopped the medication after consulting her doctor. As each symptom went away, she weaned off the medications. She learned that she should wait for the symptoms to go away and then she needed to ask her doctor how to get off the medication, since some medications can't just be stopped and must be weaned slowly. Her doctor helped to get her off the pharmaceutical drugs.

"After about 3 months, she started using the cane instead of a walker. About 5 to 6 months after starting her new lifestyle, she was not dependent on the cane at all. By 5 months, she was able to use her husband's arm because her body and legs were getting stronger. Also, she no longer had the pains in her legs and body that she used to have.

"Before the lifestyle change, she didn't get a lot of restful sleep at night because of the pain and the bouncing and jerking of her legs. When her legs stopped bouncing and jerking, she started getting a good night's sleep. It was about 3 to 4 months before this activity slowed down, and by the 5th month, it was completely gone. Then she was able to sleep through the night and get more rest. With MS, the immune system begins to be compromised and stress becomes a key factor. By then, she had been taught stress management by Bill, and that helped a lot.

Counseling Is Needed
"Judy believes that the body can heal itself, but it has to be given the proper treatment. She says, 'You can't eat the SAD diet (Standard American Diet) and get rid of MS.' She also believes now that healing MS is partly psychological, that a lot of people don't want to give up things, like resentment, which they hold onto. Anger and other issues need to be redirected and a counselor can help with this. Curing MS is a long slow process that needs to happen on the spiritual, physiological, and psychological levels, and all at the same time, which leads the patient to learn to live life in God's balance. For instance, if she got angry she would be in bed all day, so she needed to learn to control her anger. Judy believes that the diet alone won't cure anything and counseling alone won't cure anything either. Both are required, and both define the healing process.

"Sometimes Judy was jealous because she would see other people well and they could walk and go places, her world was shut down. Judy relates how one friend just couldn't relate to what Judy was going through. 'Once I knew I was sick and had symptoms every other day, what I would call a trigger day, I noticed that it started affecting my life and I started getting frustrated.' This frustration led her to not wanting to go out into the public, which made her anxious and jealous.

"Bill was actively involved with counseling Judy on issues like her anger. He was also counseling her and Ernie on issues that they were struggling with as a couple; to understand and come to grips with. One issue was that the MS affected their romance and sex life. The feelings of electric shocks in her legs and sensitivity of her body would make it such that she didn't want to make love or have sex. There were times that it was almost four to five months that Ernie could not get near her.

"Bill was very instrumental in dealing with the emotional issues that were holding her back. She learned to let go and let God! One issue was that her husband had started to take care of her totally and she lost control of her need for power: he was in charge. This hindered her from moving forward. When this issue was resolved, her healing moved forward rapidly.

"Both Bill and Judy strongly believe that good counseling is absolutely necessary to deal with personal issues or the healing process will never move forward. Since the disease is neurological, these issues could stop any progress that would otherwise not be a determining factor.

Reduction in Drugs
"By the fifth month, Judy went from taking 14 medications to taking 5. The 5 she still took were not taken every day but were for relapses and she only took them when she had a problem. Within 8 months, she dropped 11 of the 14 medications. She was using only three of the original 14 medications on an 'as needed' basis. She dropped all of them later on. She says, 'The doctors could only suppress my immune system to keep me from getting sicker.'"

"Judy was diagnosed at age 40, and the progressive symptoms of late-stage disease occurred when she was in her 50's. She just got sicker and sicker during that time period. She noted that even though she was taking the pills, she kept getting progressively sicker, and she commented, 'The medical field meant well by giving me drugs but nearly killed me in the process.'

"Judy learned from having MS that if you think you'll get better you'll take anything that they suggest. After her healing of MS through an extensive lifestyle change rather than drugs, Judy became skeptical about the drugs doctors freely prescribe. She discussed this with her doctor, saying that the medical field gives out drugs freely to make people feel better, and that a person goes to a doctor because they want something and the doctor is going to see that they get it. The doctor replied, 'If people come here and don't get a drug, they're angry, so we give them a drug!'

The Mountain to Climb
"To conquer any disease is to climb three mountains. The first mountain is the human spirit, to climb it means to never give up hope and trust in God explicitly! The second mountain is the soul (psyche) that can be climbed with good counseling. The third mountain to be climbed is the body that can be climbed through a dramatic lifestyle change.

"About 13 months after she started her lifestyle changes, Judy and Ernie climbed a mountain. She climbed 2,300 feet to the top of South Turner Mountain at Baxter State Park in Northern Maine. Five years into the plan, at age 60, she climbed Mount Katahdin which is 5,267 feet high. They did this on June 21st, the longest day of the year. They started at 8:00 AM, climbed to the top and then came back down at 8:30 PM, that evening. It was over 12 ½ hours of straight up and straight down. Now, in 2010, they average climbing about 5 mountains a year!

"Judy says: 'Now I get up every morning to face the new day well and happy. I go hiking, kayaking, canoeing, fishing, swimming, and any other sport I choose to do without a single thought of never being able to do these activities again!'"

The Neurologist Report

"Judy's neurologist was skeptical about her progress with MS at first. She didn't want her to get her hopes up. But Judy discussed with her what she was going to do before she did it. 'After 2 years into my health change, she noticed such a difference in my gait that she decided to do another MRI on my brain.' That was in 2004.

"That MRI showed just 4 lesions on her brain which was down from the 9 lesions on the brain shown in the MRI done in 2002. At that time, her neurologist wouldn't say that her disease was 'cured,' but that she now had control over it, instead of it having control over her.

"The neurologist report October 13, 2004 stated: 'The patient states that over the past year she has made substantial changes in her diet, and to some degree in her lifestyle, and feels that this has made a dramatic difference in terms of her MS. She has switched over to having carrot juice supplementation and barley supplementation daily. She has become vegetarian. Eighty-five percent of what she eats is raw food. She has cut caffeine and refined sugars out of her diet and drinks only distilled water . . . The patient is alert, oriented, and appropriate. Speech is fluent. Extra-ocular muscle movements are full. Gait is stable. Romberg is negative. We will hold off any primary MS treatment right now.'"

"The neurologist's report of March 25, 2009 stated: 'Last note from April 2006 is reviewed for disease progression. Overall, patient is doing extraordinarily well. She feels her disease has been entirely asymptomatic for the past several years. She has followed the diet with high amounts of regular carrot juice and barley supplementation. She is not taking any medications for MS. She has continued an active lifestyle over the past year with hiking, kayaking, and any sort of activity without limitations. Fatigue is not an issue. She does not have vision problems. Bowel and bladder function have been good . . . Patient is alert, oriented, and appropriate. Speech is fluent. Cranial nerves II through XII are grossly intact. Gait is normal. Patient has a past history of relapsing-remitting multiple sclerosis, but clinically appears fully recovered with stable, persistent white matter lesions which are years old. At this point no further neurodiagnostic testing or treatment is suggested. I have encouraged her to continue to be active.'"

"In 2009, Judy was climbing a mountain when she fell and injured her shoulder. She had a minor shoulder repair and the doctor noted that she was doing about 3 times better than somebody that isn't in as good of shape as she was, because they're not as healthy as she is. An MRI on the brain was done and it showed no lesions on her brain at all. It appears as if all of the lesions she once had have now healed.

"In July 2011, Judy has had no more symptoms for over eight years. The chronic progressive MS is completely gone and the MRI ordered by the neurologist showed that the brain lesions were completely gone in 2009. Thus, it can be stated that at age 40 Judy was diagnosed with MS, it progressed over the next 15 years and that, in 2011, she is 63 years old and has been free of MS for over eight years.

Judy's Talks
"Judy started giving talks and shares her experience of this: 'When I share the idea about eating raw with anyone, I can usually tell less than 10 minutes into the conversation whether or not they're going to accept it. For some people, even though eating this way may be helpful for them, they're still going to be skeptical.'

"Judy states, 'There are people who saw me very sick in the past, and know that I'm well now, who still can't apply this to their life. According to them, it's too strict of a regimen to follow. It's too much for them. They want a pill that's going to make them better. They don't want to work for the results. I had to work to get where I am; I could not take a pill and get better. The medicines never made me any better, they simply masked the symptoms.'

"'What I try and offer people is an open door that can make them completely healthy again. And it's not just with diet, but through other choices also. You can't just have a good diet, but also have stress and anger and frustration in your life and still be healthy. You have to make healthy choices in those areas too.'

"'I would tell skeptics that if they want something to make them healthy, then they have to be committed to this. I really, really wanted to get better. I'm sure other people want to get better too, but they need to know that they can often get better without drugs and stay healthy.'

The Raw Vegan Diet and Juicing
James continues, "The raw vegan diet that Judy was taught was the Hallelujah Diet, which is a standard raw vegan diet based on the Bible verse in Genesis 1:29.

"Many other raw vegan or Living Foods diets can be found that are good at helping bring into remission degenerative diseases such as: the Hippocrates diet, the Rainbow Green diet, the Raw Revolution diet, the Hallelujah diet or the Alleluia diet and others. These and others would all emphasize at least 80/20 raw vegan. Some of these emphasize juicing and juice fasting. There are many testimonials of MS being helped and cured with this approach.

"In the beginning, Judy did use Fiber Cleanse to help her detoxify her body for about six months. Judy's diet has stayed about the same over the last eight years since she started it. She allows herself, maybe one or two items a year that are not part of a strict raw 80/20 diet and knows that she can be fine with this. She definitely doesn't want to go back to the way that she was with MS, so she is going to continue her current lifestyle.

"In the morning, she eats fruit, and varies the types of fruit eaten. She may have just an apple, sometimes with some sunflower seeds or ground flax seed. She has 8 oz of carrot juice and 1 teaspoon of barley powder mixed with 6 oz of water every morning.

"For lunch, she has salads, any kind of vegetables, and mixes them together. Sometimes she has bread to go with the salads. Judy and Ernie also have smoothies: blueberries, raspberries, and other fruits in a soy milk or other nut-based liquids (such as almond milk), with ice cubes.

"When she had MS she needed to have six glasses of carrot juice and six teaspoons of barley grass powder a day. She kept the six going until about a year into it. Now she has three glasses of carrot juice a day plus three teaspoons of barley grass powder mixed with water. If she is climbing mountains or hiking or doing some other sport that requires huge energy expenditure, she has an extra teaspoon of barley grass powder and an extra serving of carrot juice. She has a glass of carrot juice and a teaspoon of barley grass powder mixed with water, about 30 minutes before lunch and dinner.

"For Dinner, sometimes they have a cooked meal, usually just a potato and a cooked vegetable. She steams it a little bit so that the vegetables are still crunchy. The potato is baked in the oven with the skin on it. Sometimes they just have a big piece of watermelon, or other fruit with it.

"During her first year, she was very strict with her diet. She noted that Ernie was not as strict since he worked and found it difficult to always stay raw. Her strict raw vegan diet and juicing routine were kept religiously for the first year. After that, she did back off a little bit and was not so strict, but still kept it up.

"Judy has talked with others who had MS, and heard about others who had MS and were healed on this lifestyle, but then fell away from it and their MS came back with a vengeance. So Judy has determined that she will be on this lifestyle for the rest of her life and she is perfectly Ok with that. She never wants to go back to the way she was, and she praises the Lord for her new found life.

"Judy says, 'To me this is a miracle from God and I pray that my experience will be an encouragement to other Multiple Sclerosis' sufferers who feel there is no hope!'"

m. Crucify all Self-indulgent Passions

The examples of healings give above are good examples of people who were able to Crucify all Self-indulgent Passions.

Self-indulgence is a big obstacle for curing any type of degenerative disease. As the Holy Book states:
- "But now, - it is Yahweh who speaks - come back to me with all your heart, fasting, weeping and mourning."   Joel 2:12
- "If you listen carefully to the voice of Yahweh your God, and do what is right in his eyes, if you pay attention to his commandments and keep his statues, I shall inflict on you none of the evils that I inflicted on the Egyptians for it is I, Yahweh, who give you healing."   Ex 15.26
- When self-indulgence is at work the results are obvious: "fornication, gross indecency and sexual irresponsibility; idolatry and sorcery; feuds and wrangling: jealousy, bad temper and quarrels; disagreements, factions, envy; drunkenness, orgies and similar things. I warn you now, as I warned you

before: those who behave like this will not inherit the Kingdom of God. What the Spirit brings is very different: love, joy, peace, patience, kindness, goodness, trustfulness, gentleness and self-control. There can be no law against things like that, of course. You cannot belong to Christ Jesus unless you crucify all self-indulgent passions and desires."
Galatians 5:19-24

- "And they who belong to Christ have crucified their flesh with its passions and desires." (Gal 5:24)

Chapter 3
The Evidence of Parkinson's Cures

Theophan the Recluse, (d. 1894), was a well-known hermit and author, and says, "Flee from satiety – the state when the heart says cunningly to itself: Enough! I need nothing more, I have worked hard; I have established order in myself, now I can allow myself a little rest. It was said about Israel, 'Thou art waxen fat, thou art grown thick, and thou art covered with fatness' (Deut. 32:15). In its original context this verse refers to physical satiety and to satisfaction with one's external conditions. But it is equally applicable to spiritual satiety and to satisfaction with one's inner state. The result is the same – forsaking of God. When there is enough of everything, why pray to God and think of Him?"[130]

a. Positive Connection between Diet and PD

Are there any studies showing a positive connection between diet and Parkinson's disease? There was a major study done in China where they found a positive connection between diet and Parkinson's disease. Many, if not most of the people in China, eat a primarily plant-based diet.[f]

In *The Better Brain Book*, David Perlmutter, MD, a neurologist, states: "I am often asked what I think is the single most important thing you can do to keep your brain functioning at its peak and prevent brain aging. The answer is easy. If you want to perform at the highest levels and maintain a lifetime of optimal brain health, you must be vigilant about what you put on your plate. It's as simple as that. Nutrition is the most important tool for staying mentally and physically fit and it is by far the most underutilized tool.

"From the perspective of a neurologist, the standard American diet is a nightmare. It is loaded with poor-quality fat that can make your brain cells sluggish but is scarce in healthy fat that can keep your brain cells flexible and "smart." It is packed with highly processed, nutrient-deficient food that is laden with sugar and chemical additives that practically invite free radicals and inflammation to invade your brain. If I were to design a diet with the sole purpose of creating an epidemic of poor brain function, accelerated brain aging, mood disorders, and other neurological problems, it would be the one that most Americans are already following."[131]

Parris Kidd, PhD, an expert in nutrients notes in his journal article, 'Parkinson's Disease as Multifactorial Oxidative Neurodegeneration: Implications for Integrative

---

[f] The prevalence of PD in a nutritionally deficient rural population in China.' Out of a large population (16,488) being studied they found 2,819 possible PD people and ended up with 617 PD patients at various stages. Their neurologists found that The diagnoses given to the remaining 617 patients (Table 2) were 86 definite PD (41 men and 45 women), 203 probable PD (106 men and 97 women), and 175 possible PD (64 men and 111women), 139 essential tremor (58 men and 81 women), 12 vascular Parkinsonism (six men and six women), and two drug-induced Parkinsonism (one man and one woman). They found a positive connection between diet and PD. Many if not most of the people in China eat a primarily plant based diet. (See the book, *The China Study*, by Colin Campbell, PhD for a detailed scientific account of plant-based nutrition in China.)

Management', *Alternative Medicine Review*, "With the evidence steadily accumulating that Parkinson's disease is a multifactorial oxidative disease, there is an urgent need for integrative management. The allopathic model that currently dominates Parkinson's management is obsolete. The major adverse side effects of the various drugs currently in use for the disease, combined with the limitations for the dopamine replacement strategy, dictate the need for alternatives."[132]

b. First Case of Curing Parkinson's

Who is the first doctor to cure Parkinson's and what is the story? The first recorded healing was by Herbert M. Shelton, PhD, DC, ND. He had a doctorate in Physiological Therapeutics (1920, Chicago), a Doctorate from the American School of Chiropractic (1924, New York) and a Doctorate from the American School of Naturopathy (1924, New York). He published his own monthly magazine, *Hygienic Review* for forty-one years and was the author of over 41 books. He had supervised over thirty thousand fasts at his facility in Alamo Heights, Texas. He is considered by many to be one of the great figures in water fasting in the US in the 20th century.

The first Parkinson's healing using this dietary approach found happened in the literature is in 1941 by Dr. Herbert Shelton. He cured Monica B. Monica B., age 39, had been diagnosed with Parkinson's disease. She fasted three times under the supervision of Dr. Shelton: 30 days, 14 days and later another 14 days, over a period of 9 months. Dr. Shelton wrote: "The developments in this case are typical with the exception that Monica completely recovered. Full recovery is not the general rule. The majority of fasters make sufficient progress to become useful again but retain part of the tremor. Monica was at the health school for 9 months and had previously suffered with Parkinsonism for 6 years. After she had fasted 30 days, the tremor immediately reoccurred, but not as severely as before the fast. After the second fast, the tremors were less and after the third fast, the tremors were gone. For more than ten years, I remained in contact with Monica and she has had no recurrence of the tremor."[133]

This health school promoted a Living Foods diet, which she was on during the 9 months, in-between her fasts. She most likely continued with the diet she learned at the health school (or close to it) after her third fast. How long she continued or how intensely she continued is not known, but for 10 years after she had no more tremors.

This is a simple case study which is very important because it occurred long before there were any drugs for Parkinson's or other therapies as mentioned in this book. It was by a leading medical expert in the field with a therapy of fasting and a Living plant-based diet as found in this book. It actually becomes a format that other PD clients can pattern a therapy on: first go on this Live Plant-based diet, second over the course of a year go on three long fasts, preferably under supervision. Third stay on this nutrition therapy!

There is one minor problem, even though Dr. Shelton cured thousands of patients in his lifetime at his clinic he could not cure himself when he got Parkinson's! On speaking with his personal assistant, Dr. Virginia Vetrano, She said he tried everything and finally he did a 30 day water fast. During and after the fast he keep seeing clients which exhausted him further, this was a mistake, and he should have rested during the fast to gain strength. He never recovered and later died. This is a very good lesson on how the body cures Parkinson's or any major disease, a person needs to rest to heal and concentrate on the healing process, but Dr. Shelton keep working seeing his many desperate clients, until it was too late the disease overcame him and he died! A second thing that we learn here is all these supplements and therapies that he used did not work back then, and do not work today to cure a major disease like Parkinson's.

The one client we know of that he healed with Parkinson's rested at his facility, ate raw foods and did three fasts before being healed.

c. Recent Testimonials of PD Cures

Are there any recent cures in the last 10 years? James says, "Yes, several. I spoke with a Hallelujah Acres Health Minister who had four or five people with Parkinson's try a raw vegan diet and three or four of them improved greatly, yet only one was completely healed. But because of confidentiality laws, I couldn't contact them. If a person doesn't follow the nutritional therapy correctly, it doesn't work."

Are there any doctors or other health professionals that have cured Parkinson's with this approach?

The important teaching about the next four testimonials is that the doctors and health professionals involved in the cures are all raw vegans: Tosca Haag, MD, Fred Bisci, PhD, Ray Kent, and psychologist Bill Irwin, MSW. All four of them emphasize a raw vegan approach, and fasting and juicing are also used. This same basic method was used way back in 1941 and is still used today by later practitioners (who were contacted in 2008, 2009, 2010 and 2011). There are about 9 testimonials of cures of PD, all involving a raw vegan or a Living Foods diet!

Tosca Haag, MD - An Elderly Parkinson's Patient
Tosca Haag, MD is a student of Herbert Shelton and a long-term raw vegan, teaching this lifestyle to others at her retreat center. She reported that: 'I had an elderly man in the beginning stages of Parkinson's who arrived in a wheelchair, took a mere 10 day fast, regained some strength, and left walking. Unfortunately, his family did not want to feed him all raw. They were more interested in making sure he adhered to orthodox fare during all the Jewish holidays, and

when he got worse, they took him to a doctor and he was put on drugs' (Letter August 2009).[134]

Fred Bisci, PhD - Intervention for PD

This is a testimonial at the end *Your Healthy Journey* (2008), a book written by Fred Bisci, PhD. Dr. Bisci has a PhD in Nutritional Science and is a nationally-known raw food speaker. Dr. Louise Priolo, MD wrote, "My father has been using the services of Dr. Bisci for almost one year, in an attempt to reduce the symptoms of Parkinson's disease. Dr. Bisci placed my father on a lifestyle designed to detoxify his body of impurities. This lifestyle eliminated dairy products, red meat, and alcohol, and relies on vegetables, fruits, and freshly-squeezed vegetable juices. Since starting this lifestyle, my father has lost weight, he is more alert, and he is more energetic. The trembling of his hands, as well as other associated symptoms of Parkinson's disease, has dramatically diminished. Even his eyes, which were yellowish in color, have become clear. It appears that my father has benefited and continues to benefit from Dr. Bisci's expertise in the field of nutritional healing. We Thank You. Dr. Louise Priolo, MD"[135]

Fred Bisci has a Ph.D. in Nutritional Science and is retired now. He has been active in the greater New York City area for over forty years and worked with over 35,000 people, all over the world. He has been a raw vegan for over 40 years and helped many people to change their diet to a real, fresh food approach. Dr. Fred emphasizes "making a commitment and setting realistic parameters" when changing their lifestyle as the key to optimum health. He also emphasizes the use of digestive enzymes and sells his own line of these enzymes.

In talking with Fred Bisci, PhD, I asked him if he has worked with people with Parkinson's. He said he has worked with people who have Parkinson's and other neurological diseases. He stated, "Seventy-Five percent of the time people do not comply and follow the dietary protocol. Some can be helped in the early stages, but in later stages, when the neurons are dead, it becomes very tricky. Neurological diseases are very difficult to heal."

Fred Bisci, PhD, (nutritionist) is quoted as stating: "I personally only eat raw foods, and have done so for 45 years with phenomenal results. There is no doubt that an all-raw lifestyle is the ultimate approach, but I do not generally recommend it to my clients because very few of them would be capable of sustaining it. A mainly raw diet provides excellent results and is a more realistic objective for most people. The worst thing for your health is to bounce in and out of different lifestyle parameters, and so it is better to adopt a mainly raw food diet and stick to it than to attempt to go 100% raw and slip back. . . . Eating Guidelines: It's What You Leave Out then it's What You Put In. The system really works, but you have to draw on deep reserves of determination, awareness, and commitment in order to achieve your goal of a healthier life. Your part is to understand that intelligent living is a process of lifestyle change, which involves personal accountability and responsibility."[136]

Ray Kent – Nutritionist
Ray Kent refers to himself as a nutritionist and has been promoting plant-based diets for 50 years, about half of that as a raw vegan. He travels worldwide, teaching and doing clinical work. He advised a patient with Parkinson's for several years to follow an approach that emphasizes fasting, juicing and a raw vegan diet to help his Parkinson's to be put into remission. Ray responded to several questions that I asked. On his website, he deals with the psychological element in-depth (Email June 2011).
- Question: "For the Parkinson's patient that you helped with fasting and diet, what did you do?
- Answer: Well, I educated him as to his disease, and told him that this very complicated cause has to be removed, because the body cannot stand the tension anymore and the tension that he applies will eventually form a palsy. He must understand

Parkinson's. It became a chronic problem after years of accumulated tension. So, there is a cause and we should not treat the symptom.

- Question: How long did you fast the Parkinson's patient and how many times did you fast him? What kind of diet did you put him on, was it a raw food diet?
- Answer: I fasted him once for 10 days, and that's it, and I had him eat 90% raw, and cut his food intake to 2 meals a day.
- Question: Did you have him doing juicing? If so, how much?
- Answer: Well, it's a standard practice. We practice that each of my students studying under me, has 2 glasses of juice per day, fresh from the juicer.
- Question: How did you know that his Parkinson's went away?
- Answer: Observation."[137]

Bill Irwin Psychologist/Chemist - Two Parkinson's Cures

Bill Irwin, MS, MSW was a chemist with his own lab. He had a medical condition which caused him to go blind. He then became a psychologist. He learned the Halleluiah Diet and taught a modified version as a health coach during his counseling. He has helped cure several people with MS and two with Parkinson's. He cured Judy Livingstone, the subject of the earlier case study in this work. The two Parkinson's patients were both from New England; yet both wanted to remain anonymous and did not want to write a testimonial or case study. They were both put in remission but one still had some hand shaking. Yet since we have nothing in writing these two cannot be counted.

Anne Wigmore diet - Several Cures of Parkinson's

Two Anne Wigmore Institutes (Hippocrates in Florida and Optimum Health in Texas) both have had people with Parkinson's greatly improve, perhaps put into remission, through their Living Foods diet approach including wheatgrass juice. They both promote an 80/20 to 100% raw foods diet with wheat grass juice. Because of confidentiality issues, testimonials are not given.

Ellioit Gallin, age 68 was healthy when he found out he had lung cancer which he went through chemo and radiation to get rid of it, then he found out he had stage 4 brain cancer which they operated on and cut out. Throughout those three years he suffered from seizures and was diagnosed with Parkinson's disease. He was vacationing in Florida and found out about the Hippocrates Health Institute and went through their three week program. He learned a lot and "Elliot said he and his wife continue to drink green juice and wheatgrass juice and eat as much live-raw vegan foods as they can."[138]

Gerson Diet - PD and Breast Cancer
Andrea Proudfoot had been suffering from Parkinson's disease for three years when a golf-sized tumor was removed from her breast and she was diagnosed with breast cancer. Reluctant to 'poison' her body with chemotherapy, Andrea researched alternative options, and in November of 1986, she sought treatment of a Gerson Therapy hospital. Later, she started the Halleluiah Diet. More than twelve years later, she is alive and well. Despite having been diagnosed with two degenerative diseases, she has outlived three of her High School boyfriends!
Last contacted by Halleluiah Acres: 2003.

Sherry A. Rogers, MD - Parkinson's Remission/Cure
Pam T., a client of Sherry Rogers, MD, was waiting in her office. Another client was also there and they started talking. Pam said that the other person explained how she had Parkinson's, and was shaking a lot, and by going to Dr. Rogers, she was completely cured of her Parkinson's. This client said she wasn't the only one with Parkinson's that was cured by Dr. Rogers. Sherry Rogers, MD from New York has been in practice for over 26 years, a Diplomate of the American Board of Family Practice, is a Fellow of the American College of Allergy and Immunology, and a

Diplomate of the American Academy of Environmental Medicine. She is a world lecturer and has published 17 scientific articles and 10 books. Dr. Rogers promotes a plant-based lifestyle orientation.

Halleluiah diet claims of healing Parkinson's
"The doctors say I am a WALKING MIRACLE' - 10/24/2002 Harriet, who lives in Tennessee, shared her testimony, not only for the incredible improvement Harriet has experienced with her Parkinson's disease since going on The Hallelujah diet, but also that you might remember her and her family in prayer: 'Dear Dr. and Mrs. Malkmus, I've been following The Hallelujah Diet for a year, because I wanted to boot Parkinson's disease out of my life, and be the Mother and wife God intended me to be! (I have and home-school seven children!) The first year on The Hallelujah Diet enabled me to reduce Parkinson's meds by 33%, to lose 50 pounds, to practically eliminate lower chronic back pain, to boost my energy, and most of all, TO GIVE ME HOPE!"[139]

Jim relates, "I had an e-mail communications with Olin Idol, (around 2008) one of the leaders behind the Halleluiah diet. He said that they only had five people with Parkinson's try the Hallelujah diet that he knows of and they were not having great success with them. As noted earlier the Halleluiah diet has had good success with MS and other diseases, that were not specifically brain diseases, like Parkinson's and Alzheimer's. The *Alleluia Diet* is very similar to the Halleluiah diet yet is more advanced in its historical analysis. They do have the nutritional approach to help cure, to a degree, diseases like Parkinson's and Alzheimer's and have a greater degree of success with MS and related diseases."

Parkinson's Remission - Alex Bernstein
In 1981 Alex Bernstein of White Plains, New York came to the United States from Russia where he was a medical doctor. He founded a company and did a lot of traveling and sales. In 2005 one of his hands started shaking

and he found out that he had Parkinson's. Several neurologists all gave the same diagnosis and one professor said "in five years you will be in a wheelchair." He went to the Hippocrates Health Institute in West Palm Beach, Florida for three weeks, had natural chelation therapy and he learned the Living Foods lifestyle. Seven years after his diagnosis he still has a little tremor but is doing great. He walks 3-4 miles a day and works out. His diet is mostly raw and he enjoys wheatgrass juice and green drinks every day.

d. The Spirit is Willing

"Be on guard and pray that you may not be put to the test. The spirit is willing but the flesh is weak." (Mk 14:38)

"If you live according to the flesh you shall die, but if by the Spirit you mortify the deeds of the flesh, you shall live." (Rom 8.13)

Judas Maccabee, was a Hebrew revolutionary in 167 BC and he had a willing human spirit in his time. We find that, "Judas, called Maccabaeus, who with about nine others, withdrew into the wilderness and lived like wild animals in the hills with his companions, eating nothing but wild plants to avoid contracting defilement." 2 Maccabeus 5:27

Another early example of vegetarianism is found with Daniel and his three friends: <u>Hananiah, Mishael and Azariah</u> were Judaeans would not eat meat and the Kings delicacies, they had a willing spirit! For ten days (possibly longer) they were vegetarians and then they were presented to the king and "The king conversed with them, and among all the boys found none to equal Daniel, Hananiah, Mishael and Azariah." Daniel 1.19

Chapter 5
The Evidence for Alzheimer's Cures

St. Augustine of Hippo (cir. 430) wrote in a sermon for the Lenten Season: "An appropriate solemn sermon is your due so that the Word of God, brought to you through my ministry, may sustain you in spirit while you fast in body and so that the inner man, thus refreshed by suitable food, may be able to accomplish and to persevere courageously in the disciplining of the outer man. For, to my spirit of devotion, it seems fitting that we, who are about to honor the Passion of our crucified Lord in the very near future, should fashion for ourselves a cross of the bodily pleasures in need of restraint, as the Apostle says: "And they who belong to Christ have crucified their flesh with its passions and desires." (Gal 5:24)"[140]

a. Dr. Doug Graham

Doug Graham, DC is a well-known raw fooder and author. He emphasizes fasting and had his own fasting center in Florida for 10 years he supervised thousands of fasts and was in private practice as a chiropractor for twenty years. He got married and moved to England where his wife is a biology professor. He promotes the 80/10/10 diet which is a raw vegan, Live-food diet.

In e-mailing Doug Graham (2/09) and asking if he had worked with Parkinson's, or Alzheimer's or MS patients he replied: "Jim, I have worked with Alzheimer's clients with excellent success. The same for MS. I have only seen a few cases of Parkinson's, to be honest. My experience with all three of these conditions, and several others, is that compliance has been extremely difficult to obtain. In other words, it seems that most of the people that I have met who suffer from these conditions aren't particularly interested in food-style modification. I actually had one guy with MS tell me, "Doc, I will do whatever you say. Just don't mess with my diet." Best to you, *Doug*

I e-mailed Doug (3/2014) and asked him if he could send me a paragraph on anyone that he worked with who had Alzheimer's and he send back this wonderful testimonial.

"Pam used to work as a nurse but was currently interning at my fasting facility. She had to cut her internship short, she informed me, in order to become a full-time caretaker for her aging mother. Her mom, it turned out, could no longer care for herself. She had a day-carer, but that too had proven insufficient. Her mom would leave the house and get lost, or would fill her grocery cart with candy bars. She'd lost all ability to be responsible for herself, her personal hygiene, her diet, etc. Pam left to care for her mom. I next saw Pam six months later, at a festival. "How's your mom," I asked. "Fine," said Pam. "I put her on a low-fat raw vegan diet, and since she was long past knowing what she was eating anyway, she didn't object. Within weeks, she was doing much better, and now, after six months, Mom's totally living on her own, with no problems at all." The number of people who have reported vastly improved mental clarity after adopting the 80/10/10 diet has been nothing short of astonishing."   (by Dr. Doug Graham)

Doug Graham emailed this testimonial (3/2014).

"I've fasted several people with MS, all with good results. Most notable was Jim, who could not walk without two canes, often fell backwards when standing still, could no longer read, was incontinent, and suffered with a host of related neurological issues. A young man still in his thirties, he'd suffered the progressively debilitating symptoms of MS for more than a decade. He fasted 21 days, by which point he could read effortlessly, was perfectly continent, and seemed far better coordinated. A week after initiating refeeding, Jim was walking up and down steep hills without any support and never falling down. He walked through immigration, baggage, and customs at a large international airport without any use of the wheelchair he had used at the same airport a month prior. I have stayed in touch with Jim for more than a decade and he is still doing well."   (by Dr. Doug Graham)

b. Dr. Scott's clients

The late Dr. Scott of Cleveland had a fasting facility there. See the section on fasting and his write up. I (Jim) was visiting him and asked him if he had ever cured Alzheimer's and he replied once a husband brought his wife who had Alzheimer's. The husband had to stay there and go on the fast with her. Dr. Scott put them on a long water fast and on the 21st day of the fast she started speaking for the first time in over a year. She wasn't always clear or made sense but she was speaking! In fact, she couldn't stop talking all day long. The next day the husband got sick and so Dr. Scott broke the fast with juicing over the next couple of days. Dr. Scott told the husband to bring her back to do another fast in a few months since this first fast started the process of healing but a second fast would be needed to continue it. Unfortunately the husband never brought his wife back.

c. Dr. Schulze clients

The following are excerpts from the book: *Curing with Cayenne* by Sam Biser. The book is a dialogue between Sam Biser and a Dr. Richard Schulze, a medical herbalist who ran a clinic before starting his herbal company. Dr. Schulze was a student of Dr. John Christopher a well-known herbalist with a product line.

Dr. Schultz developed a whole program of curing the incurables (www.herbdoc.com) and in his programs documents he has several testimonials of people with neurological diseases. One person with Parkinson's, living in Alaska, claims that he has recovered 75% by using this methodology. The program is similar nutritionally to what is in this book and has other activities, these have been related in the testimonial of Joanne S. of Maine who followed much of his program.

Sam Biser wrote, "I asked Dr. Schulze what kind of results he saw using cayenne with Alzheimer's. He started by telling me about a case in which he gave some strong cayenne tincture to an old woman who hadn't spoken a word in years. Immediately after squirting it down her throat as the family's request, she stammered, 'Stop it, you son of a bitch.' He worked with the woman, using cayenne and cleansing her bowels – and she began to get better. She began to emerge. One day, she was motioning toward a chest of drawers, knocking against it. Someone opened it and found what she was trying to communicate. Inside it were love letters she had discovered – from her husband, to his secret lover. She had caught him having an affair, and writing passionate love letters, to another woman. That's what broke her heart – and four months later, to escape her pain, she began to depart into the netherworld of Alzheimer's."

"Her emergence from the deep did not please everyone in her family, because they had re-arranged their lives around her assets – and she had been written out of their lives around her assets – and she had been written out of their lives, except as a deranged patient with a nurse. At that point, Dr. Schulze got an attorney letter ordering him to never come near their mother again – or else they would have him arrested. The family wanted things to remain just as they were, her money in their hands. And so the death shroud of memory loss closed again around this Mom, at the will of those who loved her ... money."[141]

A second story related is: "It was about a woman with Alzheimer's who ran a business, but her disease got to where she couldn't remember anyone's name, couldn't remember who they were, and wondered who the strangers were coming in." He told me, "We got her right back to normal in a little over a week, to where she remembered anything she wanted. Specifically, what we used on her was the brain tonic. That has the cayenne in it. I used it on many Alzheimer's patients. People told me their whole memory was fading. It was like a bad disk on a computer; they couldn't bring up any information. But after using the formula for three, four or ten days in the individual cases, people had their memory back."

"What's the formula?" I said. "It's just: One part Cayenne pepper, Three parts Ginkgo Biloba leaf, One part

Rosemary, the leaf or stalk (optional), and One part Kola Nut (optional). A 'part' is just a measure of volume. It could be a tablespoon, a cup or a barrelful of herbs, whether dry or fresh." I asked, "What's a good dose of this brain formula for anyone with Alzheimer's disease?"

"If you have Alzheimer's disease, or serious memory loss, the dosage would be two full dropperful's, three times a day. This is a dosage of the brain formula made properly, with organically-grown herbs, and packed with those herbs to the brim while soaking in alcohol." (in making a tincture)

I asked him, "That's enough for Alzheimer's?" He said, "No. This is the dose to start with for a few days. Then you can take it from two dropperfuls to four dropperfuls per dose. On timing, you could go up to every other hour, if you wanted to really crank it up."[142]

For depression and memory-loss: A study from Holland showed that dementia patients had 108 milliliters per minute less blood flow in their brain. And get this: "A reduction in blood flow precedes the decline in cognitive function in Alzheimer's patients, said Berislav Zlokovic, M.D., Ph.D, Alzheimer's researcher at the University of Rochester Medical Center—and a neurovascular expert.

The brain is only 5% of body mass, yet it consumes 30% of the oxygen in your blood. When the blood flow and thus oxygen level in the blood decreases it's problematic. A report in the medical journal *Radiology* says, "Old age is associated with a decrease in cerebral blood flow. These observations strongly suggest that decreased cerebral blood flow indeed causes brain damage." Blood also brings nutrients to the brain. According to a study from the *Massachusetts Institute of Technology*, blood may help you think. That's because blood affects how your brain cells transmit information to each other.

According to Dr. Zlokovic, "People used to say, well, the brain is atrophying because of the disease, so not as much blood as usual is needed. But perhaps it's the opposite that the brain is dying because of the reduced blood flow." Therefore, make a brain-repair remedy that combines cayenne (the artery-expander) with a common spice that's a brain activator.

Capsaicin one of the active ingredients in hot peppers could have implications for diabetes prevention and management. A research team at the Toronto Hospital for Sick Children found that capsaicin injected into diabetic animals caused their diabetes to disappear "virtually overnight." Furthermore, researcher Dennis J. Selko, MD, from Harvard, has connected high blood sugar to Alzheimer's. Some scientists now call Alzheimer's a kind of Type 3 Diabetes.

Reversing Early Onset Dementia

Question: An 81-year old woman, a former nurse, was recently diagnosed with early onset dementia. She was concerned about her diminishing short-term memory. She failed to recall her friend's names and forgets some of her appointments. Her G.P. prescribed Aricept but the side effects (vomiting and diarrhea) were terrible. He then put her on the Exelon Patch and the results were similar but not as bad, she ceased using the patch. She asked what he would recommend for her memory loss and to prevent further memory loss?

Answer: (His blog 2/2012) Dr. Schultz give her a long reply; The brain like every other organ or group of cell, it must have nutrition going IN and it also must eliminate waste OUT. So, great circulation is a fundamental here if we want the brain, or any organ to function at its best. So how do we get more blood to the brain? Well, this is not very difficult. The first way is simply by reversing gravity. As we age, gravity takes more of a toll on us and the flow of our bodily liquids. It can simply make it harder for you to get good circulation to all of your extremities as you age, especially your brain. Slanting the bed is good, yoga inversions are good or other methods to have gravity bring more blood to the brain.

Dr. Schultz goes on to promote his herbals, Herbally, you can drive a lot more blood to you brain, and two of the greatest herbs to do this are *Cayenne* and *Ginkgo biloba*, both of which he has in his "Brain Tonic" herbal. Then he goes onto recommend his "Super Food Plus" saying, "After all, driving blood filled with sugar and chemicals is not going to help your brain function. We need to make sure that your blood is supercharged with nutrition and the best way to do that is to eat a food program that is loaded with organic fresh foods." Next he recommends a detox with his Bowel Detox Program and a month later his Liver Detox program. He moves onto talking about walking and exercises like yoga as another way to stimulate blood flow in and out of the brain.

He concludes, "Finally Dottie, please don't pay any attention to this diagnosis of Early Onset Dementia. Nothing POSITIVE will ever come from being told you have this, nor you thinking about this. It is NEGATIVE garbage, so please Let This Go. Instead focus on getting healthier, and creating a really healthy lifestyle." Dr. Schultz does emphasize a plant-based diet, but a healthier lifestyle is going to need a strict vegan or raw vegan diet with juicing and fasting.

d. Dr. Gerson's clients
Getting evidence of Alzheimer's cures is very difficult since those with AD can't remember to follow through with any kind of plant-based nutritional therapy approach such as the Living foods, raw vegan presented here. The Gerson diet is one of the oldest forms of this approach and it has claimed to have cured Alzheimer's in its list of healings. See Jim Tibbetts book *Starving Cancer to Death*, for a more complete listing of all the cancer healings and testimonials.

Let's face reality few in the medical community believe in this approach and the drug companies do not make any money on these methods. What kinds of diseases has raw vegan diet therapy healed over the last 30 years? Claims by those who use the Gerson diet have cured such things as: Cancer; Lymphomas; Melanoma; Multiple Myeloma; Hodgkin's disease; Heart disease; Diabetes; Hypertension; Atherosclerosis; Lupus; Arthritis; Alzheimer's; Candida; Crohn's Disease; Chronic Fatigue Syndrome; Migraine headaches; Liver disease; Kidney disease; Paget's disease; Thyroid disease; Allergies and other Degenerative diseases.

In a published study (1995) University of California at San Diego's, *Cancer Prevention and Control Program*. They compared 5 year melanoma survival rates of Gerson therapy patients to rates found in comparable, conventionally- treated groups in the medical literature. The study examined 153 white adult cancer patients, 25- 72 years old, in various stages of melanoma. The study found the following:

- (localized), 100% of Gerson therapy patients survived for 5 years, compared with 79% of patients receiving conventional treatment.
- Stages IIIa melanoma (regionally metastasized), 82% of Gerson versus 39% conventional
- Stages IIIa and IIIb melanoma (regionally metastasized), 70% of Gerson versus 41% of the conventionally treated patients.
- Stage IVa melanoma, 39% of Gerson versus 6% of conventional medicine.[143]

A second study (1996) showed even higher rates for those with surgery plus Gerson Diet Therapy for a five year survival rate, since about a third of Gerson-treated patients had surgeries as well. (IIIa - 92% versus 41%; IVa - 57% versus 6%).[144]

Dr. Gerson during his fifty years of practice published 55 scientific works. In the introduction in his last book on curing cancer through diet he states: "The history of medicine reveals that reformers who bring new ideas into the general thinking and practice of physicians have a difficult time."

Parkinson's, Alzheimer's and MS disease can be brought under control, minimize the symptoms and stop further progression through the Live plant-based nutrition therapy in this book, which is a modified version of the Gerson and other raw and live food diet therapies. This approach can work to a great degree with Alzheimer's to put it into remission. The list of raw food nutrition therapies, mentioned earlier, will all yield similar results. The important thing to remember is that Parkinson's and Alzheimer's are very similar and what will work for PD usually works for AD and vice versa in the area of nutritional therapies.

e. The Narrow Gate

A verse in Matthew 7:13,14 points out: "Enter by the narrow gate, since the road that leads to destruction is wide and spacious, and many are those who travel on it. O how narrow is the door and how difficult is the road which leads to life, and few are those who are found on it." Also the parallel verse in Luke 13:23, 24 states: "And a man asked him whether they are few in number that will live, and Jesus said to them, 'Strive to enter through the narrow gate. For I say to you many will seek to enter and will not succeed.'" To achieve the Culture of Life is a narrow road, or to conquer degenerative diseases, involves a narrow nutrition Living Foods therapy.

Chapter 5

The Evidence of Not Being Interested

St. Benedict (480-526) in his Rule writes: "Renounce yourself in order to follow Christ; discipline your body; do not pamper yourself, but love fasting."[g] St. Benedict opens his rule in chapter one discussing four kinds of monks. The first kind of monks are those who live in monasteries and serve under a rule and an Abbot. The second kind are the hermits who have prepared for this life after a long time in the monastery and have learned to fight against the devil, the vices of the flesh and evil thoughts. The third kind of monk has no experience with any rule or experienced guidance of a teacher. "Their law is the desire for self-gratification: whatever enters their mind or appeals to them, that they call holy; what they dislike, they regard as unlawful." The fourth kind of monk spends their life tramping from province to province, staying as guests in different monasteries. "Always on the move, with no stability, they indulge their own wills and succumb to the allurements of gluttony."[145]

a. Three Levels of Interest

The monks are like health-food seekers, who are those who have renounced the ways of the world (standard American degenerative diet) and its meat-based diets. These health-food seekers are the semi-vegetarian, vegetarians, vegan and raw vegan groups. The first group are those who establish themselves in the various plant-based schools of thought. The second group are a few people who are more like hermits with training and experience in vegan and raw vegan to make it on their own. The third group of health seekers are those with the desire for self-gratification: whatever enters their mind or appeals to them they will eat. The fourth kind of health food seeker spends their life tramping from one diet guru to the next diet guru. They are "Always on the move, with no stability, they indulge their own wills and succumb to the allurements of gluttony."

Only the first two plant-based groups of monks succeed in putting into remission and curing PD, AD and MS

---

[g] (Mat 16:24; Lk 9:23; 1 Cor 9:27)

through the body and soul. Another way or a simpler way to look this is that in the U.S. three main groups of personality traits can be found in the area of diet. This is not set in stone and but it gives some structure. The first group, about a third of the population, doesn't want anything to do with changing their diet. As one patient said to the nationally-known raw fooder Doug Graham DC, "Doc, I'll do anything you say just don't touch my diet!" They are the *apathetic* people and just don't care and won't change.

The second group is the *curious crowd* of people, which makes up about another third of the population. They will listen and ask a lot of questions, pondering the topic, may even try something, but never move forward and always find some excuse to back away. They never get in the pool and swim but only put their big toe in the water to test the temperature, then splash around.

The last third of the population are the *affirmative crowd* of people. They will listen, learn and decide to try it, and they will move forward. They will make a serious effort to change their diet. So we're down to 33%. But probably 8-13% will fall away within the first six months because it is expensive (organic foods), it is time consuming, difficult and involves a big learning curve. So we're down to 20-25% that can be healed through this method. Usually these people need some type of coaching or counseling along the way in order to succeed.

Educational level is linked to both income and nutritional status. Several studies have indicated that level (years) of education is associated with the dietary intake of several nutrients, such as protein, iron, calcium, and several of the B vitamins.'[146] [147] [148]" (*Geriatric Nutrition* citing journals: *Journal of American Dietetic Association*) but in the following examples their education did them little good to be able to listen to the Word of the Lord and change. Following are a few examples:

b. Individuals on the Three Levels

Tried it for a week

A lawyer I met at a conference had a golfing partner;
Rudy, with Parkinson's and he bought my book to give to
this person. A few months later, I was in contact with this
lawyer and he informed me that this person tried the diet for a
week and then said it was too difficult.

People want a cure to be easy; they don't want to
work for it! Remember the story of Darlene mentioned
earlier, and how her doctor gave her testimonial to all his MS
patients and no one followed through. They all thought it
was too difficult! It's not too difficult, but it is the vices or
sins of gluttony, sloth and omission which blind them and
hold them back. They need to repent and change their life
and make the nutritional changes. This Plant-based nutrition
therapy can work at home but it takes a lot of work.

Founder of an MS foundation

Another example of someone who did not follow the
diet is Arthur a successful businessman who has MS. I e-
mailed Arthur, the founder of an MS foundation on the East
Coast and told him that I had found a nutritional cure for MS.
He e-mailed me back that he wanted to see 3 case studies of
people cured before he would believe it, or even take the time
to consider it since he is very busy. After that e-mail, he
retired from the foundation, still with MS and went back into
the financial world to make money. Harvey, who also has
MS, is a member on the MS board Arthur founded. I spoke
on the phone with him for over 30 minutes, but he didn't like
the idea of having to give up meat. He was willing to look at
a copy of my book on Parkinson and MS, so I sent him one,
but I never heard from him.

The typical I don't want too elder

Another example is a woman named Kim who sent
me a letter and then I called her on the phone. She had been
a raw fooder for five years and wanted to know if it could

heal her father who had Parkinson's but he didn't want to get into a plant-based diet. I told her that unless he went raw and was strict about it, he could not be helped. She was a bit discouraged because she said her father would not change his diet, and would not go raw vegan.

Helen's husband with AD

I (Jim) was getting a haircut and in talking found out that woman's husband had early stage Alzheimer's and they were setting up with a new house for her and her daughter to take care of him. So I sold her my book on PD, AD and MS and other books and over the new few months went to her for a haircut talking each time about her husband and this approach. In the end she was not interested because it was too much of a change and her husband wouldn't like the food. The apathy of this woman shocked me. She's going to spend the next ten to fifteen years of her life taking care of him as he degenerates and gets worst, making it more difficult for her and her daughter. Here I'm telling her of a method that can change his condition, sure its work but he can be trained into doing the work; doing the juicing, the smoothies and raw food prep. This apathy and sloth amazed me but it's part of the American society problem. In European and Asian countries there's more emphasis on nutrition and fasting and more success.

Theologian's friend with AD

A theology teacher (PhD) at a University knew another theology professor in California who had beginning stage AD and had to go to a nursing home. I gave him copies of my books to send to his friend which he did but nothing happened with it. Obviously a nursing home is not going to do that program and the theologian didn't study the book or the approach to confirm it and figure out he or someone else would have to do this nutritional approach for his friend.

University President with MS

I met with an ex-University President (17 years) who had MS for over 17 years, had a PhD in physics and belonged to a religious order. I spoke with him gave him my book but said he had read Dr. Swank's book (low fat diet for MS) 17 years ago when he first was diagnosed with MS, but he didn't want to deal with healing through nutrition! So he continues to get worse and exercises a lot to try and overcome it. Exercise only helps so much and the disease marches on!

Two University employees with PD

I talked with two people in a religious order connected to a University, one retired who had PD. I gave them my books and met with one of them twice but neither was interested. One is now in the religious orders nursing home, going downhill.

University Chaplin with PD

I met three times over several months with a university Chaplin, a priest who had Parkinson's. I gave him copies of my books and he actually read some of them and had great interest, but in the end, he fell away. He now has serious dementia (beginning Alzheimer's) and is in the religious orders nursing home. He was very bright had a doctorate in ministry but did not follow through, which is sad because he like the others mentioned in this section, could have put the disease into remission and lived out a normal life except eating a Live-Food plant-based diet, instead of the standard American degenerative diet (S.A.D.).

Jane the health food store owner

Let me relate a story about Jane who was 69 years old when I interviewed her in 2010. She has had Parkinson's for over 20 years. Jane had a health food store that she ran herself for over 25 years; then in 2004, she closed it down. During that time, she gave classes on health and healing through using different diets and supplements. For about 15 years, Jane did yoga and walked 4 to 5 miles a day. After about 17 years of healthy success with Parkinson's, she fell and broke her leg in 2007, and the doctor put her on a drug that only made the Parkinson's worse, much worse. After that, she started going downhill fast; now she can only walk with help and she shakes all the time.

Obviously most people take drugs for their Parkinson's; Jane in the beginning tried drugs but it made her worse. She made her own tinctures, smoothies, and mixtures. She said at one point, "It is damn hard work, to do all this!" She used nutritional methods and other physical methods, like massage and physical therapy, yoga and walking on the beach, which was nearby, to maintain her state of remission. Jane was very successful in slowing down Parkinson's for seventeen years but it did not stop the progression, it finally caught up with her.

Her knowledge and experience in the health food field is what helped her to progress in health and a near normal life for a long a time. Her knowledge was strong, but her living situation and support system were weak and she had very limited financial resources. Also, she never ate a strict vegan diet which was one of her downfalls. If she had the financial resources, a stronger support system and living situation and avoided animal products, she could possibly have become completely cured of her Parkinson's, or at least put it into complete remission.

So it's more than just changing to a plant-based diet. The Live-Food nutritional therapy is only one part of being successful. There are financial resources needed to follow a Living Plant-based nutrition approach. There is the person's living situation to consider as health care facilities usually will not accommodate the person following this difficult diet. Finally, a support system is needed for the person following the diet, since a health care facility will not do it.

This Living Plant-based diet sounds easy, but dying to sloth, gluttony and laziness is not always that easy! Having a facility to do this would be ideal. If the author was about the need of starting a health-care facility or tying it in with an existing one? His answer would be yes, he would like to start three of them, one on the east coast, one in the mid-west and one on the west coast for this nutritional approach.

c. Sloth, Gluttony and Rebellion!

Darlene's story and Judy's story are powerful. And the fact that her doctor gave out Darlene's testimonial and no one was interested is a witness to the sin of sloth, and laziness, the sin of gluttony, and the sin of rebellion that people are involved in and addicted to. They don't want to change even when their health and their life is at stake! Judy and Darlene shook off the sloth and rebellion to win.

It is hard for Darlene to pinpoint exactly when she became symptom-free, the process was slow and measured in tiny increments. Her best guess is that it was at least six years from when she started the diet, which places her full recovery about 1980. Over twenty years later, she doesn't consider herself to have MS. She eats carefully, still following the basic diet at home. She juices vegetables and wheatgrass and is careful to get enough of the essential fatty acids (omega-3, -6 and -9, found in fish and some vegetable oils like flaxseed, olive, sunflower, and safflower). According to Darlene, living with deep faith and trust in God, she was free to move forward, unimpeded by her own negative thoughts and moods that could have blocked her healing path. She like others overcame Sloth, Gluttony and Rebellion in order to get rid of her MS.[149]

"Such as these will end in disaster! Their god is in their belly and their glory is in their shame. I am talking about those who are set upon the things of the world." (Phil 3:19)

Fr. Johann Roten, PhD an internationally known theologian said to J. Tibbetts upon their first meeting, (cir. 2004) "Oh, you Americans you live a comfortable armchair spirituality." In a journal article J. Roten refers to the scholars relying upon the "principle of convenience, ... to generously."[150] This is found with most diets and diet therapies which are comfortable armchair diets that are convenient for both the nutritionists and the patient.

In other words the purification practices that are necessary for each human being to be cured of their degenerative disease are not the "comfortable armchair spirituality" practices based on "convenience theology" lacking a solid concrete foundation. These meat-based diet therapies are trying to please the client and are convenient dietary recommendations by the nutritionists.

"One day a farmer went out sowing. Part of what he sowed landed on a footpath, where birds came and ate it up. Part of it fell on rocky ground, where it had little soil. It sprouted at once since the soil had no depth, but when the sun rose and scorched it, it began to wither for lack of roots. Again part of the seed fell among thorns, which grew up and choked it. Part of it finally landed on good soil and yielded grain a hundred- or sixty- or thirty-fold. Let everyone heed what he hears." Matthew 13:4-9

Part III
The Nutritional Therapy Used

Chapter 6
Hypothesis to Theory: a New Evolution

St. Nilus of Sinai (d. 460) says, "It is right to pray not only for one's own purification, but for the purification of every man, imitating the angelic order." "Prayer frees the mind of all thought of the sensory and raises it to God Himself. St. Paul teaches us to continually be 'constant in prayer' (Rom 12:12), grounding ourselves in it by long perseverance (Col. 4:2; Eph 6:18). He also commands us to 'pray everywhere' (1Tim 2:8)."[151]

a. Cultural Revolution of Wild Ducks Needed

Vegetarianism dates back thousands of years. During biblical times, the emphasis on Live-Foods or raw foods was found in a few groups such as the Jewish Essenes. In biblical times, everything was organic, natural, ripe, raw and fresh! The standard vegetarian diet today includes a lot of processed foods (healthy junk foods) and the quality varies widely. The Live-food, plant-based diet approach is a whole new evolution in the plant-based field.

People in the New School of Plant-Based Thought are those promoting mostly raw vegan foods, and Live Plant-based foods. Some of these groups include: The Gerson Diet; The Hippocrates Diet; The Rainbow Green Cuisine Diet; The pH Miracle Diet; The Sunfood Diet; The Raw Food Revolution Diet; The Healthy Journey Diet; The Hallelujah Diet; The Alleluia Diet; the Natural Hygiene Diet and the 80/10/10 Diet. Some of these are mentioned in this book. This new dietary platform is an evolutionary step in nutrition, which is leads to greater degree of healing.

Furthermore the New Schools of Plant-Based Thought approach has optimized nutrition in the body, soul and spirit. This group is superior in healing degenerative diseases, both on the nutritional level and the psycho-spiritual level. The truth is Live-Foods and fasting are counter-cultural. Cooking is perceived as normal but it will be explained that cooking is a problem. Eating dormant grains is another problem. These are all counter-cultural.

Colin Campbell, PhD, professor emeritus of Cornell University, was part of the famous Women's Health Study and once asked the lead doctor of the study why they didn't show the real facts that the use of the plant-based diet orientation was a success in this study. This professor replied, "Because that's not what the public wants to hear."[152] This is common with research, it's geared to what the public wants to hear.

There is a retired CEO electronics executive, who has Parkinson's and who was written up in an article for *Newsweek.* He said, "the pressure to conform [to prevailing ideas of what causes diseases and how best to find treatments for them] means you lose the people who want to get up and go in a different direction. There is no place for the wild ducks. The result is more sameness and less innovation. What we need is a Cultural Revolution in the research community, academic and non-academic. We need to give wild ducks the opportunity to emerge and quack their way to success. But cultural change can be driven only by action at the top."[153]

Those in this new evolution of Live Plant-based foods are the wild ducks! This text is continuing the Cultural Revolution by promoting a plant-based nutrition and fasting therapy. Of course, there are those 'greats' who have preceded this book, like Anne Wigmore, Max Gerson, MD and the water fasting expert Dr. Scott in Cleveland. But we are taking this 'Cultural Revolution' in curing degenerative diseases to a whole new level.

Reformers and new thinkers often times have a hard time promoting their discoveries. Max Gerson, MD, a medical doctor in the 40's and 50's, published 55 scientific works during his fifty years of practice and created the Gerson diet. He became famous for curing cancer and in his cancer book he states, "The history of medicine reveals that reformers who bring new ideas into the general thinking and practice of physicians have a difficult time."

This Live-Food nutritional approach is a whole new level or paradigm. By presenting some of the theory will help to understand it.

b. NeuroInflammation

Two leading experts on Parkinson's in Europe are Dr. Geoffrey and Lucille Leader who write, "Parkinson's disease is associated with increased inflammation at the cellular level."[154] They have developed a theory that is very conservative and allopathic in its model.

Another "wild duck" is Sue T. Griffin, PhD[h] who is a leading expert in the role of neuroinflammation in Alzheimer's. This is a common theory which can help explain why Live-Foods can cure so many different degenerative diseases. "Alzheimer's patients' symptoms have led the majority of researchers to conclude that amyloid plaques are the pathogenic entity of the disease. But there is still no smoking gun that definitively singles out the plaques

---

[h] W. Sue T. Griffin, PhD is Professor and Vice Chairman for Research in the Donald W. Reynolds Department of Geriatrics at the University of Arkansas for Medical Sciences, and Director of Research at the Geriatric Research, Education, and Clinical Center of the Central Arkansas Veterans Healthcare System in Little Rock. Dr. Griffin and associate Robert E. Mark established the BMC online publication, *Journal of Neuroinflammation*, as editors-in-chief.

as the causative agent. Amyloid is the scientific equivalent of a culprit assumed guilty until proven innocent. Although many pharmaceutical companies vigorously took aim at amyloid, so far there is no unequivocal evidence that clearing plaques in Alzheimer's disease results in cognitive improvement,[155] suggesting that amyloid plaques may be end-stage rune stones of neuronal damage initiated by genetic variations, brain trauma, and aging.

Today, a new crop of investigators is looking at Alzheimer's pathogenesis with fresh eyes and finding that neuronal stress and the consequent overexpression of proinflammatory proteins are the likely instigators of neuropathological changes, including both plaque and tangle formation. The idea that amyloid plaques are more likely to be a response to the disease, rather than its initiator, is gaining acceptance."[156]

Dr. Griffin explains that after researching the evidence, "I couldn't help but wonder why no one had thought to look at the role of inflammation in this disease." She goes on to give a long technical explanation on the research of Alzheimer's in the brain and she states, Professor Griffin cites studies and evidence that seems to indicate inflammation might be a primary cause, ". . . suggesting that neuroinflammation plays an important role early in the disease, and could, in fact, be a driving factor."[157]

An MIT researcher, Dmitry Goldgaber,[158] identified with Sue Griffin's work on neuronal development, that inflammatory cytokines were involved in—and probably driving—neurodegeneration. Dr. Griffin wrote, "Together our studies added credence to the idea that neuronal stress and excess inflammatory cytokine production is a driving force in neurodegeneration and genesis of amyloid plaques." "In neuroinflammation we had a viable suspect—and a potential therapeutic target—which everyone seemed to be ignoring."[159]

Other studies, including a John Hopkins' study[160] on identical twins use of anti-inflammatory drugs (NSAIDs); and a Dutch study comparing a large group of Alzheimer's patients who were taking NSAIDs for other ailments to those who were not, showed a reduced risk or delayed onset of Alzheimer's disease. In a 2008 report from the Department of Veterans Affairs on 50,000 Alzheimer's patients and 200,000 control patients, researchers showed that those who took ibuprofen for as long as five years had a reduced Alzheimer's risk of almost one-half.[161] A more direct approach in a clinical trial (ADAPT) of NSAIDs, including naproxen and celecoxib, revealed a protective effect of one of the drugs, naproxen.[162] There were other related studies such as at the Scripps Research Institute.[163] [164]

"Neuroinflammation encapsulates the idea that microglial and astrocytic responses and actions in the central nervous system have a fundamentally inflammation-like character, and that these responses are central to the pathogenesis and progression of a wide variety of neurological disorders. This idea originated in the field of Alzheimer's disease[165] [166], where it has revolutionized our understanding of this disease[167]. These ideas have been extended to other neurodegenerative diseases[168] [169] [170], to ischemic/toxic diseases[171] [172], to tumor biology[173] and even to normal brain development." Dr. Griffin's inflammation theory would explain why others who don't have the disease have amyloid plaques, and also why most, if not all, degenerative diseases have neuroinflammation. This gives a common theory as to why the Live-Food's nutrition protocol works for all these different degenerative diseases.

Furthermore, "Neuroinflammation is a new and rapidly expanding field that has revolutionized our understanding of chronic neurological diseases. This field encompasses research ranging from population studies to signal transduction pathways, and investigators with backgrounds in fields as diverse as pathology, biochemistry, molecular biology, genetics, clinical medicine, and epidemiology. Important contributions to this field have come from work with populations, with patients, with postmortem tissues, with animal models, and within vitro systems."[174] Neuroinflammation in Alzheimer's and Parkinson's disease is found in articles in journals such as: *Neurobiol Aging; Progr Neurobiol; J Neuropathol Exp Neurol; Neuropathol Appl Neurobiol; J Neuroimmunol; J Neuropathol Exp Neurol, Neurology, J Am Geriatr Soc, Alzheimers Dement*, and a paper at the Proceeding of the National Academy Sciences, USA. "Scientists now widely accept her theory that this chronic inflammatory response in the brain is an important factor in the development of Alzheimer's disease."[175]

An earlier school of thought on inflammation is the early pioneer of Natural Hygiene, Dr. J.H. Tilden developed the Toxemia Model in his 1926 book, *The 7 Stages of Disease*. Stage 1 is Enervation (Nerve Energy is extremely reduced or exhausted), 2. Toxemia (Nerve Energy is too low to eliminate metabolic wastes and poisons); 3. Irritation (toxic build-up); 4. Inflammation (low-grade, chronic inflammation from toxicants that have amassed); 5. Ulceration (tissues are destroyed, body ulcerates); 6. Induration (long-term inflammation causing damage); and stage 7. Chronic, Irreversible Degeneration (cellular integrity is destroyed, cellular degeneration and death).

Victoria BidWell, PhD explains, "The role of raw foods in the climb out of disease, regardless of the Stage, early or advanced, is 3-fold. 1. They are free of Exogenous Toxins. 2. They provide the human body with the superlative nutrition the body needs to perform its basic, metabolic tasks. 3. They provide this nutrition in an energy-conservative package, being easy and energy-efficient to digest. Less Nerve Energy used to process the food ingested = more Nerve Energy for detoxification and repair. Remember: 'It's all about Nerve Energy, first and foremost!'"[176]

c. Neuron's Natural Cleansing is Dysfunctional

A few other "wild ducks" are noted in this section, one of them is R. Douglas Fields,[i] PhD, a recognized expert on neuron-glial interactions, brain development and memory. He wrote a book, *The Other Brain* (2010).[177] He states, "Back in the 1800's, the paradigm that scientists thought of the brain was that of a series of tubes for water flowing through them controlling muscles and other parts of the body. The new paradigm today in the computer age, is that scientists think of the brain as a computer, with the nerve cell, or neuron, as the microprocessor of the brain." Dr. Fields notes, "How sure can we be that our microprocessor analogy of the brain is accurate? Thoughtful neuroscientists are beginning to wonder - could our fundamental concept of how the brain works be naïve?"[178] "Most of the cells in your brain are glial, not neurons. Glial cannot fire electrical impulses nor do they have characteristic features of neurons, they do not have wire-like axons and root-like dendrites. Some scientists thought that they were just connective tissues. Scientists called them 'astrocytes' because of their protoplasmic legs extending in all directions. This name prevails for the four major types of glial cells known today."[179]

"A revolution in our understanding of how the brain is built, how it functions, how it fails in mental illness and disease, and how it is repaired has been ignited with the recent exploration of these long-neglected brain cells. Glial are the key to understanding this new view of the brain." In a study on Albert Einstein's brain, the only difference between Einstein's brain and an average brain was in these nonneuronal cells. He had twice as many of these nonneuronal cells, as Dr. Martin Diamond, a neuroanatomist at the University of California, Berkeley, has reported."[180]

---

[i] R.D. Fields is the Chief of the Nervous System Development and Plasticity, at the NIH. Editor of journal *Neuron Glia Biology.*

In a study published in 1993, "Francis Collins and colleagues announced that they had purified a neurotrophic factor that increased survival of the dopamine neurons of the type that die in Parkinson's disease. The researchers named this new growth factor Glial-Derived Neurotrophic Factor (GDNF), reflecting its cellular origin in astrocytes. At the present time, there are more than two thousand scientific papers on GDNF in the *PubMed* database of scientific medical studies. These studies show that the glial-derived factor sustains neurons in the central nervous system and also some neurons in the peripheral nervous system in association with many medical conditions."[181]

Dr. Fields new paradigm of the brain is still being developed, all because they had purified the glial cells. It was the purification that showed new light and a new direction, just like fasting purifies cells in the body and even in the brain. Purification is the key to this new paradigm! It also compliments the NeuroInflammation theory just noted.

Long term memory is separate from short term memory and it's been found that people with brain damage and severe short term memory problems can have excellent long term memory. Physicists are finding auras around the body which contain an energy field and hypothesize that this is where long term memory and the intellect really lie. Theology would confirm this since the mind or intellect exists in the soul (psyche or psychological), which is something separate from the body, yet part of it. These glial nonneuronal cells in the brain and nervous system could be the connection for this energy matrix of the soul.

Dr. Fields says, "The *substantia nigra* neurons die in Parkinson's disease because they become clogged with abnormal proteins that should have been destroyed by the neuron's natural cleansing process. Many other neuro-degenerative diseases show similar abnormal accumulations of junk proteins, including Alzheimer's, ALS (Lou Gehrig's disease), and Lewy Body disease. Until recently, scientists fixated on the protein inclusions inside patients' neurons, and overlooked the fact that the nearby astrocytes are filled with the same blobs of abnormal proteins. On an anatomical level, astrocytes are a part of these neuro-degenerative diseases, and it is quite reasonable, given the new awareness of neuron-glial interactions, that these abnormal astrocytes may be a root cause of these diseases."[182]

Dr. Fields concludes, "As recent studies of ALS and Parkinson's disease illustrate, neuro-degenerative diseases can often result directly from glial dysfunction. It is the strict intellectual segregation of neuron and glial also prevented most scientists from appreciating the converse - which known 'glial' diseases, such as multiple sclerosis, could result in the death of neurons. The recent realization that this could be so did not spring from late-breaking clues: the evidence was there in plain sight all along, but prejudicial thinking fueled the ignorance. The alternative view was regarded as controversial because it ran counter to current thinking. Now, however, neuroscience is turning the corner. As a result of this new direction in research we are beginning to reach a new basic understanding of nearly all neuro-degenerative diseases, from Alzheimer's to stroke, arising from an enlightened attitude toward glial."[183]

Purification is the key to the cure of Parkinson's, Alzheimer's, MS and many other brain diseases. Using fasting and/or a purified vegan diet, such as a Live plant-based diet, for the neurological processes helps cure all of these diseases which have Neuro-Inflammation. The neuron's natural cleansing is dysfunctional and needs purification.

Parris Kidd, PhD cited an important fact that neurons in the brain can regenerate. "The mind-body medicine Renaissance coincides with exciting new discoveries about how our brains age and how we may keep our brains young. Of all these brain discoveries, the most significant is neurogenesis (literally, birth of neurons), the process of brain cell regeneration. First identified in a landmark 1998 study,[184] neurogenesis disproved the century-old belief that neurons only regenerated during brain development. In addition to its obvious potential to boost cognitive performance, neurogenesis opened an intriguing new door to peak cognitive longevity - adults as old as 72 have been shown to regenerate neurons."[185]

Dr. Brian Clement notes, "Antioxidants have been studied for their effectiveness in reducing these deleterious effects and neuronal death in many in vitro and in vivo studies. Increasing number of studies demonstrated the efficacy of polycpenolic antioxidants from fruits and vegetables to reduce or to block neronal death."[186]

See section c. Normal Healthy pH for Gabriel Cousens, MD who promotes this Biological Terrain Theory, along with other experts like Dr. Antoine Bechamp, Professor Gunther Enderlein, Dietrich Klinghardt, MD, PhD, and Robert Young, PhD. The basis of the Biological Terrain Theory, is the key motto: "Germs don't cause disease; they develop in a diseased environment." The cornerstone of Bechamp's theory was that maintaining a healthy terrain and biological physiology is the key to health.

d. The Energy Matrix of Food

Talking about food as energy and life giving and as human life force or energy fields has been around for over a hundred years especially with early pioneers like Dr. Herbert Shelton. In fact biblical times and scriptures have the same recurring "life" and "living" terminology. The difference is that now this terminology is much more scientific and not as philosophical in its understanding.

A major paradigm shift occurred when Albert Einstein proved that $E=mc^2$ showing that it is all about energy. Victoria BidWell, PhD an expert in Natural Hygiene explains, "Nerve Energy in Natural Hygiene, refers to the low-grade electricity generated by the brain that supplies current to the body and regenerates and repairs all tissues: bone, blood, skin, muscles, nerves, and glands. The Health Seeker best appreciates the human body as a wondrous, electro-chemical power system! It is Nerve Energy that runs the whole show."[187] Toxemia or auto-intoxication is the toxic involvement of the cells which results in a depletion of Nerve energy. See, i. The Sevenfold Path of Purification for levels of energy distribution that are purified.

The natural hygiene of the cellular system is capable of cleansing and eliminating this toxicity bringing remission and healing. Foods from the Standard American Diet (SAD) are often "quasi-food" substances typical of the refined, chemicalized, and processed, often with poisons and toxins are health-threatening and reduce Nerve Energy. Many health promoters have a list of healthy life-style enhancers, Victoria BidWell's, The 10 Energy Enhancers are: 1. Cleanliness, 2. Pure Air, 3. Pure Water, 4. Adequate Sleep, 5. Natural Hygiene diet, 6. Right Temperatures, 7. Adequate Sunlight, 8. Regular Exercise, 9. Emotional Balance, 10. Nurturing Relationships. The opposite of these are the 10 energy robbers.

The Natural Hygiene School includes such notables as: Dr. J.H. Tilden, Dr. Herbert Shelton, Dr. Keki Sidhaw, T.C. Fry, Dr. William Esser, Dr. Vetrano, Drs. Tosca and Gregory Haag, Dr. Burton, Dr. David Scott, Dr. Alan Goldhamer, Dr. Doug Graham, Dr. Victoria BidWell and others. Cure is understood by this group as body-initiated, body-conducted, and body-maintained in their philosophical understanding. The body is its own self-healer this is the cure and the natural therapy or treatment. The body-as-healer provides the conditions for health and healing through the above mentioned 10 points on energy; especially a raw vegan diet and fasting are key.[188]

A modern understanding of energy is found by Gabriel Cousens, MD who is a medical doctor, an MD and a MD(H) in holistic medicine and is a doctor of homeopathic medicine, and a Diplomate in Ayurveda. He explains; "People have been eating live foods for thousands of years. Those who continue to eat live foods, in this tradition, seem to have an extended life span, higher quality of health, abundant vitality and even joy, and significantly less chronic disease. Recent research into calorie restriction has supplied some evidence as to why those who are on a high percentage of live food see to have such superior health and longevity. In my clinical experience, the minimum percentage of live food in the diet to have this healing and energetic effect is 80%. As we go deeper into the physics of it, we begin to understand that live food has the highest amount of quality nutrient concentrates, the highest amount of phytonutrients, vitamins and minerals, the highest amount of bioelectrical energy, the highest amount of biologically active water, the highest amount pi electrons, the highest amount of biophotons, and the highest amount of subtle organizing energy field energy. In other words, from the physical to the electrical to the subtle organizing energy field level, live foods are superior for our health and well-being than any other type of food."[189]

Humans are body, soul and spirit; the soul is a matrix of energies that is foundational for the physical body. Gabriel Cousens explains, "Live foods, because of their high energetic structural integrity, give the healthiest food-source nutrients on the physical plane." The human soul is the subtle organizing energy field and this energetic matrix which has life and personality. When "this matrix is energized, it becomes more coherent and serves as a better energetic pattern for the different levels of the physical formation." "Live foods or raw foods contribute the most energy to our subtle organizing energy fields, as compared to cooked and other forms of processed foods, and therefore have the greatest ant-aging effect. Processed foods and junk foods actually decrease and often disrupt our subtle organizing energy fields."[190]

A Dr. Szekely discusses four categories of foods divided according to their energy effects. The highest degree of life force is the biogenic foods which enhance the human life force or energy fields, they reverse entropy and aging. They are the ripe, raw, living, high enzyme foods like sprouts and baby greens. The second lower degree is supportive of the first and it is the fresh raw fruits and vegetables. The third are the biostatic foods that are organic and cooked; they are marginally life sustaining. The fourth are the biocidic foods which are life-destroying foods. They are the highly processed commercial foods, which have additives, preservatives, chemicals, pesticides, hormones and include animal foods. The biogenic and bioactive foods are what the raw and living food movements are all about; and which bring healing.[191]

Dr. Joanna Budwig with degrees in medicine, physics, pharmacy and biochemistry concluded that "not only do electron-rich live foods act as high-power electron donors, but electron-rich foods also act as a solar-resonant field in the body to attract, store, and conduct the sun's energy in our bodies." The phontons of the sunlight, she called "sun electrons," or "pi electrons." Dr. Budwig believes "that the energy we absorb from these solar photons acts as an anti-entropy factor or anti-aging factor." As a result of her theory, she believes that live-foods bring a lot of pi electrons into the system. Dr. Cousens concludes, "Our health and consciousness depend on our ability to attract, store and conduct electron energy, which is essential for the energizing and regulation of all life forces. The greater our store of light energy, the greater the power of our overall electromagnetic field and, consequently, the more energy available for healing and maintenance of optimal health. Metaphorically, a strong solar resonance field promotes the evolution of humanity to reach our full potential as human (sun) beings. Light supports evolution, and a lack of pi electrons in our bodies hinders it."[192]

There is an expression of the genes that indicates inflammatory stress and other types of physiological stress. This stress grows old with age, but diminishes with calorie restrictions. Dr. Cousens notes, "The medical community is noticing that chronic inflammation plays a more important role in chronic disease than we originally thought."[193]

Dr. Cousens continues, "From a live-food point of view, research such as that discussed above is extremely exciting and validating. Eating live foods is the simplest and most powerful way to achieve this healthful caloric effect, without even having to diet. This is because cooking foods usually results in destroying 50% of the protein, according to the Max Planck Institute, and approximately 60-70% of assimilable vitamins and minerals, up to 96% of the B_{12} and 100% of enzymes and phytonutrients. In other words, one need only eat approximately half the amount of food and calories on a live-food diet as on a cooked-food diet to get an equivalent amount of vitamins, minerals, protein, and phytonutrients. On a healthy live-food regime one automatically gets the anti-aging calorie-restriction effect without having to diet."[194]

Healing occurs on three levels or dimensions; body, soul and spirit, all three could be described as different levels of energy interactions. Bruce Lipton, PhD is a stem cell biologist who taught at the University of Wisconsin's School of Medicine, he writes, "Once I realized the nature of the complex interactions between matter and energy, I knew that a reductionist, linear (A>B>C>D>E) approach could not even come close to giving us an accurate understanding of disease. While quantum physics implied the existence of such interconnected information pathways, recent ground-breaking research in mapping protein-protein interactions in the cell now demonstrates the physical presence of these complex holistic pathways. (Li, et al, 2004;[195] Giot, et al,

2003;[196] Jansen, et al, 2003;[197] Barry 2008[198]). Clearly, biological dysfunctions can result from miscommunication anywhere within these complex pathways. . . . Newtonian research scientists have not fully appreciated the extensive interconnectivity among the cell's biological information networks."[199]

Dr. Lipton continues, "Hundreds upon hundreds of other scientific studies over the last fifty years have consistently revealed that 'invisible forces' of the electromagnetic spectrum profoundly impact every facet of biological regulation. These energies include microwaves, radio frequencies, the visible light spectrum, extremely low frequencies, acoustic frequencies, and even a newly recognized form of force know as scalar energy. Specific frequencies and patterns of electromagnetic radiation regulate DNA, RNA, and protein synthesis; alter protein shape and function; and control gene regulation, cell division, cell differentiation, morphogenesis (the process by which cells assemble into organs and tissues), hormone secretion, and nerve growth and function. Each one of these cellular activities is a fundamental behavior that contributes to the unfolding of life. Though these research studies have been published in some of the most respected mainstream biomedical journals, as of 2010 their revolutionary findings have not been incorporated into the medical school curriculum.[200] (Liboff 2004,[201] Goodman and Blank 2002;[202] Sivitz 2000;[203] Jin, et el, 2000;[204] Blackman, et al, 1993;[205] Rosen 1992;[206] Blank 1992;[207] Tsong 1989;[208] Yen-Patton, et al, 1988).[209]

It is very difficult to understand Live-Foods with just linear thinking; a person needs to move into holistic thinking to understand the complex web of interactions. Furthermore there is a psychological level and a spiritual level that are involved in Live-Foods Nutrition which is part of this holistic complex. The Living Foods matrix involves the body, soul and human spirit. Today in medicine and nutrition they are only taking into account the physiological body (as matter and not the energetic body) and not the psychological self, nor the spiritual self of humans.

e. Live-Foods Nutrition Blueprint

There was a summit called The International Living Foods Summit, which was held at the Hippocrates Health Institute in West Palm Beach Florida on January 14, 2006. The summit convened to try and establish scientifically-based common standards for optimum health. The author, Jim Tibbetts and Gabriel Cousens were among the twenty-three leaders[210] from eight countries who gathered to develop a set of standards that day. In later years, at other gatherings, and also by the author, these standards were updated and modified slightly, but the basic outline is as following:

Live-Foods Nutrition Blueprint[211]
The Optimum Diet for Health/Longevity

- Vegan   (no animal products of any kind, cooked or raw)
- Raw   (At least 80% raw/Live-Foods)
- Organic   (as much as possible)
- Whole Foods   (sprouted and soaked grains, nuts, and seeds)
- Contains adequate complete proteins from plant sources
- Contains adequate carbohydrate intake from plant sources with moderate yet adequate caloric intake
- Contains all essential fats, including Omega-3 fatty acids from naturally-occurring plant sources
- Contains only low to moderate sugar and exclusively from whole food sources (fruitarianism is strongly discouraged)
- Contains a significant quantity of chlorophyll-rich green foods
- Contains a large proportion of high-water

content foods
- Highly mineralized; low amounts of naturally-sourced salts; no highly-processed salt
- Nutrient-Dense, containing vitamins, minerals, antioxidants and phytonutrients
- Includes supplements as needed (vitamins including B12, superfoods, protein powders)
- Includes raw vegetable or grass juices
- Includes water or juice fasting at least once per year
- Provides adequate hydration
- Is nutritionally optimal for detoxification and rebuilding the body

We (the leaders) also agree that a Live-Food diet:
- Is in recognition of government nutritional standards and studies supporting this blueprint
- Is in recognition of Live-Food standards, studies and criterion as presented above
- Is lovingly prepared, holistic and avoids toxins
- Is environmentally friendly
- Has sunlight and fresh air
- Has natural personal care products and clothes
- Recognizes addiction, bad behavior, vice and the need for psychological health
- Recognizes the need for physical exercise
- Recognizes that there is an evolution or maturity in the body as it becomes more purified.
- Recognizes body types, transitions and schools of thought for tailoring to individual needs.

'All leaders agreed that the main objective of eating in the above mentioned fashion is to promote health, and equally to prevent and minimize disease.' This is the basic blueprint of nutrition needed for the body to cure AD, PD and MS.

As the purification becomes greater in a person's body it evolves and reaches another plateau or level. Usually people go from the semi-vegetarian level to the vegetarian level to the vegan level to the raw vegan level as they purify their body and its ability to transition to a higher level. In the psalms it talks about going from height to height up Mount Zion. As purification becomes greater so does healing.

Eating meat is on one of the lower plateau's of the mountain of optimum health. Eating meat three times or less a week is the lowest plateau, the next plateau is once a week, then lacto-ovo-vegetarians, and finally to vegans. This moves to the next higher, healthier plateaus of raw vegans and Living Foods.

One thing that needs to be noted is the natural personal care products and clothes mentioned above. Those that are not natural can be a source of chemical toxins that enter the body. In the book, *Killer Clothes,* by Anna Maria and Brian Clement, the author's state, "Permethrin-soaked clothes are not the only source of large exposures to the insecticide. The chemical is found in many personal-sized mosquito sprays and commonly shows up in residential bug sprays that are used by exterminators. It appears in lice shampoos for pets and people, along with flea dips and household foggers. It kills insects by disrupting their nervous systems."[212]

"For persons whose jobs involve handling permethrin, there is already a well-documented three-fold increase in the risk for developing Parkinson's disease. A September 2009 study published in the *Archives of Neurology* compared 519 people with Parkinson's to 511 people without, and determined that those whose jobs involved exposure to the insecticide tripled their risk for developing the disease compared to those reporting no exposure to the chemical agent."[213] Other chemicals in clothes can also be a problem.

e. A Nutritional Approach for PD and MS

A basic Living plant-based food diet for PD, AD and MS would consist of various nutrition factors, found in the raw food diets mentioned, this approach is called Six Sigma Nutrition and could be summarized in the following overview:

Plant-Based Nutrition
1. Animal fat intake and animal products are excluded from the diet.
2. Junk foods are excluded from the diet, including the five whites: sugar, salt, white flour, milk, and the fat on meats (any animal products).
3. No grains or beans unless they are soaked and sprouted.
4. An 80/20 to 100% raw vegan diet is the basic diet, Living Plant-based Nutrition is best.
5. Limiting fruit in the beginning stages (usually 3 to 6 months to reduce intake of sugar in order to minimize yeast/fungus growth.
6. Including cold-processed oil (coconut, olive oil, etc.)

Fasting, Smoothies and Juicing
7. Fasting and detoxification methods catabolize unwanted cells and normalize healthy cells.
8. Green Smoothies daily are essential, except on a juice fast.
9. Fresh juice on a daily basis to avoid dehydration and provide nutrients.

Supplements - as needed
10. A nutritional supplement regime as needed.
11. Vegan Protein powders
12. Green powders

Complementary Therapies - that influence physiology
13. An exercise and relaxation routine is needed.

14. Prayer and Meditation to reduce stress and increase healing.
15. Various other adjunct therapies, like massage, reflexology, energy healing can be very helpful.
16. Counseling to deal with the psychological issues, and/or coaching for guidance.

Key points in this diet for Parkinson's and MS are:
- ✓ High liquid intake through juices or water, avoid dehydration
- ✓ High nutrient intake through the raw vegan diet
- ✓ High chlorophyll intake through greens and powders
- ✓ Low fruit intake in the beginning to avoid yeast and fungus growth
- ✓ pH levels need to be alkaline in the intercellular fluids
- ✓ Potassium/sodium cellular levels need to be balanced appropriately, very low salt intake (avoid common table salt or iodized/processed salt)
- ✓ Nutrient density in the blood needs to be maximized for the immune system to work properly
- ✓ Oxygen intake needs to be maximized; high oxygen intake is best which is achieved through eating raw fruits and vegetables and exercising."

f. The Alleluia Nutrition Therapy for AD, PD, and MS

The Alleluia diet (Six Sigma diet - the commercial version) is founded by Jim Tibbetts who is a scholar (historian, theologian), vegetarian, and who does fasts (since 1970's). He is also a lecturer/writer on these topics and, his wife, Anne Marie Tibbetts, is a registered dietitian with over 23 years' experience and expertise in geriatric nutrition. Jim Tibbetts called their diet the Alleluia diet or Alleluia Nutrition Therapy (or Six Sigma Nutrition Therapy)! People can get healed in their body, soul and spirit, and then can shout with joy, "Alleluia!"

One of the greatest therapies for Parkinson's, Alzheimer's and MS is to enter the Alleluia Green Zone or for those not religious, the Six Sigma Green Zone. For degenerative diseases especially PD, AD, and MS, a person needs to enter into and stay in the, Alleluia Green Zone! To help achieve and remain in the Alleluia Green Zone, the Alleluia Nutrition therapy recommends at least two or three of these every day:

- o a green smoothie
- o green superfoods
- o a shot of wheat or barley grass
- o a glass or several glasses of green juice
- o a large salad with Kale and/or other greens

❖ Several glasses of green juice, Super Greens every day, a large salad with greens daily, green smoothies, juices and powders daily, green superfoods, low-fat raw vegan and emphasizing fruits.

Green smoothies contain green vegetables and fruits. There are many variations. The benefit of green smoothies to PD, MS and Alzheimer's patients is not just in the extremely healthy mixture just mentioned above, but that it gives a place to add supplements in a tasty way. Throw a lot of the daily nutrients, flax oil and protein powder into the green smoothie and blend it up, then drink it down!

When a person with Parkinson's, AD, or MS enters into the Alleluia Green Zone, they will feel better and want to continue in that space. But at first they may have to go through cleansing on their way to getting into the Zone.

The term 80/20 Raw is internationally accepted to mean, 80% raw and 20% cooked in a raw vegan diet. It is the "80/20 raw vegan threshold" that is the doorway to healing most degenerative diseases, as evidence suggests from various health professionals and case studies. This is especially true for brain and neurological diseases like Parkinson's, Alzheimer's, and MS.

The following raw vegan diets have a nutritional therapy emphasis that can possibly heal AZ, AD and MS. The founders are listed to identify each of these:

- Hippocrates Diet: Anne Wigmore, Brian Clement, PhD
- Gerson Diet: Max Gerson, MD and Charlotte Gerson
- pH miracle Diet: Robert Young, PhD & Shelly Young
- Rainbow Green Diet: Gabriel Cousens, MD
- Raw Revolution Diet: Cherie Soria, RD, MS, Brenda Davis RD, Vesanto Melina, MS, RD
- Sunfood Diet: David Wolf, MS, JD
- Healthy Journey Diet: Fred Bisci, PhD
- Alleluia Diet: Jim Tibbetts, STL, MBA and Anne Marie Tibbetts MS, RD
- Hallelujah Diet: Rev. George Malkamus, DMinistry
- 80/10/10 Diet: Doug Graham, DC
- Natural Hygiene Diet: Herbert M. Shelton, PhD, DC, ND; Gregory and Tosca Haag, MD's
- Transitional Vegetarian approaches

There are other raw vegan/living foods diets that could also be noted but these all have published works and the author has met the founders or key leaders. Transitional Vegetarian approaches are the grain-based vegetarian approaches that are going through a transition to try to incorporate the paradigms and principles of the raw vegans and living foods approaches noted above.

The Alleluia diet (Six Sigma) emphasizes a nutrition therapy approach from a review and incorporation of these approaches above and it is as follows:

- A 100%/95% Live-Food diet is the ideal.
- "An 85/15% raw vegan diet, usually one meal is a large salad; this is a 100% vegan, 85% raw plant-based foods, which has less than 15% cooked foods.
- Six 8 oz glasses of freshly-juiced carrot juice daily; freshly-juiced apple or cucumber juice or other veggie juice may replace part of the carrot juice

- Six teaspoons of a green powder like barley grass powder (taken 2 to 3 times) a day
- Breakfast should be juice, a smoothie, some fruit, or a light meal (fermented foods could be at this meal)
- Lunch and Dinner consists of two large raw vegan meals (one is a large salad and some fermented foods)
- Exercises like yoga, Pilates or walking at least ½ hour a day to help digestion; include some sunshine, fresh air and prayer daily.
- Finally, a weekly meeting with a health professional, counselor or health coach is needed to work through the issues, both past and present."

So in summary:
1. Two to three raw vegan meals; lunch and dinner one is a large salad, some fermented food or drink
2. Six 8oz glasses of freshly juiced carrot and/or apple, cucumber and/or fresh juice (not pasteurized)
3. Six teaspoons of a barley grass or wheat grass or a mixture of green grasses as a powder, a day."

h. The New Adam and Eve

The New Testament texts that connect Jesus and Adam include: Rom 5:14-19 also the verse "Just as in Adam all die, so in Christ all will come to life again." 1 Co 15:21, 22 "Scripture has it that Adam, the first man, became a living soul; the last Adam became a life-giving spirit. ... so shall we bear the likeness of the man from heaven." 1 Cor 15:45-49 The parallel of Adam to Jesus is presented nine times in the New Testament and led to the association of Eve to Mary. The post-apostolic Fathers St. Justin (155) and St. Irenaeus, (circa 177) both write on the Eve-Mary parallel. Other Church Fathers also compare Mary with Eve.[j]

---

[j] Citing: St. Jerome, St. Augustine, St. Cyril of Jerusalem, St. John Chryostom, St. John Damascene. This is stated in the *Documents of Vatican II* (LG 56); and in the *Catechism of the Catholic Church* (494).

Irenaeus sees both Christ and Mary as untying the very knot that Adam and Eve had bound together through their disobedience, which started with food.[214]

Mary belongs to an "Order of Eden" which is about the line of succession and linage from Adam and Eve to Mary's Jewish Essene parents and her uniqueness as the New Eve, and as the Daughter of Zion (Zephaniah 3.14-17) because she qualifies as a personification of the elect people, the "kosher woman." The Order of Eden is found in those Jewish and Christian communities and individuals that followed the dietary lifestyle of the original Adam and Eve which was a plant-based or Living Foods diet and the new Adam and Eve, a less strict plant-based diet.

The Professor Roberta Kalechofsky Ph.D.,[215] points out (book: *Vegetarian Judiasm*) that: "The first law of kashruth is, in fact, the commandment to be vegetarian: 'I give you every seed-bearing plant that is upon all the earth and every tree that has seed-bearing fruit; these shall be yours for food.'" This is a Genesis 1:29 diet that could be called an Alleluia diet since it is the diet of the old Adam and Eve and it approximates the diet of the new Adam and Eve.

Chapter 8

Fasting Normalizes and Detoxifies

St. Augustine wrote: "The solemn season has come which reminds us to humiliate our souls by prayer and fasting and to chastise our body to a greater degree than at other periods of the year."[216] "For forty days Moses, the guardian of the Law, fasted; for forty days Elias, the most excellent of the Prophets, fasted; for forty days the Lord Himself, to whom both the Law and the Prophets gave testimony, fasted. Hence, it was in company with these two that He revealed Himself on the mountain."[217]

For a more complete understanding of juice fasting see Jim and Anne Marie's book: *Juice Fasting Simplified a Practical Approach*, which this is an edit of it.

a. Fasting Detoxifies

Fasting implies resting which we do every night. Every morning we terminate the fast with our first meal, break-the-fast or breakfast. The fastest way to bring your body back to health is too fast. The body heals and purifies itself rapidly during a fast, often recovering decades of abuse in just a few weeks. Two key concepts need to be understood about fasting are: that fasting normalizes and detoxifies the physiology of the body.

How is fasting helpful to Parkinson's and MS? Parkinson's and MS are partly a detoxification problem. AS previously noted there is inflammation in the brain caused by several different factors. Do you know what they are?

First, heavy metal toxicity has been found in most Parkinson's patients. Heavy metal is found in most Parkinson's patients, and aluminum is found in most

Alzheimer's patients. What are the other things mentioned in the journal articles on Parkinson's?

Pesticides in the brain are mentioned in many of the journal articles, and the second thing? Seondly Lewy bodies are found in Parkinson's brains; most scientists aren't sure why, but they never made the connection to meat proteins. Lewy bodies are found in every Parkinson's patient and these are abnormal protein clumps, probably animal protein clumps; animal proteins have a double-helix bond which are more likely to clump, while plant-proteins have a single-helix bond molecule. White lesions are found in MS patients. This also adds to the inflammation. Alzheimer's patients also have toxic proteins in the brain.

Detoxification is one of the main answers, fasting or other detoxification methods are needed for the cleaning out the brain. Both juice and water fasting can be used for this. In addition to these, the internal chemistry in the brain is messed up possibly by internal cellular toxins given off or food poisons, or additives (excitotoxins), or fungi. People with PD and MS need detoxing and fasting (juice or water) to clean out their cells of mucus, toxins, poisons and related unnecessary materials in the body and in the brain; these get flushed out through the kidneys.

What about the blood-brain barrier? This is a problem if you wanted to use a drug, but if you stick with natural food-based supplements for chelating heavy metals, they would be able to pass through the blood-brain barrier. Synthetic drugs cannot pass through, under normal conditions, the blood-brain barrier; after all, drugs are low-level, legal doses of poisons. The blood-brain barrier is designed to keep these poisons out of the brain.

Is fasting a good way to detox drugs? Yes, it is an excellent way to detox you from pharmaceutical drugs. If you want to get fully healed, eventually you have to detox yourself of all drugs, especially those in the brain and nervous system.

Fasting is one of the best ways to get rid of poisons, toxins, pesticides, waxes and other synthetic chemicals that can be found in the food we eat. Other chemicals can have toxic effects on the body such as cleaning compounds, detergents, insecticides, gasoline, etc. Fasting catabolizes the dead, diseased and pesticide-ridden cells and flushes them out of the body. Fasting is the best way to get rid of pesticides and other poisons and toxins that are lodged in the body or the brain. These get lodged in our cells and eventually cause cancer and other diseases. During a fast, the body first burns up or get rid of the cells which are dead, aged, damaged and diseased tissues, tumors and fat deposits. Catabolism during fasting gets rid of the inferior cells and keeps the essential ones.

One of the main reasons for fasting is that it is the primary means of detoxification.

b. Fasting Normalizes

Fasting detoxifies the biochemistry and it also "resets" or "normalizes the biochemistry." Fasting is a "reset" of the body's biochemistry; it normalizes the biochemistry back to its original standard settings. Everyone knows that fasting detoxifies the body, but most do not understand that it resets the biochemistry. It normalizes or 'resets' the biochemistry back to what is the ideal and proper biochemical parameters, connections and chemicals, in the healthy optimal state. This is very important since it is the brain biochemistry that needs to be reset and normalized. This is extremely important for anyone with a degenerative disease and it is very little understood.

The human biochemistry has its own parameters, biochemical levels and ranges such as cholesterol levels. The brain also has these biochemical parameters and in

Parkinson's, Alzheimer's and MS and other neurological diseases these biochemical problems need to correct. Fasting can help to do this by resetting the parameters.

It's sort of like a computer with a reset button, we just press the button and it resets the computer in a few seconds. It is a lot more complicated and slower in the body but it does basically the same thing.

Fasting takes weeks to do, and it will do a reset on the biochemistry in small increments or amounts. Like a computer that can reset itself, so can biochemistry but the computer does it in a few seconds while the biochemistry can take weeks or months. Then a person will have to go on another fast to reset it even more and, later, a third long fast will finally get it back to its normal biochemical parameters. Every individual will be different. This reset mechanism, along with the detoxification, is what is very important for the cure for Parkinson's, Alzheimer's, MS and other neurological diseases. The Live-Food nutrition therapy program is the support mechanism that helps to rebuild the brain cells and biochemical environment.

Is found in clinical experience too? Gabriel Cousens, MD explains in his book, *Conscious Eating*, "In my clinical experience with juice fasting, although people may get transitory healing crisis for several days, the fasts provide a controlled and safe situation where one can 'reset one's dietary dial' to a healthier diet. After a few positive experiences of fasting on a purer diet, one has enough positive feedback that the transition to the next step goes much more smoothly. After each stage of the transition, people seem to rise to a new level of well-being, energy, love and light."[218]

c. Water and Juice Fasting

Water fasting is the oldest, the most well-known and widely used type of fasting. Water fasting is the classic form of fasting. As a science it was popularized in the U.S. around the turn of the century. Obviously fasting on water means drinking only water. Dr. Bragg recommends an alternative to just drinking water is to add one teaspoon of lemon juice and half a teaspoon of uncooked honey to each glass of water. Make up a quart or two and refrigerate it. By adding these two ingredients, they act as mucus and toxic dissolvers. By dissolving the toxic poisons they can be more easily flushed out through the kidneys.

Jim Tibbetts notes, "I have spoken with some of the top water fasting experts in the country on using juice fasting and they all disagree, they consider it a juice diet. But the experts that do juice fasting, like Dr. Cousens and others agree that juice fasting is a real fast."

Leading nutritionists and detoxification experts agree that fresh vegetable and fruit juice cleansing is superior to water fasting. Indeed, juice cleansing is an evolution in detoxification methods. Fresh juices, broths and herb teas help deeply cleanse the body, rejuvenate the tissues and guide you to a faster recovery from health problems than water fasting.

Traditional water fast can be harsh and demanding on your body. Deeply buried pollutants and chemicals from our tissues can be released into elimination channels too rapidly during a water fast. Sometimes, the physical and emotional stress of a water fast even overrides the healing benefits.

One writer Linda Page, ND, PhD writes, "Vegetable and fruit juices are alkalizing, so they neutralize uric acid and other inorganic acids, better than water, and increase the healing effects. Juices support better metabolic activity for fasting, too. Metabolic activity slows down during a water fast as the body attempts to conserve dwindling energy resources that further reduce productive cleansing. Juices are very easy on digestion - easily assimilated into the bloodstream. They don't disturb the detoxification process."[219]

Juice fasting involves drinking fruit and vegetable juices, vegetables and herbal teas. These are easily assimilated into the upper digestive tract and do not stimulate the secretion of hydrochloric acid in the stomach. Dr. Airola (European doctor) presents a list of scientific justifications for juice fasting which he bases on physiological facts and professional opinions.

1. Raw Juices and broths "are rich in vitamins, minerals, trace elements and enzymes."

2. "These vital elements are very easily assimilated directly into the bloodstream, without putting a strain on the digestive system - thus they do not disrupt the healing and rejuvenating process of autolysis, or self-digestion."

3. Juices "do not stimulate the secretion of hydrochloric acid in the stomach."

4. "The nutritive elements from the juices are extremely beneficial in normalizing all the body processes, supplying needed elements for the body's own healing activity and cell regeneration, and, thus, speeding the recovery."

5. "Raw juices and vegetable broths provide an alkaline surplus which is extremely important for the proper acid-alkaline balance in the blood and tissues, since blood and tissues contain large amounts of acids during fasting."

6. "Generous amounts of minerals in the juices, particularly in the vegetable broth, help to restore the biochemical and mineral balance in the tissues and cells."

7. Numerous fasting clinics and experts make scientific claims as well:

a) "According to Dr. Ralph Bircher, raw juices contain an as yet unidentified factor which stimulates what he calls a micro-electric tension in the body and is responsible for the cells' ability to absorb nutrients from the blood stream and effectively excrete metabolic wastes."[220]

b) Dr. Ragnar Berg a leading authority on nutrition and biochemistry states; "During fasting the body burns up and excretes huge amounts of accumulated wastes. We can help this cleansing process by drinking alkaline juices instead of water while fasting. I have supervised may fasts and made extensive tests of fasting patients, and I am convinced that drinking alkaline-forming fruit and vegetable juices, instead of water, during fasting will increase the healing effect of fasting. Elimination of uric acid and other inorganic acids will be accelerated. And sugars in juices will strengthen the heart...Juice fasting is, therefore, the best form of fasting."[221]

c) Dr. Otto H.F. Buchinger at his clinic has supervised over 80,000 fasts and employs only juice fasting. "He told me that, in his experience, fasting on the fresh raw juices of fruits and vegetables, plus vegetable broths and herb teas, results in much faster recover from disease and more effective cleansing and rejuvenation of the tissues that does the traditional water fast."[222]

When all is taken into account, we recommend juice fasting as the best way for a person to learn and experience fasting and to get the benefits thereof. Water fasting works but is more advanced and difficult to do.

d. Seven to Twenty-One Day Fasts

A seven day juice fasting program is a standard time around the world. In biblical times the Jews used to fast for six days and break it on the seventh day, for the Sabbath. Coming off a seven day fast may last for one or two or three more days, making it an 8, 9 or 10 day fast.

Dr. Airola (juice fasting) and Dr. Bragg (water fasting) both emphasize 7 to 10 day fasts. Most people who read this book are just learning to fast and have little experience in long fast. Seven days on a fast is enough for the average person starting out. After gaining some experience for several seven day fasts, you can try for a few days to a week or two more if your body and your spirit

139

encourage you too. A seven day fast is sufficient for most people, longer fast over 12 days is deeper and more therapeutic if done right. It is recommend that for fasts longer than 10 days a person should either be experienced or under guidance or have some very good fasting books.

A therapeutic fast is a fast undertaken for the purpose of healing and should be done under a doctor's supervision. A therapeutic fast is usually between 10 days and 40 days. Dr. Airola states that for therapeutic fasts, "The most common length of fasts in European clinics is 14 to 21 days. It would not be advisable to undertake a do-it-yourself fasting program for longer than one week or ten days.[223] There are several hundred so-called biological clinics in Europe, most of them directed by medical doctors, where drugless, biological medicine is practiced."

An expert on fasting for cancer is Rudolf Breuss who has a good insight into the need to have a positive attitude towards fasting, "A positive outcome of this treatment is closely tied to a person's attitude. People who go through with (his program) have a strong will and are convinced and determined that they will heal themselves with natural methods. Since attitude influences the whole metabolism, these people are truly taking their health into their own hands. The fast is often the beginning of a physical and spiritual awakening, compelling people to ensure their future health by turning their lives around, adopting positive habits and living closer to nature."[224]

Some fasting experts recommend enemas and colonics others like Paul Bragg, do not. Dr. Airola points out that; "The main purpose of fasting is to help the body to cleanse itself from accumulated toxic wastes. By the process of autolysis, a huge amount of morbid matter, dead cells and diseased tissues are burned; and the toxic wastes which have accumulated in the tissues for years, causing disease and premature aging, are loosened and expelled from the system. The alimentary canal, the digestive and eliminative system, is the main road by which these toxins are thrown out of the body. Since, during fasting, the natural bowel movements cease to take place, the toxic wastes would have no way of leaving the system, except with the help of enemas and colonics."[225] For the average fast this is not needed, for someone really sick it could be helpful.

Paul Bragg states; "Your tongue is a 'Magic Mirror'. Your tongue can reveal how much toxic material is stored in the cells and vital organs of your body....A few days of fasting will coat the tongue with a thick, white, rancid, toxic material that has a terrible odor. This heavy coating of toxic material can be scraped off and examined. In a fast, you can scrape the tongue clean, but in a few hours, the heavy toxic coating will return.[226] On a long 7 to 21 day fast I have seen this white coat slowly move backwards to about the middle of the tongue, or sometimes clear up completely."

For the best fast it needs to be individualized and suit their needs as to the length. The best length for a juice fast is usually between 7 to 21 days. Longer fasts should be under professional supervision; although some say over 10 days on a water fast should be under supervision.

e. The Physiological Phases of Fasting

There are three physiological phases of fasting. The first stage they call the gastro-intestinal phase which includes everything from the mouth to the rectum that processes and digest food. In this phase a person is getting energy for the last meal or two. This is going to last between 6 to 12 hours or more. Then the person has used up most if not all of the fuel from the last meal and they go into the second phase of fasting which is the glycogen phase.

Glycogen is stored up sugar or glucose which is the

141

primary fuel for our body. Glucose is stored mostly in the liver and in the skeletal muscle cells. Our body uses up some reserves of glycogen and this can last a day or two, depending on how much glycogen is stored in the cells of the muscles, liver and elsewhere.

During the first stage of the fast, the stomach and digestive tract are emptied and the pH changes to become more alkaline. Weight loss which is mostly water loss is greatest the first few days of the fast. Headaches and hunger pains often occur during the first three days. This first stage is one to three days usually.

Next the intestines and liver start to purge themselves of toxins and poisons. The elimination is mostly through the urine and the skin from the bloodstream. The physiological purgation on this level excretes toxins and poisons trapped in the organs, glands and muscles. Symptoms like a flu may be experienced such as diarrhea, nausea, muscle aches, etc.

In the third stage tissue and cellular cleansing occurs, blood toxins are removed and poisons deeply embedded in the kidneys and intestines are released. The process of catabolism breaks down the diseased and poisoned cells and eliminates them. Usually this third stage has positive emotions connected to it, giving a high or euphoria feeling but there can also be negative feelings as well.

Elimination on the cellular level is important and a long fast helps this to happen. A long fast once or twice a year is needed to keep the body clean at the cellular level. The beneficial effects of a long fast decrease over time. Six months to a year down the road another long fast will be needed to detoxify the inner body once again.

These three phases of fasting are why a seven day fast is important, a one to three day fast does not enter into cellular cleansing in the third phase of fasting.

f. Charts of Fasting Cures for Diseases

"Yet, when they were sick, I put sackcloth on,
        I humbled my soul with fasting." Ps 35:13

One of the greats in the use of fasting is Dr. Herbert Shelton. In his book; *Fasting for the Health of It* he presents 100 case studies of patients from 11 different doctors and Hygenic practitioners, that have been cured through fasting. Most of these cases are serious medical cases which were healed either partially or totally.[227] Some of the conditions that were cured or improved were as follows. The days fasted for each individual case is indicated.[228]

In the following studies, multiple sclerosis can be found helped and even cured through fasting. Looking at this chart, it took three long fasts to cure Parkinson's, but only one fast to cure or put into remission multiple sclerosis.

Parkinson's disease (30, 14, 14 days)	insomnia (21 days),
multiple sclerosis (14 days),	bursitis (21 days),
colitis (10, 21, 10 days),	abdominal tumor (7 days),
depression (18 days),	alcoholism (26 days),
hypoglycemia (days),	gonorrhea (12 days),
high blood pressure (10 days),	brain tumor (8 days),
	headaches (22 days),
arthritis (10, 14, 10 days),	back pain (7, 8, 7 days),
diverticulitis (14, 21 days),	eczema (28, 10, 10 days),
obesity (10 days),	hemorrhoids (14 days),
drug addiction (10 days),	intestinal disorder (21 days),
high cholesterol (10 days),	angina (28 days),
kidney stones (10, 14 days),	cerebral stroke (25 days),
acne (10 days),	glaucoma (21 days),
Crohn's disease (29, 10, 10 days)	Hodgkin's disease (12, 7, 7, 7 days),
spinal injury (25 days),	parasitic disease (41 days),
	spinal meningitis (7 days),

cigarette smoking (10 days), schizophrenia (10,10, 10 days), arthritis (10, 10, 10 days), enlarged prostate (10, 10 days) cataracts (14 days), bronchitis (39 days), pneumonia (4 days), typhoid fever (8 days), sterility (10 days), syphilis (16 days), ulterine fibroid (28 days), Bright's disease (14 days), blindness in one eye (30 days), malnutritional edema (40 days), nasal polyps (24 days), gastric ulcer (19 days), nymphomania (16 days), mental condition (insanity) (39 days),	overactive thyroid (7 days), gout (7, 7, 8, 6 days), arteriosclerosis (14 days), appendicitis (5 days), acute lymphatic leukemia (14, 8, 12, 20 days), anemia and lupus (14, 16, 26, 16, 14 days), muscular dystrophy (15, 8, 11 days), chicken pox (4 days), herpes (12 days), intestinal tapeworm (14 days), menstrual problems (21 days), rheumatoid arthritis (22 days), epilepsy (21 days), diabetes (7 days), Chronic gastritis (29 days).

It is really amazing that so many different diseases have been cured or put into remission through fasting and this therapeutic approach.

Weight Lost and Fasting
Today medical doctors and researchers have studied prolonged fasting in-depth with modern scientific methods. In one professional journal prolonged fasting among obese patients is discussed. It was found that physiological problems can occur in fasts over forty days. "Metabolic changes that occur in fasting patients were studied with special reference to those metabolic disturbances that might adversely affect the health of the patient. "Fasting is an effective method of treating obesity, and no serious metabolic

disturbances were encountered when the fast lasted less than 40 days. However, in prolonged fasting (i.e. periods greater than 40 days) electrolyte disorders, protein deficiency, normochromic anemia and mal-absorption of vitamin B12 were encountered."[229]   (*Am Journal of Clin Nut*)

In this study, 714 cases were carefully supervised by Dr. Gerald Benesh, D.C., and Dr. James McEachen, D.C., from 1952-1958 in Escondido, California."[230]

Disease	Number of cases	Cases Remedied or Improved	Cases Not Helped
High blood pressure	141	141	0
Colitis	88	77	0
Sinusitis	67	64	3
Anemia	60	52	8
Hemorrhoids	51	48	3
Arthritis	47	39	8
Bronchitis	42	39	3
Kidney Disease	41	36	5
Benign Tumors	38	32	6
Heart Disease	33	29	4
Asthma	29	29	0
Ulcers	23	20	3
Hay Fever	19	17	2
Goiter	11	11	0
Pyorrhea	8	6	2
Gallstones	7	6	1
Cancer	5	5	0
Multiple Sclerosis	4	3	1
Total	741	654	60

It is amazing, that of 4 cases of MS, 3 were remedied or improved. The evidence is overwhelming for the number of people that recovered in each of these cases!

This is another fasting facility run by Dr. William Esser, N.D., D.C., who supervised 225 cases from 1945-1947 in Lake Worth, Florida.[231] The following is the breakdown of the results of those fasts is as follows.

Disease	Number of Cases	Cases Recovered	Cases Improved	Cases Not Helped
Dyspepsia	21	18	3	0
Pyorrhea	20	8	12	0
Asthma	19	16	0	3
Eczema	18	11	4	3
Benign Tumors	18	14	3	1
Insomnia	17	13	2	2
Ulcers	14	8	4	2
Diabetes	14	12	2	0
Kidney Disease	12	10	2	0
Sinusitis	12	9	3	0
Gallstones	11	6	5	0
Anemia	11	7	4	0
Gonorrhea	8	8	0	0
Poliomyelitis	8	6	2	0
Appendicitis	6	6	0	0
Epilepsy	5	3	2	0
Acne Vulgaris	5	3	2	0
Multiple Sclerosis	4	0	2	2
Tuberculosis	2	2	0	0
Total	225	160	52	13

Almost every case was helped, out of 225 cases only 13 were not helped by fasting!

In this study 447 cases were carefully supervised by Dr. Robert Gross, D.C., Ph.D., from 1957-1963 in Hyde Park, New York.[232] There are 29 cases of mental disorders with 19 recovered and 10 that improved.

Disease	Number of cases	Cases Recovered	Cases Improved	Cases Not Helped
High Blood Pressure	54	38	16	0
Arthritis	42	28	10	4
Nasal Catarrh	39	36	2	2
Constipation	36	31	3	2
Hepatitis	36	34	2	0
Goiter	33	18	12	3
Psoriasis	32	18	10	4
Heart Disease	31	18	13	0
Mental Disorders	29	19	10	0
Bronchitis	24	22	1	1
Colitis	23	11	12	0
Hemorrhoids	23	18	5	0
Varicose Veins	23	20	2	1
Hay Fever	22	7	15	0
Total	447	318	113	17

These are very significant numbers showing statistical significance through fasting.

"As in previous studies by Bloom(1), Drenick et al. (2) and Thomson et al. (3), we found fasting an effective treatment for obesity, and one of our patients who fasted for 14 weeks lost 84 lb. In some cases the weight loss produced a dramatic improvement in the well-being of the patient."[233]

It is strange that modern medicine doesn't use fasting? But then using pharmaceutical drugs is easier, and the drug companies oppose fasting since they don't make money by getting people to do fasting.

g. Dr. Herbert Shelton on Fasting

Herbert M. Shelton, PhD, DC, ND. He had a doctorate in Physiological Therapeutics (1920, Chicago), a Doctorate from the American School of Chiropractic (1924, New York) and a Doctorate from the American School of Naturopathy (1924, New York). He published his own monthly magazine, *Hygienic Review* for forty-one years and was the author of over 41 books. He had supervised over thirty thousand fasts at his facility in Alamo Heights, Texas. He is considered by many to be one of the great figures in water fasting in the US in the 20th century.

As previously noted Dr. Herbert Shelton cured someone who had Parkinson's but it took three fasts (30, 14, 14 days) and living at his institute for 9 months eating a Live-Food diet. Three fasts caused enough purification to get rid of the chemicals or vaccines or poisons that were the problem. This fast was reported on earlier in, The Evidence for Parkinson's Cures talk but is repeated here at length because it is such an important.

"Monica B., age 39, had been diagnosed with Parkinson's disease. She fasted three times under the supervision of Dr. Shelton: 30 days, 14 days and later another 14 days, over a period of 9 months. Dr. Shelton wrote: 'The developments in this case are typical with the exception that Monica completely recovered. Full recovery is not the general rule. The majority of fasters make sufficient progress to become useful again but retain part of the tremor. Monica was at the health school for 9 months and had previously suffered with Parkinsonism for 6 years. After she had fasted 30 days, the tremor immediately reoccurred, but not as severely as before the fast. After the second fast, the tremors were less and after the third fast, the tremors were gone. For more than 10 years, I remained in contact with Monica and she has had no recurrence of the tremor."[234]

This health institute promoted a Living Foods diet, which she followed, during the 9 months, in-between her fasts. She most likely continued with the diet she learned at the health institute (or close to it) after her third fast. How long she continued or how intensely she continued is not known, but for 10 years after she had no more tremors.

There are other related healings worth mentioning but first let's review the clients listed who had improvements in MS from fasting in the above charts.

- Gerald Benesh, DC, and James McEachen, DC, did a study from 1952-1958 in Escondido, California.[235] They had 4 MS clients who fasted and 3 of these cases were remedied or improved after the water fast.
- William Esser, ND, DC, did a study and he supervised 225 cases of people with various diseases and health concerns from 1945-1947 in Lake Worth, Florida.[236] He records that 4 MS clients were fasted and 2 cases improved and 2 cases were not helped.
- Robert Gross, DC, PhD, is another doctor who uses fasting. From 1957-1963, he fasted clients in Hyde Park, New York.[237] He had 29 cases of Mental Disorders, 19 cases recovered and 10 improved.

Multiple Sclerosis
"Ms. W.O., age 34, fasted for 27 days in 1982 under Dr. Robert Gross, DC, PhD, who had cared for over thirty thousand clients in his facility since 1959. Wanda had suffered from Multiple Sclerosis for four years and was now advised to use a wheelchair because of her inability to walk without staggering. She had blurred vision in one eye and was unable to read with that eye. Her entire body felt numb, and Wanda had tremors in her hands, feet, and legs. At the

end of her fast, her walking was normal and she could read with both eyes. After seven weeks at Shalimar, (Dr. Gross' Institute), Wanda was walking two miles a day and could jog for a few minutes."[238]

Mental Condition, Insanity
"Mr. S. A., age 35, fasted 39 days under the supervision of Dr. Shelton in 1940. 'Hygienic care (Natural Hygiene therapy) greatly improved Stan's mental condition. I have used fasting in cases of mental disease and have no doubt that fasting is distinctly beneficial. I am convinced that when the insane person refuses food, this is an instinctive measure designed to assist the body in its reconstructive work. Many people have lost their abnormal mental conditions while fasting. All who have had extended experience with fasting have seen cases of insanity recover health while on the fast and many others make great improvements while fasting.'"[239]

Schizophrenia
Dr. Herbert Shelton wrote about Lynn S. who was age 21 and had schizophrenia. She was fasted for 35 days, then 18 days, then 6 days in 1961 and 14 days in 1962. "Lynn had been hospitalized, had been administered five electric shock treatments, and had been taking antidepressant drugs. On arrival, her behavior was illogical, bizarre, and erratic and she was ambivalent toward those trying to help. During her thirty-five day fast, her mental condition fluctuated from psychotic to remissions indicating 'normality.' At the termination, there were no signs of obvious abnormal behavior. After three subsequent fasts, a practical recovery was achieved, although some intellectual and emotional limitations remain. Since her fast, Lynn has married and has given birth to three children."[240]

Advanced Multiple Sclerosis
Dr. Shelton wrote, "No two cases of multiple sclerosis are identical because in no two cases are the same parts of the brain and nervous system affected." Dr. Herbert Shelton

says, "I recall a case of an optometrist, Dr. F. J., age 38 (1954), whose condition became so bad that he had to give up his work and turn his office over to someone else. For a few years, he had been under the care of several of the best neurologists in the East Coast and, as they had warned him at the outset, he had grown progressively worse. They had frankly told him that they had no cure for Multiple Sclerosis."[241]

"Previous drug treatments make me progressively worse." His condition was so severe that he had to be carried into the Health School. After a two-week fast, and an additional five weeks at the Health School, on a raw fruit and vegetable diet, Dr. J. so greatly improved, he walked out of the School under his own power. He returned home and resumed his professional activities. He was not a well man at the end of seven weeks. It is too much to expect a full recovery in such a short time. But he had made such great improvement that he felt justified in returning home and getting back to work. This is often a wrong position to take [returning to work too soon], especially with a condition like Multiple Sclerosis, but it is a mistake that the sick frequently make."[242]

Dr. Shelton continued, "Many patients seem to be satisfied to stop their efforts in recovering health when they have been freed of their most annoying symptoms. They are often unwilling to go on to full health, and are convinced they can take care of themselves. After having made a certain amount of initial improvement, they expect to take charge and they feel they can carry on, from that point, and their professional adviser also agrees. In a few cases it works out; generally they fail. In cases, watched and controlled, results of fasting can be established."[243]

Dr. Shelton continues: "I have never had the opportunity to care for a case of Multiple Sclerosis in the early stages; hence I can only suggest that if these cases were given Hygienic care at the outset of their trouble, the percentage of recoveries would be high. All of the cases I have had the privilege of caring for have been in advanced stages and I do not consider these favorable cases. The fact that I have been able to return some of these, even in helpless conditions, to a state of usefulness speaks volumes for the efficiency of the Hygienic program in restoring normal tissue and functional condition."

Dr. Herbert Shelton wrote, "Let us review the general picture of the fasting experience, as applied to a Multiple Sclerosis case. The first fast brings about remarkable improvement in the general health of the individual, with considerable increase in his control and use of his limbs, often enabling the bedridden patient to get up and walk about. He manages to hold this improvement and not infrequently to add to it, while eating a carefully planned diet and taking regular exercise and sun baths following a fast." [244] [A Living Foods diet is the type of diet they promote and what Dr. Shelton is referring to here.]

Dr. Shelton continues: "A second fast adds to his control and use of his limbs. I have employed as many as three fasts in these cases. Each fast has resulted in increased control of the limbs and has made it possible for them to be used with greater ease.

"I continue the rest in bed following the fast, adding a period or two of daily light exercise of a type that requires increasing skill in their performance. The purpose of the exercise in these cases is not so much that of increasing the size and strength of the muscles as to increase the individual's skill in their use. Heavier exercise may come later if desired." [245]

"I am convinced that daily sunbathing in these cases is especially helpful in furthering the evolution of nerve health. The diet is one of fresh fruits and vegetables with moderate quantities of fats, sugars, starches and proteins. I prefer the vegetable proteins - nuts and sunflower seeds are good in these cases."

"The important thing for us to remember is that the sclerosis does not belong to the initial stages of the disease. In these early stages, recovery is most likely to take place, providing only that all impairing influences are removed from the life of the individual and his blood and flesh are freed of their toxic load."[246]

"It is the initial stage that full recovery is or should be possible, not the advanced stages when irreversible changes in the nerve structures have taken place. The ancient adage: "A stitch in time" - in this case, action in time, can make the difference."[247]

These are interesting comments and analysis by Dr. Shelton who used his methods back in the 1940's, 1950's and 1960's before there were any real drugs for Parkinson's or MS, and he was successful.

h. Allen Cott, MD on Fasting

A powerful witness about healing Schizophrenia is by Allen Cott, MD in his book, *Fasting: The Ultimate Diet.*[248] It gives a remarkable account on cases of schizophrenia and fasting. He writes how in the Moscow Psychiatric Institute they use long fasting (25 days); 70% of schizophrenic patients treated by fasting improved so remarkably that they were able to resume an active life!

This is a totally remarkable finding that 70% of the schizophrenic patients were treated by long fasts and improved so remarkably that they could resume an active life! Think of all those suffering from mental illness, who, like schizophrenics, could possibly be treated by fasting and recover some, if not most, of their mental abilities, as well as getting off the drugs too!

153

Dr. Cott writes: "My experience with fasting mentally ill patients began in 1970 on my first visit to the Moscow Psychiatric Institute. I went there at the invitation of Dr. Yuri Nikolayev, the director of the fasting unit, who was the first to suggest that schizophrenia may be caused by a biochemical imbalance that can be corrected through the restorative powers of fasting and revised diet. Dr. Nikolayev himself fasts several times a year in 10-to-15-day stretches. 'I usually fast for prophylactic reasons,' he told me. 'I have fasted several times with a scientific purpose in view, to make an experiment. I always feel excellent when I fast. It is always a happy occasion and a rest for me.' Dr. Nikolayev is fond of quoting an old German proverb: 'The illness that cannot be cured by fasting cannot be cured by anything else.'"[249]

Dr. Cott continues, "Fasting per se is not a 'cure' for anything - and I cannot repeat this too often - but we know that it permits the considerable healing powers of the body - and of the mind - to assert themselves. An epochal breakthrough in the treatment of schizophrenia came when Dr. Nikolayev discovered that his patients responded to the fasting treatment after all the other forms of therapy had failed. The patients had been chronically ill and felt hopeless about the future. Most of them would never have functioned again. Some would have committed suicide. Many would have deteriorated and lived out the balance of their lives in the bleak backwards of a mental hospital. *Seventy percent of those treated by fasting improved so remarkably that they were able to resume an active life.* I was particularly impressed with one of Dr. Nikolayev's successes. At the Institute, there was a nuclear scientist whose case was diagnosed as senile psychosis. His memory had lapsed to the point where he could not recall his own name. But after an extended fast his memory was completely restored and he regained full possession of his intellectual powers."[250]

Dr. Cott goes onto describe one of his case histories: "The 25-day fasting treatment for schizophrenics that I

154

instituted at New York's Gracie Square Hospital was in accordance with procedures used in Moscow . . . I started him (19 year old boy) on the fasting program, and by the fifth day, phased out the heavy medication he had been taking for several years. In the beginning, he did not have an easy time of it . . . By the tenth day of his fast, my patient began to have what he described as 'happy feelings.' He said they were the first happy feelings he had experienced in years.

"His periods of feeling well became successively longer. His fast lasted until real hunger returned, which was four weeks. He took easily to the re-feeding diet. Four years later, this once 'hopeless' youth still feels well and is functioning effectively . . . I should like to stress that the schizophrenic person must fast only in a medical setting."[251]

i. Abram Hoffer, MD on Fasting

Abram Hoffer, MDin his book *Healing Schizophrenia*, gives his theory of schizophrenia and also his treatment approach. He explains that diseases have multiple causes and can be divided into two main groups: "primary or immediate causes (often the most readily modifiable causes); and secondary or contributing factors. We can divide the causes or factors that lead to schizophrenia in the same way. The most readily treated factors are biochemical. The secondary or contributing factors are psychological and sociological."[252]

Dr. Hoffer writes, "In about 1965, Dr. Allan Cott observed a fasting treatment used in Moscow for the treatment of schizophrenia. When he tried the same program in New York on a few patients, he observed the same results. Following this, I began to fast a few of my intractable patients. To my surprise, I found that they were well in five days and did not need the 30-day fast that the Russians were using. I was asked to see a chronic schizophrenic woman who was unable to come to my office because she was rigid and catatonic. I visited her in her home. She had been ill at least 10 years and had not responded to treatment. I had her

155

delivered to hospital by ambulance. She agreed to try a 30-day water fast, and to my amazement, she was well on the fifth day. She completed the fast and lost about 30 pounds, but a few days later, her psychosis recurred. During her fast, she had felt so well that she begged me to allow her to do another long fast. I agreed to do so, but only after she had regained some weight. Once again, five days into her fast she was well."[253]

"By this time, I was becoming more knowledgeable of cerebral allergies and clinical ecology. I terminated her fast and began testing for food allergies. She was allergic to all meats: as soon as she ate meat her major symptoms recurred. She then went on a vegetarian diet and remained well. Since then I have fasted at least 200 schizophrenic patients. More than 60 percent were well after the fast."[254]

Dr. Hoffer continues, "During our study with fasting, over a four-month period 60 patients went through a fast, usually at home. They took no food, no medication, and did not smoke, but consumed 6-8 glasses of water per day. Forty were well at the end of the fast and have remained well since. They do not need any medication but must avoid the foods which they are allergic. The other 20 did not improve whatsoever. The 40 who recovered have remained well since. Thirty were allergic to dairy foods. Two were also allergic to beef. One was allergic to smoking, one to aspirin, and the rest to sugar and other foods. Other orthomolecular physicians have found similar recoveries."[255]

j. Dr. David J. Scott on Fasting

There is another fasting expert that I (Jim) knew personally, that needs to be mentioned. Sadly he passed away October 2011. Dr. David J. Scott, D.M., N.D., D.C. of Cleveland had a degree as a Chiropractor and had several other specialized degrees and was the founding president of the International Association of Hygienic Physicians and taught physiology at Great Lakes College. He was in practice for over 50 years and he water fasted, under direct supervision, some 20,000 patients.

Dr. D. J. Scott was unique in that he used the latest technologies to demonstrate the status of health by physiological parameters. Dr. Scott's office had a fully functional and modern scientific laboratory. From there he provided standardized testing to determine multiple indicators used to monitor a persons' progress during the fasting process. These extremely sensitive but standard medical technologies, including blood work, can discover early and even late signs of disease. He was the only one in the country that used these kinds of measurements during a long water fast.

Dr. Scott states, "Many conditions may be uncovered through our testing. The many treating methods available frequently only relieve the symptoms. While utilizing these methods, in time one may move from acute disease into suppressed chronic disease. Left unhealed, the chronic disease in time may move from chronic inflammation into degeneration and even end in malignancy. By our methods, we clearly document when your disease markers are brought into remission or healing. If you go back to your old habits, we most likely will find you are only beginning to re-feed those same diseases again."[256]

The following are some of the many patients conditions benefited in over 50 years by therapeutic fasting and fasting over 20,000 people at his facility.

Acholasia	Constipation	Heart Disease	Prostate
Acid Reflux	Crohn's	Hemorrhoids	Disease
Acne Rosacea	Disease	Hiatal Hernia	Pruritus Ani
Acne Vulgaris	Cystitis	High	Psoriasis
Allergies	Depression	Cholesterol	Pulmonary
Anemia	Diabetes	Hyperacusis	Fibrosis
Angina	Digestive	Hypertension	Pyorrhea
Pectoris	Disorders	(High Blood	Rectal
Arrhythmia	Disc	Pressure)	Prolapse

Arteritis	Herniation	Iritis	Rheumatoid
Arthritis	Diverticulitis	Irritable Bowel	Arthritis
Asthma	Diverticulosis	Kidney	Sciatica
Atonic Bowel	Emphysema	Disease	Seizures
Blepharoptosis	Facial	Kidney Stones	(Epilepsy)
Blocked	Neuralgia	Liver Disease	Sinusitis
Arteries	Fevers	Macular	Sleep Apnea
Breast Cysts	Fibroids	Degeneration	Sleep
Breast Disease	Fibromyalgia	Migraine	Disorders
Bronchitis	Fistulac	Headaches	Stroke
Bursitis	Fracture	Multiple	Disabilities
Candidiasis	Healing	Sclerosis	Tendonitis
Catarract	Support	Myositis	Thrombo-
(early stage)	Gall Bladder	Nicotine	phlebitis
Chemical	Disease	Addiction	Tic
Sensitivity	Gallstones	Ovarian	Douloureux
Cholecystitis	Gastritis	Disease	Torticollis
Chronic	Glaucoma	Pancreatitis	Tumors
Fatigue	(early stage)	Parotitis	(Benign)
Colitis	Goiter	Paroxysmal	Ulcers
Congestive	Gout	Tachycardia	Varicose
Heart	Hay Fever	Polymyalgia	Veins
Failure		Polymyositis	Ulcers
			Vertigo

Awhile back I was talking with Dr. Scott and I asked him about his approach for healing Parkinson's and if he would accept patients. He told me, "James do not send me anyone unless they are willing to totally change their diet!" He believes it would take at least two to three years to rebuild the biochemistry in the brain for a Parkinson's or Alzheimer's patient to be fully healed.

I asked him if he had healed anyone of Parkinson's or Alzheimer's? He did have someone who brought his wife who had Alzheimer's. The husband had to stay there and go on the fast with her. Dr. Scott put them on a long water fast and on the 21st day of the fast she started speaking for the first time in over a year. She wasn't always clear or made sense but she was speaking! In fact, she couldn't stop talking all day long. The next day the husband got sick and so Dr. Scott broke the fast with juicing over the next couple of days.

Dr. Scott told the husband to bring her back to do another fast in a few months since this first fast started the process of healing but a second fast would be needed to continue it. The husband never brought her back.

Are there different types of cleansing diets? Yes, there are different types of cleansing diets and fasts that can be done with juices, such as an intestinal cleanse or a kidney cleanse, etc. Dr. Norman Walker's expertise was the colon cleanse and he was an expert in these different cleanses thru fruits and juices too. The Gerson Therapy today uses a strict vegetarian or raw vegetarian diet and about 13 glasses of freshly made juices a day. The Gerson Diet is very successful for cancer. (See J. Tibbetts book, *Starving Cancer to Death*.)

m. Paavo Airola, PhD on Fasting

Paavo Airola, PhD, ND, author of numerous books has a booklet: *Cancer Causes, Prevention and Treatment the Total Approach*, published in 1972 it gives a good insight of cancer treatment before 1970 in Europe, and many of the methods are still valid today. The booklet was a paper delivered to the "Ninth Annual Cancer Convention of the International Association of Cancer Victims and Friends.[257] He writes:

"There are several hundred so-called biological clinics in Europe, most of them directed by medical doctors, where drugless, biological medicine is practiced. In my book, *There is a Cure for Arthritis*, I list over a dozen such clinics with the complete addresses and names of the doctors. The most prominent cancer specialists in Germany using biological therapies in the treatment of cancer are Dr. Josef Issels, Prof. Werner Kollath and Prof. Lampert. However, there are over 4,000 medical doctors in Germany, members of the Association of Naturopathic (Biological) Doctors, who apply biological therapies in the treatment of most diseases, including cancer. All of my statements made about causes of cancer, and to effective nutritional and other biological methods of approaching cancer treatment, are well documented. Again, I do not offer a new or any other kind of cure for cancer - I report only what various cancer researchers have found and how cancer is successfully treated in European biological clinics. In this country, [America] all harmless, unorthodox treatments of cancer are outlawed leaving only surgery, radiation or chemotherapy. I feel that the millions of people who suffer from cancer are entitled to know the truth."

Following is Dr. Airola's section on using fasting for cancer or other degenerative diseases. This juice-fasting approach, as he indicates above, is used in European biological clinics. Most American clinics utilize water-fasting rather than juice-fasting. A twenty-one day fast is considered normal for therapeutic fasting in Europe.

"One of the most important components of the total, combined anti-cancer program is the detoxification of the whole body. The underlying reason why the organism succumbs to cancer in the first place is the diminished or broken down resistance to the carcinogenic factors mainly due to the disordered metabolism, weakened activity of essential organs, such as liver, kidneys and pancreas, and general auto-toxemia. The purpose of juice-fasting is to normalize all the vital body processes, revitalize the liver and other cleansing organs, cleanse the whole body of accumulated toxins, restore the digestive and assimilative functions of the stomach and intestinal tract, and, in general, increase the body's protective and healing capacity. The success of most anti-cancer programs in European biological clinics, as well as the Gerson's cancer therapy, is attributed largely to their thorough cleansing programs."[258]

"Short, repeated cleansing fasts on raw vegetable and fruit juices are advisable. Most useful juices are red beet (from tops and roots),[259] carrot, green juice made from

160

leafy green vegetables, grape,[260] lemon, and all dark-colored juices. During fasting, daily coffee enemas are used - one cup of strong, freshly brewed coffee in a one pint of water, used as a retention enema - to stimulate the liver and increase its detoxifying activity. Although healthy persons can fast on their own, cancer patients should fast only under sympathetic professional supervision."[261]

The coffee enema is not a cure but an adjunct therapy. Today tea could be a better substitute. The coffee enema is part of the Gerson Therapy routine and has become a routine enema for detoxification of the liver, used by many people. The purpose of coffee enemas is to lower serum toxins via. the colon. It pulls the toxins and poisons out of the liver into the colon, which get expelled.

l. Rudolf Breuss on Fasting

There is another juice fasting expert in Austria who was not medically trained named Rudolf Breuss who started leading people in long juice fasts and many people were completely healed of cancer and other degenerative diseases. Later, a Fasting Institute was started in his name: Breuss Fasting Clinic Durhotel Chattenbuhl, Germany. The cures of many other types of degenerative diseases through his juice-fasting method can be given. Rudolf Breuss is one of many Nature-cure doctors in Europe that uses juice-fasting as a method of healing.

Rudolf Breuss Juice Mixture

To prepare the juice, take 3/5 beets, 1/5 carrots, 1/5 celeriac (celery), and then add a little black radish and one egg-sized potato. For example:
- 300 g (9.6 oz.) beet root
- 100 g (3.2 oz.) carrots
- 100 g (3.2 oz.) celeriac (celery root)
- 30 g (1.06 oz.) black radish root
- 1 potato, the size of an egg

He adds a Note: "It is not crucial to add the potato juice, except for treating cancer of the liver, where it is necessary. Use a modern juice-extractor, or press the vegetables the old-fashioned way, then put the juices through a tea strainer or a linen towel. There is a tablespoon of sediment for each quarter liter of juice, which must not be consumed. This sediment would make the juice more difficult to drink and, more importantly, would serve as food for the cancer."[262]

"The cancer lives only on solid foods taken into the body. If for 42 days the patient only drinks vegetable juices and tea, the cancerous growth dies while the person can live through it all very well! It is better if a few days before starting this treatment, the patient drinks approximately one-quarter liter (1 cup/250 ml) of juice per day. The patient may go up to one half liter but this is not necessary."

"Drink the juice slowly with the help of a spoon. Do not swallow it immediately but let the juice remain in the mouth for a few moments. Every now and again, the patient may have a mouthful of sauerkraut juice, which is beneficial to the patient. The juices are to be taken as indicated. A little lemon juice can be added but never apple juice! Freshly squeezed apple juice is allowed in between by itself but never mixed with the other juices. You may drink as much sage tea with St. John's Wort, peppermint and balm as you want, but do not add any sugar."[263]

"Over the years I have noticed that so-called failures of the treatment could be attributed to patients not following it in all aspects. An estimated 40,000 cancer patients and others suffering from seemingly incurable illnesses have regained their health through my juice treatment."

"I beg you to remember how many great inventions were made by lay people. The most important thing, in the end, is the success of an idea and its usefulness for humankind. Scientists should acknowledge this fact, even if they cannot yet explain it. They should not care with whom or where the invention originated. I would be extremely happy if you could improve my Total Cancer Treatment even more by combining it with other successful methods of cancer therapy.'"[264]

m. Some Reasons for Fasting

There are different schools of thought on fasting. The two main ones which are in conflict are the Water Fasters versus the Juice Fasters. Those who use juice fasting accept water fasting, but those who promote water fasting do not promote juice fasting since they call it a juice diet and not a fast. Jim T. has discussed this with a number of the top water fasting experts in the US, and their minds are set. For them, water fasting is real fasting, juice fasting is a juice diet or something else. This book promotes juice fasting but we are also open to water fasting.

We would recommend Paul Bragg, PhD book, *The Miracle of Fasting* on water fasting it is a classic book on this topic. For juice fasting, we would recommend Jim and Anne Marie Tibbetts' book: *Juice Fasting Simplified a Practical Approach.*[265] These are books to start with as they cover the different topics and viewpoints on juice fasting.

Fasting optimizes the body for maximum effectiveness, because fasting is cleansing and detoxifying the liver, the large intestine and many other organs and parts of the body on a fast. *Fasting also catabolizes dying, dead and disease cells, allowing a healthier body.* A few of the many reasons why people need to fast:
1. Fasting is a quick way to lose weight.
2. Fasting burns up all the diseased and inferior tissues.
3. Fasting will lead to a more disciplined eating habits.
4. Fasting tones up the flesh to make you look younger.
5. Fasting is perhaps the best method of cleansing the body.
6. Fasting helps build the immune and nervous system.
7. Fasting can help reduce high blood pressure.

8. Fasting is a way to rid the body of poisons in the body.
9. Fasting can help clean out the toxins of air pollution.
10. Fasting is good to build endurance for athletes.
11. Fasting can be used to treat physical illness.
12. Fasting can be used to treat mental illnesses.
13. Fasting can help break bad habits, like smoking or drinking alcohol or drugs.
14. Fasting and prayer can help cast out sin and evil spirits.
15. Fasting is found in all the world's religions.
16. Fasting is encouraged and practiced in the Bible.
17. Fasting is a requirement by Catholics and Orthodox.
18. Fasting can be a silent protest for world hunger.
19. Fasting can help reduce the desires of the flesh.
20. Fasting can help people live longer, healthier lives.

People should fast at least twice a year, a seven day or longer fast. Two or three times a year is best, once a year is good but really not enough. One long 14 to 21 day fast plus one or two seven day fast is optimal and recommended.

n. Caloric restriction and intermittent fasting

What are the only consistently proven methods of extending lifespan? A brief review of the literature shows that there are four aspects that extend life, "for the majority of cases of longevity:
1. Vegetarian diets;
2. Low calorie intake;
3. Inner Calm;
4. Fasting."[266]

One study showed that fasting (diet restriction) is the only consistently proven method of extending lifespan and it hypothesizes that it is because it reduces the total amount of oxidative stress within an animal. Technically speaking, oxygen destroys mitochondrial genomes which lack DNA repair mechanisms. Diet restriction can attenuate age-associated mitochondrial enzymatic dysfunction.[267]

Looking at PubMed.gov on the internet, caloric restriction and intermittent fasting are two potential diets found to be successful for helping brain aging diseases like Parkinson's. The journal quote follows:

> "The vulnerability of the nervous system to advancing age is all too often manifest in neurodegenerative disorders such as Alzheimer's and Parkinson's diseases. In this review article we describe evidence suggesting that two dietary interventions, caloric restriction (CR) and intermittent fasting (IF) . . . *Food restriction (FR) reduces brain damage and improves behavioral outcome following excitotoxic and metabolic insults.* ... These findings suggest that FR not only extends life span, but increases resistance of the brain to insults that involve metabolic compromise and excitotoxicity.[268]

An article on Integrative Medicine Approaches, from the *Swedish Medical Journal* (2010), by David Perlmutter, MD, is a good insight into neurological diseases' new direction. "Animal studies suggest that calorie-restricted diets are beneficial for cognitive function. In a similarly designed dietary interventional study, memory function, a hallmark of Alzheimer's disease, was assessed at onset and after 3 months in 50 healthy to overweight subjects, mean age 60.5 years placed on a 30% reduced calorie diet, compared to a matched nonintervention group. A significant increase in verbal memory scores was observed in the calorie-restricted subjects compared to those with unrestricted access to calories. The authors concluded that their study demonstrated 'experimental evidence in humans that calorie restriction improves memory,' and reasoned that this effect was likely mediated by the action of CR on enhancement of neurotrophic factors. While recommending a 25-30% dietary calorie reduction to patients may at first seem draconian, this recommendation is tempered by the recognition that in the United States, and likely in many developed countries, average adult caloric consumption is approximately 20% greater than is required to maintain ideal body mass."[269]

Dr. Perlmutter also notes: "Integrative medicine is often criticized by mainstream practitioners as lacking evidence-based underpinning for its seemingly unorthodox practices. Indeed, a level playing field should hold all participants in the game of healthcare to the same standards. Requiring scientifically-validated evidence to support specific recommendations for patient care represents the current standard and assures patients the highest quality of care in terms of efficacy and safety. At present, the recommendations for caloric intake reduction and physical exercise are the only meaningful evidence-based therapies available for individuals with early dementia. Adhering to evidence-based practice as it relates to early dementia will represent a massive cost savings for healthcare systems and eliminate the potential risks of medication induced negative consequences."[270]

o. Moreover, when you Fast!

There is a long history of fasting in the Church and a few of the early Church Fathers are worth quoting here. First for Origen, fasting is an experience of freedom, not an obligation in view of Pythagorean metapsychosis.[271] For Ambrose and Gregory of Nyssa, mortification of the flesh puts man in communion with Christ who raises him from human to a divine existence.[272] For St. Basil, fasting guarantees peace in the world and in families, because it frees people from egoism.[273] And for Ambrose, it is the angelic life that leads us back to Paradise, where 'sin entered through food'; 'those who do not believe in the afterlife indulge in food and drink.'"[274] For St. Jerome, the monk must always remain a little hungry: 'If you wish to be perfect, it is better to fatten the soul than the body.'[275] St. Basil and Cassian recommended moderation, each one adapting the fast to his own situation.[276] St. Benedict's (d. 547) *Rule* recommends us to 'love fasting' with discretion.[277] While the Monastic East explored the personal aspect, the Western communities looked to the social value. Leo the Great, who dedicated 30 treatises to fasting, said: 'the abstinence of him who fasts becomes the nourishment of the poor.'"[278]

"Moreover, when you fast..." Mt 6:16 This is a direct command to fast, by Jesus. The three practices that Jesus gives in Matthew 6 are almsgiving, prayer and fasting. After the Lord 's Prayer Jesus said, "Moreover, when you fast..."

Jesus gave an admonition telling people to fast: "Moreover, when you fast..." (Mt 6:16) If Moses, who beheld God, (on Sinai) and St. Paul, the divine apostle (Act 9:9) fasted, so must we. If the Ninevites in the book of Jonah fasted (Jonah 3:5), and this included all their children plus their 'senior' citizens, so we must. If the Church Fathers and the Christian and Jewish Saints fasted, and expected others to fast, so must we. Finally, if Rabbi Jesus Himself fasted and was hungry (Lk 4:2), who are we to introduce a 'new improved and fast-free' spirituality?

Chapter 8

Detoxification of Metals, Pesticides and Poisons

Fr. Hesychius, a pupil of St. Gregory the Theologian (d. 433), says, "Humility and bodily privations free man from all sin: first, by cutting away the passions of the soul, and second, by cutting away those of the body. And for this cause the Lord says, 'Blessed are the pure in heart: for they shall see God.' (Mt 5:8). That is, they shall see Him and the treasures that are in Him, when through love and abstinence they purify themselves; and so much the more as their purification is increased."[279]

a. What Poisons in my Body?

Now tell me have you had your daily poisons today? Are you adding to the poisons already found in your body? The next question will be OK, what poisons in my body?

Studies on tissues and body fluids and bone show the presence of numerous toxins in the body, including toxins that could be in the food or the environment: DDE & DDT &, B-BHC,[280] TCDD,[281] p-DCB,[282] Lead,[283] Mercury,[284] Cadmium,[285] PBBs,[286] 2,5-DCP & l-naphthol & 3,5,6-TCP & 2-naphthol & 3,5,6-TCP & PCP, 4-nitrophenol, (pesticide residues in urine in adults in U.S.)[287] Styrene & Vinyl chloride (packaging migrant),[288] Toluene (Solvent),[289] Xylene (solvent)[290]."

There are also poisons and toxins directly involved in the food chain: some of which we consume and some are in the environment, various studies cite these chemicals: Acetone (pesticide solvent),[291] Arsenic (arsenical pesticides),[292] Benzene (solvent for pesticide formulations), [293] Bromobenzene (fumigant precursor),[294] Carbon tetrachloride (former fumigant),[295] Ethylene

dibromide (fumigant),[296] Ethylene dichloride (fumigant),[297]
Hexane (solvent),[298] Kepone (pesticide),[299]   Methoxychlor
(insecticide),[300] Methy isobutyl ketone (synthetic flavoring),[301]
Methylene chloride (decaffeinator),[302] and studies on coal tar
dye colorings containing polycyclic aromatic hydrocarbons.[303]

Dr. Chauncey Leake, past president of the American
Association for the Advancement of Science, and one of the
nation's most distinguished pharmacologists, warned in 1963
that general use of the new chemicals in large quantities has
created a new hazard - subclinical poisoning - so insidious
that physicians cannot connect the poison with the ailment.[304]

"Added to the intentional and unintentional chemicals
in our foods are the chemicals we ingest as medicines.
Americans are the most medicated people in the world.
Every year we swallow 37 billion doses of therapeutic pills,
powders, capsules, and elixirs."[305] No one really knows what
effect the combinations of pesticides, food additives; and
medicines may have on the body?

b. Disturbed Intestinal Ecology

Dr. Burrill B. Crohn a Professor Emeritus of
Medicine at Mount Sinai School of Medicine, told his
colleagues at the Eighth International Congress of
Gastroenterology in Prague, that the current high incidence of
intestinal diseases may reflect the "disturbed ecology of the
human race." - After listing many of these diseases. - He
could not accept the view that the 'upsurge' of these
disorders could be laid to the stresses of the twentieth
century. Other centuries have also been marked by stress, Dr
Crohn stated.

"Is the causation of these diseases to be found in the
food we eat?" Dr. Crohn asked. "In the last decades of our
ecology, our foods contain multiple chemical preservatives;
our growing crops are sprayed with insecticides. We ingest
multiple new drugs never before used, such as the coal-tar

products of which aspirin and its derivatives are regular household remedies. The pollution of our drinking water might also be a factor."[306]

During the past three decades, surveillance of toxic exposure in the U.S. population has been a routine governmental practice. Since 1970, the U.S. Environmental Protection Agency (EPA) has conducted the National Human Adipose Tissue Survey (NHATS) to determine the prevalence of fat-soluble toxins in the fat cells in U.S. citizens.[307] The 1986 version of this survey, for example, analyzed 671 adipose tissue specimens to determine the prevalence of 111 toxic compounds.[308] And this is just fat tissues; they didn't analyze muscles or organs.

All these therapeutic pills, powders, capsules, and elixirs; and all these food chemicals, pesticides, food additives, coal-tar derived products and water pollution such as fluoride are affecting the animal products that we eat. In-addition, maybe the meat-based products are becoming deformed proteins because of all the chemicals found in meats nowadays. It is the deformed proteins and Lewy bodies that are found in the brains of Parkinson's, Alzheimer's and Multiple Sclerosis!

Before the industrial age, meat was a largely an uncontaminated product. Back then, few chemicals found their way into the chops, steaks and roasts you put on your table. But today, one of the fastest-growing - and most potentially dangerous - developments in agriculture is the use of a host of new chemicals in feed, livestock medication and meat processing. A recent news headline points up the new trend: "Livestock Thrive on Chemical Diet." Like a whirlwind, chemical feeding is taking over. The animals and poultry we eat have become chemicalized and are contaminated with chemicals, pesticides and pharmaceutical drugs. We don't know what effect this has on the meat products that we eat! Or what happens with these meat products and chemicals once they get into our bodies!

c. Heavy Metals Connection to PD, AD and MS

Because of the blood-brain barrier in the brain it is difficult to get into the brain. Studies show that milk consumption increases lead and cadmium absorption. The main protein in milk, casein, has been shown to increase lead levels in the brains, liver, and kidneys of animals. Researchers (Robert Hatherhill, PhD, *The BrainGate*) have not determined why this happens, but it is possible that heavy metals piggyback on the amino acids in milk to get access to the brain. Milk fat also increases uptake of lead and other environmental pollutants.[309] Milk will be discussed in a later chapter. The evidence is clear that milk is detrimental for people with neurological diseases.

The journal article: *Current Status of Metals as Therapeutic Targets in Alzheimer's Disease*,[310] (*J Am Geriatr Soc*, 2003) shows that there is accumulating evidence that interactions between Beta-amyloid and copper, iron, and zinc are associated with the pathophysiology of Alzheimer's disease (AD). A significant amount of copper, iron, and zinc has been detected, and the mismanagement of these metals induces-amyloid precipitation and neurotoxicity. This study has 43 citations and most are journal studies on heavy metals in the brain and in Alzheimer's.

Can these heavy metals in neurological patients be dealt with through chelating agents, which is basically an intravenous therapy? Yes, "chelating agents offer a potential therapeutic solution to the neurotoxicity induced by these heavy metals."[311] (*J Am Geriatr Soc*, 2003) Alzheimer's and related brain diseases like Parkinson's are very similar and used interchangeably in studies but they have different heavy metals in the brains, so the treatments would be slightly different. Chelating therapy is rather complex as a therapy but it does work and this would help Alzheimer's, PD and MS. Fasting detoxifies heavy metals and resets the biological system. Live-Foods in a nutritional program do a similar thing but it takes longer.

What about heavy metals found in the environment? Dr. Michelle Cook, ND cites in her book, *The BrainWash*, that: "Experts estimate that at least twenty-five percent of the American population is likely to suffer from heavy metal poisoning. These heavy metals include cadmium, aluminum, lead, and mercury, all of which are increasingly being linked to brain disease."[312] "The incidence of Parkinson's in the United States has risen tenfold since the 1970's. This sharp rise may indicate that the disease is severely influenced by environmental factors, since the release of many industrial toxins has also risen drastically over the time period."[313]

The heavy metal mercury can gain access to the brain and can be very damaging to nerve and brain cells. Drs. Mercola and Klinghardt state: "Mercury exposure and toxicity is a prevalent and significant public health threat."[314] Mercury is a well-established neurotoxin, which has been connected with brain diseases like Alzheimer's.[315] Research shows that people with Alzheimer's disease often have blood levels of mercury up to three times higher than people who are not suffering from the disease."[316]

Aluminum is one of the most abundant metals on the planet. It is not strictly a heavy metal but placed in that category. Forty years ago, researchers found that aluminum injected into the brain of rats triggered the same changes bio-chemically found in Alzheimer's disease.[317] The problem is that aluminum is found in many different products (creams, deodorants, shampoos, and drugs), foods (baking soda, baby formula, processed and baked goods, antacids, supplements) and even in pots (pans, aluminum foil, pie plates, and municipal water supplies). The body can detox a small amount of aluminum but large amounts can collect in the body. "A study conducted by the University of Cincinnati Medical Center indicated that if tomatoes are cooked in an aluminum container, the aluminum content per serving increases by two to four milligrams."[318]

Robert Hatherhill, PhD notes, "Aluminum can cross the blood-brain barrier and cause nerve cell death. Once aluminum enters into the brain, it promotes inflammation by causing the formation of brain-damaging free radicals[319] and induces numerous toxic reactions, including the disruption of calcium control.[320] There are abnormally high concentrations of the metal aluminum in the brains of people diagnosed with Alzheimer's. Some studies indicate that the brains of Alzheimer's patients contain thirty times the levels of aluminum to their healthy counterparts.[321] There is still debate as to whether aluminum causes Alzheimer's, or if the accumulation of aluminum is the result of the disease, but it is known that aluminum is so toxic to the brain that it interrupts over fifty brain chemical reactions, and its' relationship to Alzheimer's is undeniable. Not only has aluminum been shown to have ties to Alzheimer's, but also to the increasing incidence of Parkinson's disease."[322]

Aluminum sulfate is used by water utilities to remove fine particles from drinking water. One study found that areas in England that have elevated levels of aluminum sulfate in the drinking water have elevated incidence of Alzheimer's disease.[323] Researchers have found that aluminum also may be linked to multiple sclerosis and Parkinson's disease.[324] (The Lancet Journal)

Some of the personal care products also have aluminum in them. Such as the Roll on Antiperspirant Deodorant – Active: Aluminum zirconium gly 15.4% One obvious solution is to use products in a health food store before using the standard supermarket products which have a higher chance of taking in toxic chemicals (toxic as causing a chronic disease) from these commercial chemicals in your personal care products.

"Two fruit acids, citric acid and malic acid, have been demonstrated to facilitate the excretion of aluminum in mouse experiments. The acids are commonly found in foods such as fruit and wine, and are used as flavorings. Citric acid and Malic acid bond with the aluminum and carry it out of the body safely.[325]"[326]   (*Journal of Toxicology*)

Violent or compulsive behavior is common in autism and in some criminals. "Lead crosses the blood-brain barrier and can cause senile dementia and Alzheimer's and learning disabilities and such as attention deficit disorder and aggressive behaviors. Significant research shows that lead poisoning affects the pre-frontal cortex of the brain, the part that governs impulse behavior, and may cause someone to react violently if disrupted.[327]

It is more than just a theory but also a compilation of what everyone is saying in the scientific literature according to a technical book, *Geriatric Nutrition the Health Professionals Handbook*, (2006) citing various journals and books. "There is a strong hypothesis that aluminum is part of the etiology of various dementias. Most interest in aluminum toxicity as it relates to elderly people who are not on dialysis or parenteral feeding regimens is related to the putative connection between disposition of aluminum in the brain and the development of various senile dementias, including Alzheimer's disease.[328] [329]   There is no question that aluminum is a potent neurotoxin, both in experimental animals and in humans.[330]   Reports of elevated aluminum in the brains of individuals with Alzheimer's disease and with Amyotrophic Lateral Sclerosis (ALS or Lou Gehrig's disease) or with Parkinsonism dementia associated with regions that also contain neurofibrillary tangles have supported this putative association.'[331] It is clear 'that if aluminum does gain access to the central nervous system, it acts as a potent neurotoxin.'[332]"

So heavy metals are definitely connected with Parkinson's, MS and Alzheimer's and possibly other neurological diseases and there are a lot of journal studies done over the last two decades that show a connection. To mention a few . . . (*Mov Disord.* 1993)[333]; (*J Neural Transm.*, 1997)[334]; (*Mov Disord.*, 1998)[335]; (*Neurology.* 2003)[336]; (*Lancet Neurol.*, 2004)[337]; (*Behav Pharmacol.* 2006)[338]."[k]

Has it ever been shown that these environmental poisons are a cause of Parkinson's or MS? Yes, in the book *The Brain Gate*, Robert Hatherill, PhD, an expert in this field of biochemistry, explains: "Researchers have struggled for more than a century to figure out what causes Parkinson's disease. . . Then, in 1982, a series of bizarre events occurred. Since the disease usually occurs in older people in the sixth

---

[k] Some journal studies evidence for heavy metal toxicity in PD and MS:

"Parkinson's disease (PD) mortality rates in Michigan counties for 1986-1988 were calculated with respect to potential heavy metal exposure (iron, zinc, copper, mercury, magnesium, and manganese) from industry based on recent census data. . . . These ecologic findings suggest a geographic association between PD mortality and the industrial use of heavy metals." (*Mov Disord.* 1993)

"Excessive iron accumulation in the brain: a possible potential risk of neurodegeneration in Parkinson's disease. . . . This supports the hypothesis that excessive cerebral iron may contribute to the aetiology of Parkinson's disease (PD)." (*J Neural Transm.*, 1997)

"Recent studies have proposed a role for diet in Parkinson's disease (PD). PD is characterized by a high deposition of iron and a low concentration of ferritin in the substantia nigra." (*Mov Disord.*, 1998)

"Dietary influences on oxidative stress have been thought to play important role in the etiology of PD . . . A high intake of iron, especially in combination with high manganese intake, may be related to risk for PD."   (*Neurology.* 2003)

"Abnormal interactions of copper or iron in the brain with metal-binding proteins . . . that lead to oxidative stress have emerged as important potential mechanisms in brain ageing and neurodegenerative disorders." (*Lancet Neurol.*, 2004)

"Following recent reviews . . . Poor metal ion homeostasis is credited with pathological roles in the progression of a number of disorders including Alzheimer's disease, Parkinson's disease and multiple sclerosis." (*Behav Pharmacol.* 2006)

decade of life, doctors found it strange that young drug users started turning up at hospitals showing signs of Parkinson's disease. Scientists found a toxic contaminant present in the synthetic street heroin being used that caused this strange outbreak of Parkinson's and solved the mystery. 'Foreign' chemicals such as pesticides were actually causing Parkinson's disease. An alarming study, published in the *Journal of the American Medical Association,* claimed that environmental chemicals cause the majority of Parkinson's disease. Other published studies indicated the same troubling connection. While most scientists don't accept it, Parkinson's disease has become the first documented brain ailment of the industrial revolution. Pollutants that taint our food supply may foster new generations of brain illnesses."[339]

Dr. Hatherill continues; "Studies have shown a correlation between incidences of Parkinson's disease and industrialization, pesticide exposure, and consumption of water from wells. Heavy metals, such as iron, mercury, manganese, and aluminum – all byproducts of industry – have been shown to increase the risk of Parkinson's. These studies support efforts to address environmental causes to reduce the incidence of Parkinson's. The higher incidence of Parkinson's in rural farming areas and areas that get most of their water supply from wells correlates with the increased use of pesticides in these areas. Other studies showing the agricultural influences on Parkinson's have been conducted in the United States and Canada. One agricultural area south of Montreal uses pesticides intensely, sells more L-dopa (used to treat Parkinson's), and has a higher mortality rate from Parkinson's disease than other metropolitan locations."[340]

d. Pesticides Connection to PD, AD and MS

"The University of Rochester School of Medicine and Dentistry conducted a study of a common herbicide, parquet, and a common fungicide, maneb. Mice that were subjected to these chemicals developed the same pattern of brain damage seen in Parkinson's disease. Pesticides and herbicides are increasingly linked to other brain and neurological disorders, as well as heart, lung, kidney, and adrenal gland diseases."[341]

Pesticides are mentioned by David Perlmutter, MD who writes about Parkinson's disease in the Physicians' Committee for Responsible Medicine website: "Dr. Manfred Gerlach published research identifying N-methyl-(R)-salsolinol as a possible endogenous MPTP-like neuro-toxin.[342] The possibility that xenobiotics may act in a fashion similar to MPTP, coupled with the obvious link of Parkinson's disease risk with pesticide exposure, has encouraged research specifically focused on the role of xenobiotics as toxic agents with respect to mitochondrial function."[343]

Everyone uses pesticides on their lawn and gardens. Also pesticides are heavily used in farming. Both insecticides and herbicides significantly increased the risk of Parkinson's disease, the researchers report in the online journal *BioMedCentral* (BMC, 2008) Neurology. "The strongest associations between Parkinson's disease and pesticides were obtained in families with no history of Parkinson's. This finding suggests that sporadic Parkinson's cases may be particularly vulnerable to the toxic effects of pesticides, but the possibility of pesticides influencing risk of Parkinson's in individuals from families with a history of PD cannot be ruled out."[344] Furthermore, in another study, a lipid-soluble long-lasting mitochondrial toxic pesticide was found in six of twenty brains of Parkinson's patients and in none of controls.[345] (*Ann Neurol*)

According to Doris J. Rapp, MD, author of *Our Toxic World: A Wake Up Call* (2004), pesticides, and other chemicals found in human tissue, have been found to alter "the brain and nervous system causing headaches, difficulty thinking or remembering, inexplicable emotional ups and downs, inconsolable depression, irritability, moodiness, aggression, hyperactivity or extreme fatigue . . . [pesticides also affect] the muscular system causing twitches, tics, muscle pains or weakness; in time, possibly leading to fibromyalgia, multiple sclerosis, amyotrophic lateral sclerosis (ALS) or to Parkinson's disease."[346]

A study cited in the *International Journal of Epidemiology* (2007), analyzed data concerning pesticide use in California counties and found an increasing mortality rate from Parkinson's disease in those counties using agricultural pesticides. The same study found that California's use of about 250 million pounds of pesticides annually accounts for one-quarter of all pesticides used in the United States.[347]

Fungicides deserve special mention because we know already that they can because Parkinson's in farmers. In the small farming community of Fairfield, Montana, for example, because of pesticide exposure, the rate of Parkinson's in older inhabitants is one in every 60 people, compared with the national average of one in about 272. In a recent representative study, Parkinson's in farmers was linked directly to pesticide exposure, with fungicides being the most likely cause.[348]

"Organophosphates are the most widely used type of pesticides. At least forty different types are in use in homes, gardens, agriculture, and veterinary practice. Organophosphates were originally developed by Nazi chemists during World War II as a chemical weapon nerve agent. Once the war was over, industry found a new use for these nerve agents, in the form of pesticides for lawn 'care'. The US Department of Defense (DOD) published a 1.5 million dollar study in the journal Nature Genetics connecting neurological disorders like attention deficit and hyperactivity disorder (ADHA) and Parkinson's disease with organophosphates."[349]

e. Vaccinations Connection to PD, AD and MS

What about vaccinations which contain mercury and other metals? Vaccinations with mercury or other heavy metals having a direct cause-effect relationship with Parkinson's, Alzheimer's and MS is a real possibility. There is a very strong case that vaccinations are connected with Autism, and possibly other childhood diseases and conditions, but to go into all those studies would fill many pages if not books. This has been an ongoing debate for many decades. Do the introduction of poisons, chemicals, heavy metals and other non- organic chemicals, and virus strains and antibodies have a negative effect on the body? Yes, of course but a pharmaceutical company will never admit that and most universities receive grants from them.

There is huge money to be gained or lost over these questions. In 2005, the global vaccine market was estimated at 5.8 billion dollars. IMS Health, a company that tracks the pharmaceutical industry's sales, indicates vaccine sales are estimated to increase by twenty percent per year over the next five years.[350]

Do vaccinations with mercy or other heavy metals have a direct cause-effect relationship with Parkinson's, Alzheimer's and MS is a debated question. Some vaccinations do not seem to have a bad effect for Alzheimer's. In a journal study, "Past exposure to vaccines and subsequent risk of Alzheimer's disease" (2001)[351] they concluded: "Past exposure to vaccines against diphtheria or tetanus, poliomyelitis and influenza may protect against subsequent development of Alzheimer's disease." They also note that, "Furthermore, changes to the immune system have been implicated in age-related conditions such as Alzheimer's disease."[352] (*Canadian Medical Ass. Journal*)

There is a lot of evidence that childhood vaccinations have a connection to autism. "Pediatrician Dr. Jeff Bradstreet also cited in the Homefirst article, stated there is virtually no autism in home-schooling families who decline

179

to vaccinate for religious reasons. There is also anecdotal evidence that the Amish, who are not vaccinated for religious reasons, are virtually untouched by autism."[353] There is more evidence on autism but that is for another book on the topic of autism and ADD. Like PD, AD and MS it is another example of a neurological disease.

In the section *A Medical Antidote for PD, AD & MS!* Dr. Carley proposes that through vaccinations it affects the Allergy-Immune Diseases then through the auto-antibodies to Myelin that affects the Nervous system. Then through the nervous system the central (Encephalitis) it affects and perhaps causes things like Autism, Multiple Sclerosis, Parkinson's, Lou Gehrig's Disease and others.
Rebecca Carley, MD states, "The research I have done over the past 11 years ... my only child was brain damaged from vaccines, and I learned how to reverse it."[354]

Let's end this section looking at something different. "An article appeared in *The Townsend Letter for Doctors and Patients* indicates that 'perfumes contain neurotoxins, which have a causal link to central nervous system disorders, headaches, confusion, dizziness, short-term memory loss, anxiety, depression, disorientation, and mood swings.' The author of the article explains that fragrance inhalation through the nose goes directly to the brain where it can have neurological effects."[355]

f. Food Additives Connection to PD, AD and MS

What about food additives?   In an article on 'Food Additives,' in *Chemical and Engineering News* it noted: "The use of chemicals in foods has soared from 419 million pounds in 1955 to more than 800 million in 1968. Each of us (in 1968) eats more than three pounds of food additives a year."[356] Back in 1968 three pounds was a lot back then but what would it be in our time today?

In a book by a medical doctor and associate, *Natural Detoxification: A Practical Encyclopedia* (2000), they state: "The average person eats 124 pounds of food additives a year. There are more than three thousand additives and preservatives found in our food supply today. Food are inundated with artificial colors, flavor enhancers, bleach, texture agents, conditioners, acid/base balancers, ripening gases, waxes, firming agents, agents that enrich nutrients, preservatives, heavy metals, and other chemicals. Most of these artificial ingredients have never been subjected to long-term tests to determine their effects on human beings."[357] So it was 3 pounds in 1968 and it could be up to 124 pounds today!

In the book *Brain Wash* Dr. Cook continues, "The real issue is that for anyone with brain diseases, the food colors have been shown to cross the blood-brain barrier. The term barrier actually instills a false sense of security because chemicals like food dyes actually trick the brain into allowing their entry, putting them in a position to do harm to perhaps the most delicate organ in your body."[358]

Robert Hatherill, PhD also gives an understanding of Excitotoxic agents: "Commercially prepared foods are loaded with 'flavor enhancers,' 'stabilizers,' and other chemical additives used to make food taste better, have better 'mouth-feel,' and to extend shelf life. These additives, especially glutamate, aspartate, and MSG, are all known excitotoxins, meaning they literally excite cells to the point of death. Excitotoxins interact with receptors and overexcite nerve cells, leading to the death of brain cells. Excitotoxic agents are linked to brain diseases such as Alzheimer's, Parkinson's, and ALS. Scientists also believe that excitotoxicity can cause age-related memory loss, confusion, and mental decline. The brain uses the amino acids glutamate and aspartate as the primary excitatory brain messengers."[359]

"A variety of processed foods commonly contain the flavor enhancer MSG (monosodium glutamate). All sorts of foods, from soups and gravies to potato chips and crackers, all can contain MSG. In particular, low-calorie or diet foods containing large amounts of flavor enhancers with excitotoxic potential. Many canned and processed soups and gravies typically contain multiple types of excitotoxic additives such as hydrolyzed proteins. Hydrolyzed proteins contain high levels of glutamate and other flavor enhancers. Soups or liquid foods flood into the bloodstream quickly and can display even more excitotoxicity. Wheat gluten contains over 40 percent glutamate; casein, the primary milk protein, is 23 percent glutamate; and beef gelatin protein is 12 percent glutamate. Red meat, processed tomatoes, and cheeses are also known to contain high levels of glutamate."[360]

"The artificial sweetener aspartame (NutraSweet) contains 50 percent aspartame, an excitatory amino acid. Aspartame is almost universally present in sugarless chewing gums and desserts, and low-calorie soft drinks. The consumer needs to be wary of food additives since our food processors have disguised additives or free amino acids that have excitotoxic potential with names like hydrolyzed vegetable protein, chicken broth, textured vegetable proteins, hydrolyzed plant proteins, soy extract, casein or casein-ate (a milk protein), yeast extracts, spices and natural flavors."[361]

Russell Blaylock, MD in his widely read book: *Excitotoxins the Taste that Kills*, gives some excellent reasons why a person with Parkinson's or Alzheimer's should go raw vegan. It is the easiest and best way to get off of all manufactured foods!

Dr. Blaylock writes: "Many meals served in restaurants contain very high doses of MSG and other excitotoxic amino acids.[362] In fact, they equal or even exceed experimental doses that regularly produce brain lesions in animals. (Remember, humans concentrate glutamate in their blood following a meal containing MSG higher than any other known species of animal.) Even a single bowl of soup may contain several grams of MSG. Most salad dressings are loaded with MSG and hydrolyzed vegetable protein (also labeled as vegetable protein), as are croutons. If you use steak sauce, it frequently contains both, disguised as "natural flavoring" or "spices". Chips, creamy sauces, some gravies, rice dishes, and other gourmet foods can all be loaded with excitotoxic 'taste enhancers.'

Dr. Blaylock states, "I believe that there is enough research evidence demonstrating the harmful effects of excitotoxins in food additives that all persons having a history of one of sensitivity to MSG or a strong family history of one of the neuro-degenerative diseases should avoid all foods and beverages containing these excitotoxin 'taste' additives."[363]

"Today MSG is added to most soups, chips, fast foods, frozen foods, ready-made dinners, and canned goods. And it has been a heaven sent for the diet food industry, since so many of the low-fat foods are practically tasteless. As Dr. George Schwartz has pointed out in his remarkable book, *In Bad Taste: The MSG Syndrome*, often MSG and related toxins are added to foods in disguised forms. For example, among the food manufacturers favorite disguises are "hydrolyzed vegetable protein", "vegetable protein", "natural flavorings", and "spices". Each of these may contain from 12% to 40% MSG."[364]

"Glutamate and aspartate are neurotransmitters (the keys) found normally in the brain and spinal cord. And even though they are two of the most common transmitter chemicals in the brain and spinal cord, when their concentrations rise above a critical level they can become deadly toxins to the neurons containing glutamate receptors (the locks) and to the nerve cells connected to these neurons. This latter point is especially important. What it means is that excessive glutamate will not only kill the neurons with the receptors for glutamate but it will also kill any neurons that happen to be connected to it, even if that neuron uses another type of receptor. This will become important when we discuss Alzheimer's disease and Parkinson's disease. Both glutamate and aspartame can cause neurons to become extremely excited and, if given in large enough doses, they can cause these cells to degenerative and die."[365] With excitotoxin food additives being in virtually every manufactured food product, our brain is constantly being assaulted by excitotoxins."[366]

Dr. Blaylock lists in the appendix Hidden Sources of MSG: "As discussed previously, the glutamate manufacturers and the processed food industries are always on the quest to disguise MSG added to food. Below is a partial list of the most common names for disguised MSG. Remember also that the powerful excitotoxins aspartate and L-cysteine are frequently added to foods and according to FDA rules require no labeling at all."[367]

Additives that always contain MSG:[368]	Additives that frequently contain MSG:
Monosodium Glutamate	Malt extract
Hydrolyzed Vegetable Protein	Malt Flavoring
Hydrolyzed Protein	Bouillon
Hydrolyzed Plant Protein	Broth
Plant Protein Extract	Stock
Sodium Caseinate	Flavoring
Calcium Caseinate	Natural Flavoring
Yeast Extract	Natural Beef or Chicken
Textured Protein	Flavoring
Autolyzed Yeast	Seasoning
Hydrolyzed Oat Flour	Spices

"Additives that may contain MSG or excitotoxins: Carrageenan, Enzymes, Soy Protein Concentrate, Soy Protein Isolate, Whey Protein Concentrate Protease enzymes of various sources can release excitotoxin amino acids from protein foods."[369]

"Amphetamines are known to cause specific destruction of a group of neurons that are concerned with controlling fine and coordinated movements of the arm and legs."[370] The collection of neurons and their connecting fibers are referred to as the nigrostriatal system, which is the same nerve system destroyed in Parkinson's disease. "Further evidence comes from a recent observation involving one of the primary drugs used to treat Parkinson's disease L-DOPA. While this drug has done much to relieve the crippling symptoms of this terrible disease, and even to extend the lifespan of younger patients, there is some evidence that it may speed up the progress of the disease. Several studies have indicated that patients started early on L-DOPA therapy tend to deteriorate faster than those in which other drugs were used initially."[371]

Part of the explanation of this phenomenon may lie in the findings of Dr. John Olney who demonstrated that L-DOPA is a mild excitotoxin.[372] "It was found to be approximately half as potent as MS. A metabolite of L-DOPA, called 6-hydroxy-DOPA is about six times more powerful than MSG. From this observation it would be reasonable to assume that high doses of the Parkinson drug L-DOPA is about six times more powerful than MSG. From this observation it would be reasonable to assume that high doses of the Parkinson drug L-DOPA could kill off already weakened neurons in the nigrostriatal system, thereby speeding up the progress of the disease. Dr. Olney suggests that L-DOPA does not act alone but rather acts with glutamate to produce the damage. This is one reason why persons with Parkinson's disease should avoid all foods and drinks containing excitotoxin additives such as MSG, hydrolyzed vegetable protein, cysteine, and asparatate (NutraSweet)."[373]

A journal study (*Nature,* 2006) basically says the same thing Robert Hatherill, PhD just explained that

"Gultamate" is an excitatory neurotransmitter of the nervous system, and excessive amounts in the brain can lead to cell death by a process called excitotoxicity. Excitotoxicity occurs not only in Alzheimer's disease, but also in other neurological diseases such as Parkinson's disease and multiple sclerosis.[374]

"Research suggests that over-activity of a brain messenger called glutamate, a protein precursor that causes excitation of certain brain cells and neurons, may lead to brain cell death and Parkinson's progression. Monosodium glutamate has excitotoxic properties, which means that MSG can over-excite brain cells until they die. According to Dr. Patricia Fitzgerald, (*Neurology*, 2000) 'Ingesting MSG over the years has also been linked with Parkinson's and Alzheimer's.'"[375]

g. Mercury Fillings Connection to PD, AD and MS

What about the mercury in your mouth and all the fillings that people have. Dr. Michelle Cook points out: "Both methyl-mercury and Mercury vapors from dental amalgams have been proven to find their way into the brain. Methyl-mercury can bind to an amino acid from protein to create a complex that resembles another amino acid, thereby tricking the brain. Once mercury finds its way into the brain, numerous toxic processes take place, including the depletion of essential antioxidants that protect the brain, subsequent stress on the brain, and the blocked formation of an important brain messenger called 'acetylcholine.' Acetylcholine transmits messages that regulate nerve-muscle activity and memory through the brain and nervous system."[376]

The problem with removing dental mercury fillings is that a highly skilled dentist with specialized training is needed and that working with a health practitioner skilled in detoxification and mercury detoxification is best.

The use of dental amalgam in most developed countries is a political discussion which involves a lot of money for dental industry that uses mercury in dental amalgams. The research shows it is a clear and present danger to health in humans:

- It is known from animal research (six studies) that mercury vapor is emitted continually from dental amalgam and is absorbed and accumulated in the organs tissues.[377]
- Humans with amalgam fillings have significantly elevated mercury levels in the blood, (5 studies)[378]
- About 3 - 5 times more mercury in urine, (four studies have been done)[379]
- And 2 to 12 times more mercury in their body tissues, than individuals without dental amalgams. (six studies have been done)[380]

Many studies have been performed in the past as just noted above and new studies confirm a lot of this data. It is widely accepted that the main source of mercury vapor is dental amalgam and it contributes substantially to the mercury load in human body tissues. The modern debate is about the consequences of this additional mercury exposure from amalgam to human health. Some countries like Denmark, Norway and Sweden have restricted the use of amalgams of mercury.

What about the dental mercury connection to MS or Parkinson's? In the *Journal of Nutritional and Environmental Medicine*, (2001) "Dr. Mercola and Dr. Klinghardt state that people with amalgam fillings exceed all occupational exposure allowances of mercury in all European and North American countries. Adults with four or more amalgams run a significant health risk from the amalgam, while in children as few as two amalgams will contribute to health problems. According to Mercola and Klinghardt, a single dental amalgam with a surface area of 0.4 square centimeters is estimated to release up to fifteen micrograms of mercury per day, primarily through mechanical wear and evaporation."[381]

"The average person with four amalgam fillings will absorb up to 120 micrograms of mercury per day, just from their fillings. Compare that with the daily estimates of mercury absorption from fish and seafood, which is 2.3 micrograms, and from all other foods, air, and water is 0.3 micrograms per day."[382]

Dr. Perlmutter writes that, "some countries (Denmark, Sweden, and Germany) have started to restrict the use of mercury fillings and an advocacy group, Citizens for Mercury Relief started an international petition, Ban Mercury in Teeth Everywhere (BITE). Approximately eighty percent of American adults have mercury amalgams in their teeth."[383]

Are amalgam fillings linked with any degenerative diseases? "Numerous studies demonstrate that amalgam fillings are linked with many diseases, including Alzheimer's, autoimmune disorders, kidney dysfunctions, infertility, polycystic ovary syndrome, neurotransmitter imbalances, food allergies, multiple sclerosis, thyroid problems, and impaired immune system."[384] (*Journal of Nutritional and Environmental Medicine*, 2001) The Environmental Protection Agency and the United States military have declared the amalgams removed from teeth are considered toxic waste.[385] This is a real ethical issue!

There is evidence that the mercury is directly linked to PD and MS. In an article in the *Townsend Letter* (2004) by Mike Godfrey MD, which is on, 'Multiple Sclerosis and dental amalgams'. He points out that mercury from dental amalgams is a factor in MS. The fundamental 'proof' of this disease has been the presence of oligoclonal globulins in the cerebrospinal fluid. The presence of these proteins has been seen as a permanent and irreversible feature of the disease. Huggins and Levy published a paper in *Alternative Medical Review*[386] on Cerebral fluid protein changes in multiple sclerosis after dental amalgam removal. This was a most profound landmark study that got published in a minor indexed journal where it immediately sunk into obscurity.[387] Our recent paper on 400 patients[388] (Godfrey, et al. *Journal Alzheimer's Disease,* 2003) has revealed a potential genetic marker as to why some people could be much more susceptible to neurotoxicity including Alzheimer's senile dementia and MS. Mercury going through the roof of the nose by day and night, accumulates in the limbic brain areas and levels are proportional to the number of fillings."[389] Furthermore, mercury vapor is an industrially recognized cause of hypertension and cardiovascular disease and, according to the WHO, the World Health Organization in 1991 dental amalgam is by far the largest source of mercury vapor."[390] It is mercury poisoning and must be regarded as a medical matter. It is best done by a team approach involving several health practitioners and different modalities."[391]

There is a study into 400 consecutive patients clinically diagnosed with mercury toxicity; Biting the 'silver bullet' in *NZ Psych Soc* (1999).[392] This was authorized by the NZ Director of Dental Research and it showed that protected amalgam removal combined with effective detoxification, resulted in 95% of those who followed the correct protocol, obtaining long-term major health benefits.[393]

Dr. Godfrey continues, "I have witnessed remarkable changes in patients with proven MS after proper amalgam removal and detoxification. I have seen some justifiably angry patients who have been helped by this after being misdiagnosed and effectively mismanaged for some years at great cost. The late Hans Nieper MD, who successfully treated some thousands of patients with MS from all over the world who travelled to his clinic in Hanover, Germany always advised that amalgam and root-filled teeth had to be removed."[394]

h. Xenobiotics the Detoxification System

What about the body's defenses against all these? There is the body's detoxification system called the Xenobiotics system, which is a chemical detox system in the body, but it is limited and can only handle small amounts of detoxification. It will become overloaded with the vast amounts of pollutants that enter the body, and these get stored in the cells, later causing health problems or degenerative diseases like Parkinson's or MS, ALS or Alzheimer's.

A Live-Plant-based nutrition diet is a detox diet partly because of the high levels of antioxidants and vitamins in the fruits and vegetables. These can help and in fact some nutrients, like zinc, are necessary in the Xenobiotics system to latch onto and drag out the heavy metals, pesticides, food additives and other toxins and poisons. A raw vegan diet will greatly help in the process of detoxification. A seven day, or longer, juice or water fast is one of the best types of detox methods. A seven day fast should be done at least two or three times a year to really be effective.

So let me review this. Some of the things that could be in the brain of those with Alzheimer's, Parkinson's and possibly also those with MS, which need to be taken out of the brain and or the neurological system are:
1. Heavy metal toxicity
2. Pesticides
3. Pharmaceutical or street drugs
4. Vaccines or chemical poisons
5. Excitotoxins and other chemical additives
6. Fungi, mold, yeast
7. Bacteria and pathogenic microorganisms
8. Toxic (denatured) Animal Proteins
9. Internal Cellular Toxins (i.e. parasites)
10. External Environmental Toxins
11. NeuroInflammation in brain and CNS

12. pH &/or sodium-potassium levels are off
13. Allergy to meat and gluten
14. Food additives and/or colors (i.e. glutamate)

One expert in metal toxicity and its removal gives some good insight into this area; Dietrich Klinghardt, MD, PhD who also uses the Biological Terrain Theory in his practice writes on Heavy Metals and Chronic Diseases: "In the case of mercury the therapeutic dilemma is most clear, small doses may have a therapeutic effect in a short term, lifesaving direction, but may also cause their own illness. Most metals have a very narrow therapeutic margin before their neurotoxic, in some cases carcinogenic effect, outweighs the benefits."[395]

"So in the long run, the situation looks different: the cells of the body are harmed by toxic metals whereas the invading microorganisms can often thrive in a heavy metal environment. Research by Ludwig, Voll and others in Germany, by Omura and myself here in the US, showed that microorganisms tend to set up their housekeeping in those body compartments that have the highest pollution with toxic metals. The body's own immune cells are incapacitated in those areas whereas the microorganisms multiply and thrive in an undisturbed way. The list of symptoms of mercury toxicity alone, published by DAMS (dental amalgam support group), includes virtually any illness known to humankind: chronic fatigue, depression and joint pains are the most common."[396]

One possible way to deal with heavy metal toxicity is to use the supplement Chlorella Pyrenoidosa, or it is simply called Chlorella. Chlorella can be bought in a health food store and it is a good source of vitamins and other nutrients. Chlorella Pyrenoidosa is used for chelation therapy to bind heavy metals and drag them out. There are different types of chelating therapy for heavy metals and this is one of them. This is also good for biotoxin illnesses. There is a drug cholestyramine that does the same thing but one would be better off with a natural supplement, like Dr. Klinghardt's formula,[1] but there are others that are also good.

A possible universal answer to dealing with all these is a Living plant-based diet and juicing and fasting.

i. Obedience to God and Happiness

A scholar Fr. Antonio Martins, SJ explains "According to the Bible, there is an intrinsic co-relation between sin and affliction, between obedience to God and happiness. Down through the centuries, God has made use of all kinds of means to recall men, these are his children, the marvelous destiny for which they were created: to be holy, like unto God. 'You must be perfect, as your heavenly Father is perfect' (Mt. 5:48). But men prefer to be slaves of their own degrading and unruly passions."[397]

In the book of Judges we read: "Then the sons of Israel did what displeases Yahweh and served the Baals. They deserted Yahewh, ... Then Yahweh's anger flamed out against Israel. ... Thus he reduced them to dire distress." (Jg. 2:11-15) Similar accounts are scattered through page after page of the Book of Judges, which prove the veracity of the threatening words written down in Deuteronomy: "See, I set before you today a blessing and a curse. A blessing, if you obey the commandments of Yahweh your God that I enjoin on you today; a curse, if you disobey the commandments of Yahweh your God." (Dt. 11:26-28)

If from the Book of Judges, we pass to I and II Samuel, we find the same thesis of sin followed inexorably by chastisement. If from the historical books we pass on to the prophets, we can verify that the idea of sin being followed

---

[1] A place to get them is www.Biopure.com in California. Each tablet is 200 mg, but to get enough to do the work of chelating a person needs to work up to 2.5 g or 12 tabs a day. But start out with one tab a day and another on every day, working up to 12 tabs.

by punishment is emphasized with even greater vigor. It suffices to read Hosea 13:1-15; Amos 2:1-16; 3:11; 6:6-9; Micah 3:1-12, in order to be completely convinced. Some will obviously disagree but, "There is a way that some think right, but it leads in the end to death." (Prov. 14:12).[398]

Chapter 9

Plant-based Diets are Reconstructive

St. Basil of Caesarea (329-379) and Ephrem the Syrian, show solid evidence for a vegetarian position within mainstream Christianity in the fourth century. For St. Basil, those who desire to live their lives in imitation of the life of Paradise must make use of fruits and grains, because the diet that includes meat is a result of the fall.[399] St. Basil links the event of the fall with the eating of forbidden fruit and therefore with gluttony and the failure to practice abstinence. Elsewhere, he says it was only after the flood that wine and meat were introduced into the human food chain because in Paradise there was no wine, nor animal sacrifice, nor meat-eating. But he is careful not to condemn the eating of any one type of food, and on at least one occasion he distances himself from those who condemn the eating of meat.[400] St. Jerome argued for an essentially vegetarian fare.[401] One scholar of early Christianity wrote in his book that the regular avoidance of meat and wine, except for those who are weak or ill, is one of the most common theses of ascetic and monastic literature from the early Christian period."[402]
It looks like a significant number of early Church Fathers and early Christian communities believed in and practiced a plant-based lifestyle!

a. Greens in the Nutrition Program

Greens are the key to dealing with degenerative diseases. Gabriel Cousens, MD writes, "Primitive foods such as spirulina contain the highest food energy, the highest nutrient value, and use up the least amount of the planet's resources. Spirulina is also a powerful alkalinizing and healing food. It is an excellent support for the healing of hypoglycemia, diabetes, chronic fatigue, anemia, ulcers, and for boosting the immune system. It has been shown to repair free radical damage. Researchers have found it to contain a tumor necrosis factor. The anti-cancer power of spirulina is significant enough that at Harvard Medical School they found that extracts of spirulina were extremely effective in treating cancer in hamsters."[403]

In a study from the journal *Lancet*; a low fat diet, maintained for a period of up to 3 years, failed to lower either the mortality or morbidity of patients suffering from arteriosclerosis (a) whereas after a period of only 4 to 5 weeks a diet high in fresh vegetables caused a significant reduction in this affliction. (b)[404]   Other studies from *Environmental Nutrition*; and *The American Journal of Clinical Nutrition* have shown that greens such as kale, broccoli, and bok choy are as good as milk in terms of calcium absorbability.[405]

The problem is most people like to eat a little salad and think that it is enough, but it is not even close to being enough. You have to eat a large enough salad so that it fills you up. The salad should consist of all kinds of vegetables. Another way to get many nutrients and chlorophyll is to have a teaspoon or two of green powders mixed with water or juice.

The Alleluia diet includes the recommendation for a nutritional therapy for healing Parkinson's, AD and MS. It recommends 6 glasses of green powdered drink or 6 teaspoons of Barley Grass a day mixed with water or juice, because that is what has been found to work. Some of the people that have been cured, or put into remission for Parkinson's and MS used green powders and/or green juices. It is a lot of work to juice greens and you need an expensive juicer as most juicers are not powerful enough to break up the plant fibers of the greens.

Green food supplements or powders are one of the keys to health and healing. It is a much easier and more efficient to get greens into your diet in an optimum way. One expert on Green food supplementation wrote: "Green food supplements, if properly formulated, can provide astonishing nutrient density. The import of this is significant, for few aspects of human biochemistry can function properly if trace nutrients are undersupplied, thereby making it harder to deal with the gluttonous portions of fat and carbohydrate present in modern diets. The appeal lies in the simple fact that green foods are incredibly nutritious, with an actual power to heal. If each cell receives what it needs to function fully and efficiently, then the human body can, in many cases, re-establish normal biochemistry. Depending on the individual, the results might range from a noticeable improvement in endurance, energy or faster recovery from exercise, to the eradication of a disease. Although green foods are usually not promoted as therapeutic supplements, the good ones will end up being so simply because they give the body what it needs to correct its own dysfunctions. The body heals itself, after all. Consumers are discovering these real benefits, and passing on the good news."[406]

b. The Value of Chlorophyll

What is it that makes these green powders so important? It is the Chlorophyll which is built around a structure known as a porphyrin ring, which is common to a variety of natural organic molecules. Chief among these is hemoglobin, the substance in human and animal blood which carries oxygen from the lungs to the other tissues and cells of the body. When looking at the structures of heme (the oxygen carrying portion of hemoglobin), it's easy to see their similarities. The main difference between them is that the porphyrin ring of hemoglobin is built around iron (Fe) and the porphyrin ring of chlorophyll is built around magnesium (Mg).[407]

Brian Clement, ND writes, "You know that all life requires oxygen, but you may not know that the foods we eat can rob that life-giving oxygen from our cells, causing disease and death. That's why it's important to be sure that we select foods that feed, rather than rob, oxygen. But how

196

can we know which foods give and which foods take oxygen? Botanical food is composed of oxygen in the molecular structure of its chlorophyll content. Chlorophyll is the 'blood' of a plant. When compared to a molecule of hemoglobin (the oxygen carrier in human blood) chlorophyll is almost identical. Have you ever thought about what happens to that oxygen when we eat those foods in their living state? It feeds oxygen to our body - the oxygen we need to stay alive and healthy. Only living foods bring that oxygen into the body."

Dr. John Gainer wrote, "On a high-fat and high-protein diet, our oxygen supply is greatly reduced." He stated, "that even a moderate increase in blood-plasma protein can reduce oxygen levels of the blood by as much as 60 percent."[408]

Dr. Benjamin Gurskin, "The value of chlorophyll isn't a new discovery. In the early part of the twentieth century, chlorophyll was regarded as a top-notch weapon in the arsenal of pharmacopoeia. Many physicians used it as a treatment for various complaints such as ulcers and skin disease, and as a pain reliever and breath freshener." One report by Dr. Benjamin Gurskin, then director of experimental pathology at Temple University, was published in the *American Journal of Surgery*. Dr. Gurskin discussed more than one thousand cases in which various disorders were treated with chlorophyll. Commenting on his associates' experiences with chlorophyll, he wrote, "It is interesting to note that there is not a single case recorded in which either improvement or cure has not taken place."[409]

A lot of the health food stores sell wheat grass, barley grass and other green grass supplements. Wheatgrass, the grass grown from wheat berries (wheat seeds), is rich in chlorophyll, a substance nearly identical to the hemoglobin in human blood. Weight for weight, wheatgrass has sixty times more vitamin C than oranges and eight times more iron than spinach. It has over a hundred vitamins, minerals and

nutrients including a good source of vitamin B17.
Wheatgrass contains concentrated chlorophyll, which is
almost identical to the hemoglobin molecule in human blood.
The only major difference between them is that the central
atom in hemoglobin is iron; in chlorophyll, it is magnesium.

One of the founders of the wheatgrass movement is
Ann Wigmore, she developed wheatgrass therapy and in
most holistic clinics and health food stores it can be found.
Wheatgrass juice along with raw foods, exercise, meditation
and detoxification methods like juice fasting became the key
elements in her healing program.[410] Richard Walters stated
in his book, "Wheatgrass juice, it is claimed, helps to
detoxify the body, eliminate dead tissue, and nourish the
system. A nutritional program combining wheatgrass and
'live' foods (that is uncooked food - with enzymes and
nutrients undamaged) is said to create optimal immune
functioning, enabling the whole organism to reverse the
cancer. Wheatgrass therapy has brought about striking
recoveries from cancer."[411]

The problem with straight wheatgrass juice is that you
have to drink it right away because it degrades quickly.
Most research studies use dried products of wheatgrass.
Barley grass is a sister to wheat grass but barley is sweeter
and less bitter in taste.

Chlorophyll heals and cleanses all our organs and
destroys many internal enemies, like pathogenic bacteria,
fungus, cancer cells,[412] and others. Chlorophyll has been
proven helpful in preventing and healing many forms of
cancer[413] and arteriosclerosis.[414] Chlorophyll has a long
history and many advocates. There are numerous healing
benefits of chlorophyll, taken from cereal grass, that can be
considered. Here are a few of the many benefits and studies
done on chlorophyll and related grasses:
- Drs. F. Paloscia and G. Pollotten used chlorophyll therapy with
  some success in the treatment of **tuberculous empyema**.[415]
  Cancer [416] [417] [418] patients seem to have benefited to some

degree from chlorophyll therapy, although results are inconclusive.

- A Dr. Mahnaz Badamchian of the Dept. of Biochemistry and Molecular Biology, George Washing Univ., Medical Center found that **Anti-tumor properties** of barley leaf extract (BLE) significantly reduced human prostrate, breast and melanoma cancer. Badamchian states, this "could provide a novel nutritional approach to the treatment or prevention of cancer and present a potential breakthrough in cancer research."[419]

- A study on wheat grass showed that it caused the **inhibition of Carcinogens**. "These results are of interest for two reasons: first, the inhibition of activation of potent carcinogens is quite strong at a reasonably low level of extract and second, the wheat sprout extract is nontoxic even at high levels while most known inhibitors are toxic at medium to high levels."[420]

- **Chlorophyll is non-toxic**: Toxicity studies [421] [422] [423] have shown that chlorophyll is absolutely non-toxic when administered parenterally (intravenous or intramuscular) or by mouth to animal and humans. *Rev. Gastroentology; American Journal Surgery; Am. J. Med. Soc.*

- "In hundreds of experiments and trials on humans and animals, chlorophyll therapy has always been shown to have **no toxic side effects**. Not just low toxicity. NO toxicity – whether ingested, injected or rubbed onto a surface. This fact alone makes chlorophyll one of the most unique therapeutic substances known to medical science."[424]

- Chlorophyll heals wounds ... **stimulates repair of damaged tissues and inhibits growth of bacteria**. Medical literature is replete with reports demonstrating these effects. Surface wounds and sores due to surgery, compound fractures, osteomyelitis (bone inflammation), decubitus (bed sores), and routine cuts and scrapes all show fast and dramatic improvement with the topical use of chlorophyll. Chlorophyll therapy has saved limbs from amputation."[425]

- D.H. Collings proved that chlorophyll therapy has a **shorter healing time of wounds**, shorter than with vitamin D, sulfanilamide, penicillin, or no treatment.[426]

- **Burns caused by heat, chemicals, and radiation heal faster** with chlorophyll therapy, whether or not they are infected. Chlorophyll was used to prolong the survival of skin grafts before the development of immune-suppressing drugs which are now used."[427]

- Chlorophyll has also been shown to be extremely effective in **speeding the healing of peptic ulcers**, wounds which develop internally in the gastrointestinal tract. Several studies document the use of chlorophyll in the treatment of ulcers resistant to more conventional therapies. The results are quite impressive."[428]

- "Chlorophyll tended to '**promote regularity**' in the patients studied. According to several investigators, chlorophyll did not act simply to stimulate bowel activity, as does a laxative. Rather, it promoted bowel regularity, stimulating bowel action only when the action was sluggish."[429]
- "Japanese researchers have discovered a protein – P4-D1 – in barley grass juice that seems to protect cells from ultraviolet radiation and a specific carcinogen. This was said to be a result of the stimulation of DNA repair by this protein. Both the protein and another in barley grass juice – D1-G1 – have been shown to have **anti-inflammatory activity** when injected into lab animals. In addition, both these barley compounds are remarkably free from side effects."[430]
- Dr. Asaf Qureshi, a food consultant with the U.S. Department of Agriculture, did a study (1977) in which he "isolated an active compound in barley that suppressed the liver's ability to make cholesterol. This inhibitor is called tocotrienol – or Inhibitor 1, and two other inhibitors were found. These were found present in barley, rye and oats. All three inhibitors in barley deactivate an enzyme in the liver needed to make cholesterol. And **they suppressed the liver's ability to make LDL, the 'bad' cholesterol** which clogs the arteries, yet the 'good' cholesterol, HDL levels, remained intact. These three inhibitors in barley are also found in lesser amounts in other grains and vegetables."[431]
- In a study, "Israeli scientists tried substituting barley flour for wheat flour in biscuits and scones and gave them to 19 patients suffering from chronic constipation. Each patient was asked to eat three of the four barley biscuits a day. Fifteen of them (79%) became completely **free of constipation, had less gas and abdominal pain, and quit taking laxatives**. When they were deprived of these barley foods, virtually all the group became constipated and went back to laxatives within a month."[432]
- There is no gluten in barley grass and it can be used safely by people with gluten intolerance (celiac disease). Also the "chlorophyll in **barley grass dilutes and enhances the elimination of gluten** from the digestive system, according to one expert. According to John Heinerman, certain allergy specialists in southern California have been recommending green barley-juice powder, mixed with distilled water, to many of their gluten-sensitive patients."[433]

It is unbelievable that chlorophyll can be so beneficial and healing. The article, 'Chlorophyll Supporter of all Human and Animal Life, (2010)'[434] which is an excellent historical overview of chlorophyll. In addition to its critical role in photosynthesis, chlorophyll is also a great indicator of the health attributes of foods. The deeper the green color of a plant food, the richer the food is in chlorophyll – and the more abundant the food is in health-building qualities. Foods rich in chlorophyll can play a role in blood production[435] and protection from cancer[436][437] and from the side effects and damage of radiation.[438][439] Chlorophyll also has many therapeutic uses. Among these are wound healing,[440] intestinal regularity,[441] cholesterol reduction,[442] detoxification and deodorization. Chlorophyll is an especially unique way to address these issues because, through hundreds of experiments and trials on humans and test animals, chlorophyll therapy has always been shown to have no toxicity (absolutely zero toxic side effects) – whether ingested, injected or rubbed onto your skin.[443] The article also notes:

- Studies indicated that feeding chlorophyll-rich foods to rats triggered the **regeneration of red blood cells**.[444] Researchers demonstrated that this effect was not due to the iron or copper in the green foods.
- Dr. Rothemund discovered that porphyrins from chlorophyll **stimulated the synthesis of red blood cells** in a variety of animals when fed in small doses.[445]
- Drs. Hughes study suggested, "the chlorophyll is acting as a physiological stimulant of the bone marrow and is not really concerned with the actual chemistry of regeneration of the porphyrin."[446] This study shows that chlorophyll found in food or very small purified amounts of chlorophyll **may stimulate the synthesis of red blood cells in the bone marrow**.
- Dr. Arthur Patek conducted a study in which fifteen patients with iron-deficiency anemia were fed different amounts of chlorophyll along with iron. Iron alone had already been shown to reverse this condition, but Patek demonstrated that when chlorophyll and iron were given together **the number of red blood cells and level of blood hemoglobin increased faster** than with iron alone. As stated by Dr. Patek, "This study may serve to encourage the use of a diet ample in greenstuffs and protein foods, for it must be that over a long space of time favorably nutritious elements are absorbed which aid the blood reserve and which furnish building stones for the heme pigments necessary to the formation of hemoglobin."[447][448]
- Research indicates that some porphyrins (ringed structures in heme and chlorophyll) **stimulate the synthesis of globin (the protein portion of the hemoglobin molecule)**. This could

partially explain the effect of chlorophyll on hemoglobin synthesis.[449] Essential nutrients for the maintenance of healthy blood include iron, copper, calcium, and vitamins C, B-12, K, A, folic acid, and pyridoxine, among others. Many of these blood-building components are found in chlorophyll rich foods such as cereal glasses (wheat, oats, barley, etc.) and dark green vegetables.

- Scientific evidence has shown that chlorophyll and the nutrients found in green foods **offer protection against toxic chemicals and radiation**. In 1980, Dr. Chiu Nan Lai at the University of Texas Medical Center reported that extracts of wheatgrass and other green vegetables inhibit the cancer-causing effects of two mutagens (benzopyrene and methylcholanthrene).[450] The more chlorophyll in the vegetable, the greater the protection from the carcinogen.

- Chlorophyll can reduce the ability of carcinogens to cause gene mutations, as shown in several laboratory studies. Chlorophyll-rich plant extracts, as well as water solutions of a chlorophyll derivative (chloropyllin), dramatically **inhibit the carcinogenic effects of common dietary and environmental chemicals**.[451] [452]

- Green vegetables provide protection from radiation damage in test animals. This information has been reported in scientific literature dating back to the early 1950's. Reports showed that certain vegetables significantly reduced mortality in rats exposed to lethal doses of X-rays.[453] Dark green broccoli offered more protection than the lighter green cabbage. In the later study, the same vegetables were shown to **reduce the damage caused by radiation**.[454] These protective effects were more pronounced when even darker green vegetables such as mustard greens and alfalfa leaves were used. When two or more of the green vegetables were fed together, the positive resistance to radiation was greatest.

- Chlorophyllin is a semi-synthetic sodium/copper derivative of chlorophyll. It has been used for over 50 years as a food additive and alternative medicine because it has a longer shelf life than natural chlorophyll and it cost less than some forms of natural chlorophyll. A 2005 study was conducted in the Netherlands to compare the effects of chlorophyll and chlorophyllin. While chlorophyllin has exhibited some of the same benefits as natural chlorophyll, **this study shows that the natural option has an overwhelming advantage in at least one application**. The best way to incorporate more natural chlorophyll in your diet and reap all its wonderful health benefits is through green foods. When you eat fresh, organic, chlorophyll-rich foods and drink their juices, you're getting the best of the best. Growing your own cereal grasses and juicing

202

them costs pennies, and these foods are the richest in chlorophyll."[455]

c. Normal Healthy pH

The body needs to be kept in its normal alkaline pH range. Degenerative diseases thrive when the body is acidic, which is usually caused by all the acidic foods we eat. The standard American meat-based diet is extremely acidic; plant-based diets are very alkaline.

Robert Young, PhD, DSc (Microbiology and Nutrition), is an expert on acidity: "Multiple Sclerosis, Parkinson's, Alzheimer's, ALS are all inflammatory diseases. Inflammation is just another word for acidity that affects the central nervous system and causes a variety of symptoms including changes in sensation, visual problems, muscle weakness, depression, speech and coordination difficulties, severe fatigue, short-term memory loss, balance impairment, overheating and pain."[456]

"Thus, what is said to be MS, Parkinson's Alzheimer's, or ALS is a misunderstanding of the body's alkaline design and acidic function and the use of a throwback catch-all diagnostic category when no other present-day medically-accepted explanation or category seems to fit. Every cell in the body regenerates itself over time, especially when the body receives the proper nutritional resources. This means that the body must have plenty of living waters and foods like green vegetables and healthy fats which not only neutralize acids but provide the raw materials for building new red blood cells and, therefore, bodily cells which also include the rebuilding of nerves and the myelin sheath."[457]

Robert Young, PhD continues, "The human body requires efficient digestion and proper elimination in order to maintain health and energy. Excellent health is supported by an abundance of friendly plants (bacteria/ flora) living in the intestines. It is the consumption of animal food products, junk and processed food, chemicals, prescription and over-the-counter medicines, over-eating, and excess stress of all forms, all which compromise digestion. This disrupts and weakens the friendly flora. In turn, this causes the development of our inherent Yeast/Fungus, which is normally held in check."

"Certain drugs, including steroids, antibiotics, birth control pills and cortisone, plus chronic infections, poor nutrition, prolonged illness, emotional stress, alcohol abuse, smoking, lack of exercise and rest - all these make great demands on immune response and weaken it. One of the worst offenders is antibiotics, which play a major role in the encouragement of Y/F (yeast, fungus), by disturbing the intestinal flora and suppressing the immune system response."[458]

Gabriel Cousens, MD also promotes this theory, along with other experts like Dr. Antoine Bechamp, Professor Gunther Enderlein, Dietrich Klinghardt, MD, PhD, and Robert Young, PhD. In his 2003 book, *Rainbow Green Live Food Cuisine*, Dr. Cousens points out that, "The *microzymas* (which are ferments in the blood) are living microscopic and colloidal elements capable of fermenting in the sugar in our system. The *microzyma* is the smallest living unit in nature and in our bodies; it is much smaller than cells."[459] This became the basis of the Biological Terrain Theory, with the key motto as: "Germs don't cause disease; they develop in a diseased environment. The cornerstone of Bechamp's theory was that maintaining a healthy terrain and biological physiology is the key to health. When the biological terrain was disrupted, when people got too acid, then the natural fermentation process in the body was accelerated, and a morbid evolution of these microzymas would take place. They would coagulate and pleomophically permutate into bacteria, yeast, fungus, and eventually mold. As these morbid pleomorphic forms from the microzymas developed, they fed on our vital body substances and produced more toxins, which we call mycotoxins. This toxic process resulted in a degenerative disease symptomology."[460]

d. A Low-glycemic Approach

Gabriel Cousens, MD, in his book *Rainbow Green Live-Food Cuisine*, (2003) he acknowledges the influences of Robert Young, PhD and his book, *Sick and Tired*, which emphasized a diet that is low in fungus and mycotoxins (toxins produced by fungus) is best for our overall health. Dr. Cousens had been studying this pleomorphic science for ten years plus. This diet of a low-glycemic fruit, vegetable, nut, seed, sea vegetable, algae-based diet, helped people make remarkable changes in their health and energy levels. Dr. Cousens wrote in the introduction: "As I looked at the results, I could not help but say, 'We need to make some changes' because most of the live-food preparation in North America certainly includes a fair amount of natural sweets. Sweet foods, which have a high glycemic index even if they are natural and raw, are still very mycosis-producing."[461]

"The process of chronic disease is activated in a person who is toxic enough to push the 'composting button' (The acceleration of the rate of fermentation). Depending on the degree of toxicity, this composting process leads to chronic disease, misery, and ultimately death. The key to restoring health is minimizing or eliminating the toxic conditions so that the composting button is turned off. A low sweet, live-food, non-acidic diet and a healthy mind are the key factors in turning off the composting button and reestablishing vibrant health. These reverse the forces of entropy or composting."[462]

Foods to Avoid for Optimal Health[463]
Rainbow Green Live-Food Cuisine

All cooked foods	Corn
All processed foods including:	Yeast
canned, microwaved, refined,	Alcohol
non-organic, GMO foods	Coffee
All animal products:	Caffeine
fish, dairy, eggs	Tobacco
Grains: wheat, barley, oats,	Heated oil (except coconut)
etc. (except non-stored grains)	All soy products including
White potatoes, white rice,	nama shoyu
white flour	Mushrooms
Sugar, honey, maple syrup,	Peanuts and cashews
artificial sweeteners,	Cottonseed
fructose, maltose	Bottled fruit juices

Dr. Cousens, in *Rainbow Green Live-Food Cuisine,* gives glycemic levels and foods to avoid for optimum health. These Foods to Avoid, could also be recommended for those with neurological diseases. Parkinson's and Alzheimer's patients should focus on moderate and low glycemic foods and only eat small amounts of high glycemic foods. A cooked carbohydrate has a higher glycemic index because the starches are broken down into simple sugars. These cooked carbohydrates could become fuel for the PD and Alzheimer's fungus and bacteria conditions. The high glycemic foods when raw are not going to feed neurological diseases because their sugars (which are raw and thus molecularly different then cooked) are not going to feed these diseases.

Foods to Avoid for Optimal Health
Rainbow Green Live-Food Cuisine[464]

- First category: Cooked and Processed foods including, canned, micro-waved, refined, GMO foods.
- Second category: all Animal Products, including animal flesh, dairy, and eggs.

- Third category: Grain products such as wheat, barley, oats, corn, white potatoes, white rice, white flour.
- Fourth category: Sweeteners: sugar, honey, artificial sweeteners, maple syrup, fructose, and maltose.
- Fifth category: heated oils, except coconut oil.
- Sixth category: beverages including alcohol, coffee, caffeine, all soda, carbonated beverages, and bottled pasteurized fruit juices.
- Seventh category: yeast, brewer's yeast, nutritional yeast, all soy products including Nama Shoyu, mushrooms, peanuts, cashews and cottonseed oil.

e. Brain-fats and Neurological Diseases

In the book, *Brain Building Nutrition* (2007),[465] Michael A. Schmidt, PhD, points out the profound influence of how the brain and nervous system are influenced by the various kinds of fats. "Over the past 100 years, the types of fat we consume have changed dramatically. By some estimates, the amount of brain-fats we consume has declined by more than 80 percent.[466] This occurred because many of us switched to animal fats, warm-weather vegetable oils, and processed foods. We once consumed a balance of fat of approximately one to one. Today, scientists estimate the ratio to be as high as thirty to one."[467]

"The dietary ratio of omega-6 to omega-3 fatty acids were once approximately 1:1. Modern diets have a ratio of as high as 30:1. The breast milk of some women contains a ratio of as high as 45:1. The brain's requirement for highly specific fats, coupled with the poor dietary choices of most people living on modern diets, has us on a collision course with ourselves. We now have powerful evidence that millions of people in all walks of life consume a diet of fats that is not at all conducive to building a complex, superbly functioning brain and nervous system."[468]

One expert on the brain wrote that fatty acids and phospholipids have been associated with a surprising number of disorders of the brain, he stated, "In reviewing several thousand research papers, hundreds of lab profiles, Magnetic Resonance Imaging (MRI) reports, and case studies, we have totaled more than fifty conditions of the brain that involve fatty acids or have responded to fatty acid treatment. The following is a partial list to show the great promise for solving difficult problems. It also shows the potential for things to go wrong if we do not pay attention to proper fatty acid balance.'"[469]

Aggression	Phobia (fears)	Hostility
Alzheimer's disease	Postpartum depression	Learning disability
Anorexia nervosa	Rage	Lower IQ
Attention deficit	Reading problems	School failure
Autism	Retinal disease	Slower information processing
Bipolar disorder	Schizophrenia	
Brain tumor (glioma)	Developmental delay	Slower reaction time
Cerebral palsy	Depression	
Chronic fatigue	Diabetic retinopathy, neuropathy	Stroke (prevention, recovery)
Memory problems		
Migraine		
Multiple sclerosis	Down's syndrome	Suicide
Paresthesia	Drug abuse	Tremors
Parkinson's disease	Hyperactivity	Violence
	Head Injury	Zellweger's syndrome (and others)

Both MS and Parkinson's are affected by this issue. Dr. Julian Whitaker, MD, writes about the breakthrough discovery that Medium Chain Triglycerides (MCT's) that are found in coconut oil had a very salutary effect on restoring brain function. Dr. Whitaker recommends coconut oil for other neuro-degenerative diseases such as Parkinson's disease, Dementia, Multiple Sclerosis and ALS (Lou Gehrig's disease). Coconut oil could be used for the millions who currently suffer, from Alzheimer's disease, Parkinson's disease, Huntington's Chorea (disease), Multiple Sclerosis, ALS, Type I and Type II diabetes, as well as any number of other conditions that involve a defect in transport of glucose into neurons and other cells. Numerous studies can be cited for the connection with these diseases which could benefit from a product like coconut oil.[470]

f. L-Dopa in Seedlings, Pods, and Beans

Some foods have been shown helpful such as those that are discussed in a study that identified L-Dopa in the seedlings, pods, and beans of the broad bean, Vicia faba. The researcher "identified L-DOPA in the seedlings, pods, and beans of the broad bean, Vicia faba (VF). Since then, anecdotal cases of symptomatic improvement after VF consumption have been described in patients with PD. In the present study ... these data show that VF ingestion produces a substantial increase in L-DOPA plasma levels, which correlates with a substantial improvement in motor performance. Our findings may have implications for the treatment of PD, especially in patients with mild symptoms."[471]

Another study indicated that food can be associated with PD development: "In a case-control study, we compared the past dietary habits of 342 Parkinson's disease (PD) patients recruited from nine German clinics with those of 342 controls from the same neighborhood or region. ... These results suggest that the intake of certain foods may be associated with the development of PD."[472]

209

g. Early Jewish and Christian Communities

Professor Kalechofsky, PhD writes: "With the fall of Jerusalem in 70 C.E. came the destruction of the Temple and the disappearance of priestly slaughterers. ... A central feature of some of these ascetic groups (Nazarites, Rechabites, Essenes, Therapeutae, and Zakokites) was abstinence from the eating of meat."[473]

Rabbi Gabriel Cousens, MD wrote, "There were different sects back in the times of the early Christians. The Encratites were early Christian ascetics whose ideal was self-control. The name Encratites is derived from the Greek meaning self-control, which is alongside love, joy, peace, as a fruit of the Spirit.[m] This sect was a strict vegan community. Clement of Alexandria wrote, 'It is far better to be happy than to have our bodies act as graveyards for animals.'"[474]

In the *Encyclopedia of the Early Church*, the Church Fathers[475] wrote that certain groups abstained from particular foods: Encratites, Ebionites, Marcionites, Manichaeans, Priscillianists, who seem to have considered Jesus a vegetarian.[476] Origen says that these Jews who have received Jesus Christ were all called by the name "Ebionites."[477] And St. Epipanius (ca. 350) writes that "the Ebionite Sect was in existence (35 CE)."[478] Bishop Epiphanius (A.D. 315-403) of Constantia in Cyprus, in his book *Panarion*[479] states, "Whenever you speak to them (Ebionites) concerning flesh food, the Ebionites reply they were vegetarian because 'Christ revealed it to me.'"[480] This is another reference connecting the Ebionites as a vegetarian group, to the early Christians as vegetarians.

---

[m] (Gal 5:23; cf. 1 Cor 7:9, 9:25; Ti 1:8; Ac 24:25; 2 Pt 1:6)

According to the *Encyclopedia of the Dead Sea Scrolls* it writes: "In the second and third centuries, the church fathers Irenaeus (c. 130-200 CE), Clement of Alexandria (c. 150-215 CE) and Hippolytus (c. 170-236 CE) applied that name Encratites to a diverse array of early Christian groups adopting ascetic practices such as celibacy, abstinence from wine, and vegetarianism. Particularly important is an organized Jewish-Christian community that, according to Irenaeus,[481] was founded in the latter part of the second century in Mesopotamia by Tatian."[482]

Tatian was a pupil of Justin Martyr (c. 100-165 CE) and author of the Diatessaron (a famous harmony of the four canonical Gospels). Justin Martyr was involved in Christianity during the beginning of the early Church and surely would have known the Apostle John. The Encratite community that Tatian founded was vegetarian which means that Justin was probably a vegetarian himself or at least approved of it. This is significant to have this witness on vegetarianism so close to the original Christian community in Jerusalem. The connection here is important. Tatian was a disciple of Justin Martyr. Justin was probably a disciple of the Apostle John, and John took care of Mary, which implies that perhaps Justin, John and Mary were vegetarian or at least approved of it!

Chapter 10

Milk and Dairy Products are Problematic

St. Francis of Assisi died in 1226 and lived a life of purification and penance. One day a Franciscan brother was languishing of hunger from fasting too much and St. Francis of Assisi, set the table and they began to eat. After eating, St. Francis commented: "To deprive the body indiscreetly of what it needs is a sin just the same as it is a sin to give it superfluous things at the prompting of gluttony."[483] What the Bible calls 'the king's delicacies,' St. Francis called 'superfluous things,' and today we call these junk foods.

a. The Blood-Brain Barrier

Milk and dairy products are one of the worst things for people with neurological diseases, like Parkinson's and MS to consume. Heavy metals, toxins, poisons, and pesticides attach themselves to molecules in milk and dairy products, and they piggy-back across the blood-brain barrier, tricking the blood-brain barrier to allow heavy metals, toxins, poisons, and pesticides inside the brain.

Robert Hatherhill PhD in his book *BrainGate*, explains that studies show that milk consumption increases lead and cadmium absorption. "The main protein in milk, casein, has been shown to increase lead levels in the brains, liver, and kidneys of animals. Researchers have not determined why this happens, but it is possible that heavy metals piggyback on the amino acids in milk to get access to the brain. Milk fat also increases uptake of lead and other environmental pollutants."[484]

There are numerous reasons besides carrying heavy metals, toxins, poisons, and pesticides across the blood-brain barrier to avoid dairy products. Another major reason is that the denatured proteins in the brain are animal proteins (double- helix bonds) and that includes milk proteins. These deformed proteins are a major source of irritation and destruction of the brain cells, and the creation of Lewy bodies and scarring in the brain.

Dr. Cook points out, "lead blocks the formation of hormones like dopamine and serotonin. Mental functions such as impulse control and managing violent behaviors depend on adequate production of both of these hormones. At least seven studies have shown that violent criminals have elevated levels of lead, cadmium, manganese, mercury, and other metals in their blood, compared with prisoners who are not violent. Lead is also linked with progressive mental decline."[485]

Pesticides are also a factor in Parkinson's and possibly MS. The author Sandra Steingraber, PhD wrote, "The largest contributors to daily intake of chlorinated insecticides are dairy products, meat, fish and poultry."[486]

An article in the *Journal of Animal Science*, reported: "The lipophilic nature of dioxins results in higher concentrations in the fat of animal and fish products, and their excretion via milk secretion in dairy cattle may result in relatively high concentrations of dioxin contamination." The United Press International reported, "Dioxins are the most deadly substances ever assembled by man… 170,000 times as deadly as cyanide."[487]

b. Increased Osteoporosis Risk

Research presented at the American Academy of Neurology (2006) pointed out that, people with Parkinson's and Alzheimer's disease are at increased risk of developing osteoporosis.[488] Osteoporosis is the loss of bone mass that leads to increased risk of fractures. A study of 166 Parkinson's disease patients found that 51 percent of the female patients had osteoporosis; the rate of osteoporosis among women of the same age without Parkinson's is about 25 percent. Among the males with Parkinson's disease, 29 percent had osteoporosis, compared with about seven percent of men without Parkinson's. Large percentages of the Parkinson patients also had osteopenia, which is low bone mass, which puts them at risk of developing osteoporosis. Of the women, 45 percent had low bone mass; 48 percent of the men had low bone mass. [489]

There was a major study in the *American Journal of Clinical Nutrition* that found that by the age of 65:

- Male vegetarians had an average measurable bone loss of 3%
- Male meat-eaters had an average measurable bone loss of 7%
- Female vegetarians had an average measurable bone loss of 18%
- Female meat-eaters had an average measurable bone loss of 35%

"In this study, by the time she reaches the age of sixty-five, the average meat-eating woman in the United States has lost over a third of her skeletal structure. In contrast, older vegetarian women tend to remain active, maintain erect postures, and are less likely to fracture or break bones even with their increased physical activity. If their bones do break or fracture, they heal faster and more completely."[490] (Journal of Clinical Nutrition)

The Journal of *Science* points out that: "Osteoporosis is caused by a number of things, one of the most important being too much dietary protein."[491] The *American Journal of Clinical Nutrition* states: "Even when taking in 1400 mg of calcium daily, one can lose up to 4% of his or her bone mass each year while consuming a high-protein diet."[492] The *Nutrition Action Healthletter* notes: "Countries with the highest rates of osteoporosis, such as the U.S., England, and Sweden, consume the most milk."[493]

In a Harvard study of 78,000 women in the *American Journal of Public Health*, "women consuming greater amounts of calcium from dairy foods had significantly increased risks of hip fractures."[494] Other related studies show similar results.

While daily calcium intake is important, numerous studies have clearly demonstrated that too much dietary protein, not too little calcium, is the major cause of osteoporosis. Why? Too much protein causes an excess of hydrogen ions in the blood, which elevates blood acid levels. Because high acid levels can be dangerous, the body "buffers," or neutralizes the blood acid levels by drawing calcium from the bones. The resulting waste products, including calcium, are excreted in the urine.[495] This evidence can be found in various journals including: *American Journal of Clinical Nutrition, Journal of Nutrition, Journal of the American Dietetic Association, and Hospital Practice.*

Another journal author (*Lancet*) states: "Even the most conservative medical investigators no longer deny the connection between excess protein and osteoporosis. In a report published in the British journal *Lancet,* Drs. Aaron Watchman and Daniel Bernstein commented on work sponsored by the United States Department of Health and Harvard University. They called the association of meat-based diets with the increasing incidence of osteoporosis 'inescapable.'"[496]

One doctor who promotes a plant-based dietary approach, Neal Bernard, MD points out, "Animal proteins are high in what are called sulfur-containing amino acids.[497] These acidic protein-building blocks tend to leach calcium from the bones, and that calcium passes through the kidneys and into the urine."[498] [499] "Plant-based proteins contain all the essential amino acids needed for the body. They are far lower in sulfur-containing amino acids, and they help protect your bones."[500]

c. Milk Consumption and PD, AD and MS

In one study (*American Journal of Epidemiology*, 2007), it has been confirmed that a relationship exists between consuming large amounts of dairy products and an increase in the rate of Parkinson's disease in men. Researchers found that among more than 130,000 U.S. adults followed for 9 years, those who ate the largest amount of dairy foods had an increased risk of developing Parkinson's disease. This study and previous ones indicate that calcium, vitamin D and fat are not responsible for the link between dairy foods and Parkinson's disease.[501] So the question is raised if it not the calcium or vitamin D in the milk that is responsible, what is it in the dairy products that contributes to developing this disease?

Every single study in history that has been done on Parkinson's and dairy found that the more dairy products consumed, the higher the risk of getting Parkinson's. So a meta-analysis of all prospective studies on dairy/milk consumption and the risk of Parkinson's disease in men and woman was done and they found that dairy consumption was positively associated with the risk of Parkinson's disease.[502] (*Am J Epidemiol*, 2007)

The Wendt doctrine explains one major factor connecting excess protein consumption to some forms of chronic degenerative disease like MS, AD and PD.[503] The Wendts were able to prove with electron microscope pictures that excess protein clogs the basement membrane, a filtering membrane located between capillaries and cells. It helps regulate the flow of nutrients and waste products between capillaries, cells, and fluid in the tissues they penetrate. Excess protein lodged in the basement membrane results in a thicker basement membrane with clogged pores. It becomes harder for proteins, other nutrients, and even oxygen to get through into the cells and for waste and breakdown products to get out of the cells. This could be a major part of the problem; milk and dairy products would be involved in this build-up leading to MS, AD and to Parkinson's.[504]

There was another study done at the College of Medicine, Korea University, (*Neurology*, 2005) which had the objective of examining the relation between milk and calcium intake in midlife and the risk of Parkinson's disease (PD). The findings suggest that milk intake is associated with an increased risk of Parkinson's disease.[505]

A study on 'Diet and Parkinson's disease: a potential role of dairy products in men' found a higher risk for Parkinson's disease in men with high intakes of dairy products (roughly 3 servings per day). "Positive associations between dairy products and Parkinson's were found for dairy protein, dairy calcium, dairy vitamin D, and lactose, and not for other sources of these nutrients. Researchers suggest that tetrahydroisoquinolines found in dairy products may be a potential cause of this disease, due to their ability to cross the blood–brain barrier and induce degeneration of dopaminergic neurons in experimental models. The presence of dopaminergic neurotoxins, including beta–carbolines and their derivatives, pesticides, and polychlorinated biphenyls found in dairy products, may also be involved."[506] (*Annuals Neurology*, 2002)

One of the national Parkinson's foundations had a Registered Dietitian who wrote a book on nutrition for Parkinson's, *Parkinson's Disease: Nutrition Matters*.[507] The author Kathrynne Holden, MS, RD, did state several times in the book that people with Parkinson's who are sensitive to milk proteins should not drink milk and even those who are not sensitive to milk should not drink milk. She lists several milk alternatives and includes recipes that do not include milk. She covers food drug interactions which can be found in most books on Parkinson's. It is good to see that a nutritionist in the field, knowledgeable about Parkinson's, knows that milk is not a good choice for people with Parkinson's.

d. Neurotoxin's Violent Immune Storm

In his book, *The BrainGate*, Dr. Hatherill, PhD an expert on brain toxins explains:
- Milk increases the uptake of neurotoxic cadmium, mercury, and lead in the brain.
- The milk sugar galactose builds up in the lens of the eye, causing cataracts.
- Dairy products create an increased risk of diabetes. Diabetics are developing more serious nervous system problems, such as dementia.
- The high fat content of dairy products leads to increased intake of neurotoxic environmental chemicals like PCB and dioxin.
- Milk causes leaky gut, which does not support optimal brain health.
- Milk intake increases heart disease risk, which ultimately impacts brain function."[508]

These are further reasons that could make the Parkinson's, MS and milk/dairy connection, especially the intake of neurotoxic environmental chemicals like PCB and dioxin. Another reason is that milk increases the uptake of neurotoxic cadmium, mercury, and lead in the brain. All of this creates the neurotoxin's violent immune storm in the body which is another cause and continuation of MS and PD.

Dr. Robert O. Young, PhD, D.Sc., a biochemist and raw vegan nutrition expert, has suggested that dairy products are some of the most toxic or acidic foods one can eat and should be eliminated from any diet in order to maintain the alkaline design of the human body.[509]

Dr. Young states "that animal proteins in foods cause the immune system to react exactly the same way it does to the protein coat of bacteria, and other infectious agents. The

218

resulting antibody production results in an 'immune storm,' which (hopefully) destroys the infectious agents, but may also result in such a large overreaction of the immune system that the excess antibodies start going after healthy tissue. If the animal proteins in foods, e.g., hamburgers, milk, cheese, etc., cause the same violent immune storm and end up breaking healthy tissue (especially in older people), it could explain a whole host of autoimmune diseases which are increasing without explanation, e.g., Lupus, MS, Type II diabetes, and others."[510]

According to the microbiologist Dr. Robert Young, "An increase in lactose (a sugar) from dairy products, especially cheese and ice cream, increases the lactic acid in the body which ferments in the bowels, the blood and the brain, leading to Parkinson's and other neurological diseases. He points out, the idea that dairy products are healthy is pure hype and a cultural myth. While cheese is a product of fermentation, dairy foods also contain residues of hormones and fungally-based antibiotics, as well as yeast, fungus, mold, and mycotoxins because cows are fed stored grains. Dairy is also the leader of all foods in being mucoid-forming. It just gums you up. In addition, milk, and especially cheese contain lactose (milk sugar). Eight ounces of milk have approximately twelve grams of lactose that can break down into yeast, fungus - feeding sugars. If all that isn't enough, pasteurization (based on the fast germ theory) destroys any enzymes that might be there to begin with, and makes the milk 'sick.' Sick milk will rot and stink if left out, proving that pasteurization doesn't even work (can't kill microzymas), whereas raw milk will curdle naturally, and is still 'edible.' Last, but not least, dairy is highly acid-forming. This is all part of the immune storm attacking the body."[511]

The late Dr. Frank A. Oski, MD, Director, Department of Pediatrics, John Hopkins School of Medicine states: "It is estimated that half the iron-deficiency in infants in the United States is primarily a result of cow's milk inducing gastrointestinal bleeding. This is a staggering figure when one realizes that approximately 15 to 20 percent of all children under the age of two in this country suffer from iron-deficiency anemia. The resultant iron-deficiency anemia makes the child irritable, apathetic, and inattentive. The infant cries a great deal, the mother gives a bottle of milk to soothe him, and the condition continues to get worse."[512]

"Diarrhea and cramps, gastrointestinal bleeding, iron-deficiency anemia, skin rashes, atherosclerosis, and acne. These are disorders that have been linked to the drinking of whole cow's milk. As well as recurrent ear infections and bronchitis. Leukemia, multiple sclerosis, rheumatoid arthritis, and simple dental decay have also been proposed as other disorders that are related to consumption of dairy products. In one study on the causes of MS in the US and 21 other nations, the only significant link was between multiple sclerosis and average milk consumption."[513]

The *British Medical Journal* stated, 'Vegetarians often have lower mortality rates from several chronic degenerative diseases than do non-vegetarians.'[514] Many other journal studies make similar statements about chronic and degenerative diseases.

Some studies have linked milk consumption to children's developing type I diabetes.[515] Chickens are fed progesterone to help them grow fasters and cows are fed synthetic hormones, such as recombinant bovine growth hormone (rBGH) or insulin growth factor-1 (IGF-1).[516] Other contaminants found in milk are antibiotics, pesticides, polychlorinated biphenyls (PCBs), and dioxins.

The average American drinks and eats 29.2 ounces per day of milk and dairy products or about 666 pounds per year![517] Milk and meat products creates an internal mental "fog" that has been noticed by some people. Upon getting off these and cleaning out the body the internal "fog" will lift. Going back to the standard American diet the internal "sludge" and mental "fog" and old health problems and symptoms usually return.

In the vegetarian literature there are more scientific reasons as to why a person should not drink cow's milk. But milk relates directly to Parkinson's, in which those suffering from it have an excess of lead (or other heavy metals) in the brain, partly caused by dairy. Another interesting fact is that depleted uranium is 15x higher in milk. When after the Chenobal disaster in 1986, there was a 900% increase in prenatal mortality. How did that happen? Because I-131 uranium went up into the stratosphere, landed in the grass, the cows ate the grass and the women drank the milk and were affected by radiation.[518]

e. Do not eat of any of the fat

Keep in mind that there is the prohibition against eating dairy products with red meat in Scripture. (Ex 23.19, 34.26; Deut 14.21) Also, whole milk has animal fat; "Say to the Israelites: 'Do not eat of any of the fat of cattle, sheep or goats.'" Lev 7:23.

Gluttony is a major sin of commission. Milk and dairy products are the wrong types of foods for chronic diseases. The sin of omission is found in the book of James which states: 'To know good and not to do it, for him it is a sin.'" (James 4:17) As people of the Lord we have our 'Daily Duty' to take responsibility for our body.

Chapter 11

Meat-based Diets Clog Membranes

St. Francis of Paola (1416 to 1507) was a miracle working hermit back in in Spain. When he established a religious order he had the traditional vows of perpetual poverty, chastity, and obedience a fourth vow of abstinence from meat and animal products was taken. "Furthermore, as additional penance, he required the acceptance of perpetual fasting and complete abstinence from meat, eggs, milk, and all other animal food stuffs, except in case of illness - when a physician might prescribe a change in diet for the duration of the condition under treatment.[519] St. Francis of Paola was a vegetarian, and he even required the priests of his order to live a plant-based lifestyle. St. Francis of Paola cured the sick, raised the dead, prophesied the future, walked on water, was an influence on seven Popes and five kings, founded an order of hermits that eventually established about 500 monasteries. He died at the age of 91 and was canonized just 12 years after his death.[520]

a. Plant-based Protein is Healthy

Dean Ornish MD, published his famous study and book back in the early 1990's about reversing heart disease through a vegetarian diet, which did include eggs. He has debated Dr. Atkins several times in public on the issue of meat vs. plant-based diets. He noted that these were interesting debates, but they didn't accomplish much and were, in some ways, a waste of time, because people are set in their ways, their desires.

The journal studies show that a vegan diet is the only diet that has helped Parkinson's. This would also apply to Alzheimer's, which is very similar.

The protein issue is one of the most common topics that come up and it's one of the most misunderstood. A person can get all the protein they need on a vegetarian diet and a higher quality of protein too. All the requirements of the RDA and more can be met on a plant-based diet.

There is a long involved history behind the recommended daily allowance (RDA). The RDA is really a compromise between the government and industry. Back in the 1970's, the NIH and others did a lot of research on how much protein a person really needs and came up with the figure of 36 grams per day for the average 150 pound male; one non-government study showed 35 grams. The European studies done at the famous Max Plank institute in Germany showed 30 grams per day. Studies of the Hunzas, one of the longest lived cultures of people in the world showed 28-30 grams per day, and other studies indicate lower figures. So the US government took its 35 gram figure and bumped it up to 42 grams to add a safety factor in, which really wasn't needed. Then in the early 1980's, the government had public discussions and the meat and dairy industry got involved and by the end of the discussions the recommended amount was bumped up to 54 grams, which is close to the figure today. So the governments' figures are much higher than what is actually needed because of politics.

In separate research programs, Ragnar Berg, the well-known Swedish nutritionist, and D.V.O. Siven in Finland both concluded that 30 grams of protein per day is sufficient for good health.[521] Dr. Hegsted from Harvard University and Dr. Kuratsuen from Japan independently determined that 25-30 grams is sufficient. Dr. K. Eimer found that when athletes reduced their protein intake from 100 grams of animal protein per day to 50 grams of vegetable protein, their performance improved. Dr. Chittenden, in extensive studies on soldiers and athletes, found that 30-50 grams per day is sufficient for maximum physical performance."[522]

It is also interesting to note that the average protein concentration in mother's milk is just 1.4 percent, sufficient to supply the human organism with all the essential amino acids and protein needed during the period of most rapid growth and brain development.[523] Apes, considerably stronger than humans, live on a fruitarian diet that averages between 0.2 and 2.2 percent protein, equivalent to the protein concentration in human breast milk. Based on this humans would only need 12-15 grams but 20-25 for raw fooders has been noted. Thus 30 to 35 grams normative.

There is some evidence that high protein diets can be the cause or influence brain diseases like Parkinson's, MS, Alzheimer's or Schizophrenia. The Russians have had some interesting success in treating schizophrenia with fasting and low-protein vegetarian diets. Although they have made a clear connection between a high-animal-protein diet and certain types of schizophrenia, the exact causes are not clear.[524] This evidence concerning schizophrenia could also be applied to Parkinson's, Alzheimer's and Multiple Sclerosis, since these diseases are related brain diseases. The nutrition therapy for both PD, AD and MS needs to be a low protein diet. In the literature those who have been cured of PD and MS were on low-protein diets, primarily plant-based diets and their diets were in the Live-Food Nutrition Zone.[525]

The higher the temperature and the longer you cook meats, the more they become denatured. Proteins start to become denatured over 150 degrees, that is why pasteurization tries to stay under 150 degrees. One study showed that when you fry two eggs about 50% of the protein is denatured and you're only getting the amount of protein from one egg. Protein goes through a change when it is cooked. Protein is destroyed above 150 degrees. At this temperature the chemical body and structure of protein is 'de-natured,' and once this happens, there is nothing we can do to 'un-de-nature' protein.

One scholar wrote: "The presence of connective tissue in muscle [animal meat] is undesirable from the standpoint of its use as food. The proteins collagen and elastin are not 'complete' in terms of nutritive value. They do not contain all the essential amino acids."[526] People always associate animal meat with a complete protein. It is a second rate protein, plant-based proteins are first rate proteins.

b. Excess Protein Clogs Membranes

Excess protein negatively influences chronic degenerative disease. The Wendt doctrine, is a result of thirty years of research by Wendt, Wendt, and Wendt, a family of physician researchers, who have now received formal recognition by nutritional scientists in Germany. It explains one major factor connecting excess protein consumption to some forms of chronic degenerative disease.[527]

Dr. Gabriel Cousens writes, "The Wendts were able to prove with electron microscope pictures that excess protein clogs the basement membrane, a filtering membrane located between capillaries and cells. It helps regulate the flow of nutrients and waste products between capillaries, cells, and fluid in the tissues they penetrate. Excess protein lodges in the basement membrane, resulting in a thicker basement membrane /clogged pores. It becomes harder for proteins, other nutrients, and even oxygen to get through into the cells and also harder for waste and breakdown products to get out of the cells. Eventually, the basement membrane becomes so clogged with excess protein that the cells on the inside of the capillary walls begin to store and secrete the excess protein in insoluble forms that accumulate on the inside of the capillaries and arteriole walls, causing atherosclerosis, hypertension, adult-onset diabetes, and what the Wendts term capillarogenic tissue degeneration, the result of clogged basement membranes all over the system."[528]

"This clogged basement membrane produces cellular malnutrition and results in the anoxia of the tissues. According to Dr. Steven Levine's hypothesis, anoxia is the cause of all degenerative diseases.[529] The key understanding is that excess protein in the diet results in a protein storage disease that slowly chokes off the system. It is much harder to meditate when one is choking on a cellular level and the vitality of the system is slowly dying out. The Wendts found that this whole process could be reversed by stopping the intake of all animal protein for one to three months, and by eating a low-protein diet or by doing extensive fasting."[530]

In terms of metabolic combustion, excess protein in the diet does not "burn cleanly." It has been associated with creating acidity, because of the accumulation of toxic protein metabolic wastes such as uric acids and purines in the tissues. A hypothesis of Dr. Airola who points out that overeating protein 'contributes to the development of many of our most common and serious diseases, such as arthritis, kidney damage, pyorrhea, schizophrenia, osteoporosis, atherosclerosis, heart disease, and cancer" and that a 'high-protein diet causes premature aging and lowers life expectancy."[531] A high-protein diet increases the rate of amyloid deposit in the cells. Amyloid is a by-product of protein metabolism that is deposited in connective tissues and organs. It has definitely been linked with tissue and organ degeneration and premature aging."[532]

c. Animal Protein Pathogenic Microorganisms

It should be noted that the average American meal of animal products contains 750,000,000 - 1,000,000,000 pleomorphic pathogenic microorganisms per meal (US Department of Agriculture).[533] The average vegetarian meal, consisting of only plant food has less than 500 pleomorphic pathogenic microorganisms per meal. The body's defense system can easily handle this low amount, but the higher amounts indicated above for animal products are problematic especially for neurological diseases like Parkinson's, MS,

Alzheimer's or ALS. A plant-based diet is obviously healthier because it contains less pathogenic microorganisms per meal. These are unhealthy microorganisms, something the body does not need or want. The brain also does not need or want this influence which could lead to numerous problems such as fungi in the brain and Lewy bodies found in Parkinson's and MS. Let us look at this chart.

This chart shows Animal Foods for acceptable sale per U.S. Department of Agriculture[n]

- Milk, Grade A Pasteurized: 20,000 microorganisms/ pathogens per gram, or 5,000,000 per cup.
- Butter: 300,000 to 1,000,000 microorganisms/ pathogens per gram, or 7,000,000 per patty.
- Cheese: 300,000 to 1,000,000 microorganisms/ pathogens per gram, or 100,000,000 per serving.
- Ice Cream: 300,000 to 1,000,000 microorganisms/ pathogens per gram, or 225,000,000 per serving.
- Eggs: 50,000 to 500,000 microorganisms/pathogens per gram, or 37,500,000 per egg.
- Beef, Poultry, Lamb, Pork, Seafood: 300,000 to 3,000,000 microorganisms/pathogens per gram, or 336,000,000 per serving.
- Honey: 500,000 microorganisms/pathogens per gram.

➢ The average American meal of animal products contains 750,000,000 - 1,000,000,000 pleomorphic pathogenic microorganisms per meal (US Department of Agriculture).[534]
➢ The average vegetarian meal consisting of only plant food has less than 500 pleomorphic pathogenic microorganisms per meal. The body's defense system can easily handle this low amount, but the higher

---

[n] For microform/ pathogenic load comparison of foods, the following Microform/Symptogenic Load Comparisons of Foods by Robert Young, PhD, DSc., a biochemist, is citing the US Department of Agriculture's figures on pathogenic microorganisms.

amounts indicated above for animal products are problematic, and for some with diseases dangerous.
➢ Vegetables, fruits, legumes, seeds, nuts and sprouted grains (if uncontaminated in handling): are only 10 microorganisms/ pathogens per gram.

Pathogenic Microorganisms [535]

Honey	5 million per cup
Milk	5 million per cup
Butter	7 million per cup
Eggs	37 million per egg
Cheese	100 million per serving
Ice Cream	225 million per serving
Beef, Poultry, Fish	336 million per serving
Average American Meal	750 to 1 billion per serving
Average Vegan Meal	500 per meal

A plant-based diet is obviously healthier.

d. Fish: Biological Magnification Threat

There is mercury in almost all fish and some levels are called "acceptable" according to the government. Why gamble? Just avoid fish it's not needed!

In the book: *The Brain Gate,* Robert Hatherill, PhD, notes: "Fish and shellfish contain mercury (methylmercury), and mercury vapors have been demonstrated to cross the BrainGate. Once mercury crosses the BrainGate, a number of toxic processes occur. Mercury creates oxidative stress by depleting antioxidants. This depletion then blocks the formation of the brain messenger acetylcholine. The decrease in acetylcholine occurs mostly in the brain cortex and hippocampus."[536] In addition, Dr. Hatherill continues: "High levels of homocysteine result primarily from the intake of animal proteins, not plant proteins. Animal proteins contain an abundance of the essential amino acid methionine. If you eat a lot of methionine-rich foods, you will form higher levels of the toxic amino acid homocysteine.

Homocysteine is formed from methionine. Fish have particularly high levels of methionine. To convert toxic homocysteine back into methionine requires folic acid and B vitamins. Some researchers believe that it's elevated homocysteine levels, and not high cholesterol, that actually cause brain strokes."[537] This would also be symptomatic for Parkinson's, AD and MS."

Another example is given by Neal Barnard, MD, founder of The Physician's Committee for Responsible Medicine in Washington, D.C. who writes that: "Many people have turned from red meats to fish, encouraged by reports that fish contains 'good fats.' However, those 'good fats' are just as fattening as any other kind of fat, as the native populations of Arctic regions have demonstrated. Perhaps the worst of all, fish is by far the most contaminated food. As environmental experts monitor chemical contamination in fish, they routinely issue advisories, such as one from Virginia's Department of Environment Quality, which recently pointed out that catfish and carp had PCBs up to 3,212 parts per billion, more than five times the allowable limit. PCBs, or polychlorinated biphenyls, are chemicals that were used in electrical equipment, hydraulic fluid, and carbonless carbon paper. They linger in waterways and, like mercury and other contaminants, flow through fish gills, lodge in fish muscle tissues, and routinely show up in governmental tests."[538]

Brian Clement, PhD writes in his book, *Killer Fish* that, "There are three central reasons why one should not be eating fish and other aquatic life. First' is the fact that these creatures harbor saturated fats and disease-causing elements derived from the way we prepare them for consumption. Next, is the fact that each of these creatures is filled with our industrial waste (chemicals, heavy metals, etc.) and the globally scattered radiation from our endless wars and faulty nuclear energy endeavors. Last, but not least, are the multitude of parasites and amoebas that water-based creatures contain, which are passed to those unfortunate individuals who eat them."[539]

Dr. Clement points out that "Fish gives the wrong ratio of these fats and creates an imbalance of omega 3 to 6. There is often an 11:1 ratio of omega-6/omega-3 in some of the most commonly consumed fish versus the optimum 1:3 level found in plant-based sources. The unhealthy fatty acid ratio found in many common fish precipitates higher levels of cardiovascular disease for those who consistently eat these 'fishy foods.'"[540]

"Another common myth is that fish oil slows mental decline. A study from the *Journal of the American Medical Association* (JAMA) reports that there was no benefit derived by a group consuming fish oil since their cognitive function did not improve mild to moderate Alzheimer's disease. JAMA went on to say, 'There is no basis for recommendation of supplementation in the quest of helping those afflicted with dementia.'"[541]

Finally, Dr. Clement writes about the long legacy of people who have contracted disease by consuming aquatic life. He writes "The handful of studies that point to fish as a heart-healthy food are over-shadowed by many studies that prove their consumption actually severely increase the chances of heart attacks and strokes. As far back as 2004, *Annals of Internal Medicine* stated, 'Americans have heard less about, and have paid less attention to, various health warnings associated with fish consumption. Studies have linked over-consumption of certain popular fish to neurological deficits, cancer, auto-immune and endocrine disorders, and in addition, heart disease.'"[542]

The families of toxic contaminants in fish such as dioxins, PCBs, and pesticides are by-products of industrial processes. These and many others are found in lakes and streams all over the U.S. and Canada, even in Alaska. The following is a list of contaminants in fish from 11 studies.[543]

Toxin	Type	Effects	Fish with High levels
Dichlorodi-Phenyltri-Chloroethane (DDT)	Insecticide	Endocrine disruption, diabetes, and possibly cancer	Sockeye Salmon
Hexachloro-benzene (HCB)	Fungicide	Neurological problems, enlarged thyroid and liver	Wild Salmon Mackerel
Polychlorinated biphenyls (PCBs)	Industrial chemical used as coolant fluid	Endocrine disruption, neurological problems	Black bass, carb, channel catfish, largemouth bass, and smallmouth bass
Polycyclic aromatic hydrocarbons (PAHs)	By-products of burning fuels	DNA damage, cancer, and lower IQ	Atlantic mackerel, Atlantic salmon, blue whiting, clams, herring (smoked), mussels, rainbow trout (farmed), and shrimp

In 1969 the US Food and Drug Administration (FDA) established 0.5 parts per million (ppm) as the maximum safe level of mercury contamination in fish. In 1979 that level was arbitrarily raised to 1 ppm, despite the well-documented neurological problems in humans caused by mercury exposure.[544]

The following information is based on data compiled by the FDA from various studies. Mercury levels in fish: Shark 4.5; Tilefish (from Gulf of Mexico) 3.7; Swordfish 3.2; Chilean sea bass 2.1; Tuna (fresh or frozen) 1.8; King mackerel 1.6; Halibut 1.5; Tuna (yellowfin) 1.4; Bluefish 1.4; Snapper 1.3; Grouper 1.2; Orange roughly 1.1.

Dr. Eric R. Brown, chairman of the microbiology department of the Chicago Medical School, went fishing with his son one day. Curious about the tumors on the fish he caught, Dr. Brown initiated an investigation of the fish and of the water where he was fishing, Fox River, a typical American river flowing a few miles west of Chicago. The bacteria count ran as high as 39,000 per 100 milliliters of water. That indicated a high proportion of fecal matter. There were also herbicides, insecticides, phosphates, nitrates, gasoline, ether, and carcinogenic (cancer-producing compounds of the benzathracene group) substances. In addition, lead, mercury, calcium, cadmium, zinc, and antimony were found. "What a fish eats of elements such as mercury and arsenic," Dr. Brown points out, "the fish keeps. When a bigger fish eats several smaller fish, he keeps the mercury and arsenic that they all ate. When a human being eats the fish, he keeps these poisons and they build up in him. This process of 'biological magnification' is a major threat in the use of flesh as food."[545]

e. Poultry: Antibiotics, Chemicals, Bacteria

About half of the 31 million pounds of antibiotics produced every year in the U.S. goes into animal feed. Bruce Miller, MD stated that, "Because of health concerns over antibiotic-resistant bacteria, several European countries banned the use of antibiotics in animal feed in the 1970's. Our government is still dragging its feet due to money, power and politics, not science! Besides penicillin and tetracycline in meat, you also can get nitrofurazone (and other nitrofurans), and sulfamethazine (along with other sulfa drugs). These can increase the risk of cancer."[546]

Of the major types of disease-causing bacteria and parasites found in food, nearly all have been found in meat or poultry. "Poultry in America is commonly contaminated with salmonella. The USDA says that about one-third of raw chickens are contaminated with salmonella. But some unbiased experts say 50 to 90 percent of poultry leaving the plant are contaminated. In 1990, the University of Wisconsin screened over 2,300 laying hens from three flocks. They found only eight birds that were not infected with campylobacter, another 'bug' that causes food poisoning."[547]

One journal, *Advances in Meat Research* reported that, "Poultry seems particularly prone to contamination with campylobacters; 80% of chickens and 90% of turkeys carried through a typical slaughterhouse produced positive cultures for it.[548] Complete cooking can kill most of these microbes and bacteria that are found in poultry. But campylobacters survive freezing and "chicken that appears pink and underdone is the most likely source of infection."[549] Sandwiches and salads that have chicken and turkey meat that has not been properly cooked should be avoided.

Inspectors inspect chickens at a rate of one every two seconds or so, as they speed by the inspectors on hooks. But these inspections do not detect bacterial, antibiotic or other chemicals or toxin contamination. The USDA only uses tests that detect about 40 of the 227 different chemicals (some pesticides) that are used on meat or that come from their feed. Before 1950, antibiotics were not used but today chickens have a steady supply of sulfa drugs, hormones, antibiotics and nitrofurans. Veterinary drugs are used on every food-producing animal and many of these thousands of new drugs have not been tested. Over 90% of the chickens today are fed arsenic compounds. (1987)[550] One of the dyes injected into chickens is used so that their meat and yolks will appear to be a "healthy looking" yellow.

In 2013, the FDA said its own research shows that arsenic, a cancer causing chemical, added to chicken feed ends up in chicken meat where it is consumed by humans. Until this new study, the arsenic in the feed was given to chickens for decades. The company making this feed has agreed to pull this toxic feed chemical off the shelves in the United States, but refuses to pull it from the dozen other countries until forced to by regulators.[551]

f. Good Fish - Bad Fish Parable

Jesus used the parable of the dragnet to distinguish between the good fish and the bad fish. "Once again, the kingdom of heaven is like a net that was let down into the lake and caught all kinds of fish. When it was full, the fishermen pulled it up on shore. Then they sat down and collected the good fish in baskets, but threw the bad away." (Mt 13:47, 48) They threw away the bad fish that were non-kosher or impure. Seafood's such as shrimp, scallops, lobster are scavengers and toxic and non-kosher; fish like sharks are highly toxic and also non-kosher. Only the healthy fish are kosher. The best way to avoid all this toxicity is simple, eat a plant-based diet!

Rabbi Gabriel Cousens, MD wrote, "The historical evidence strongly suggests that Jesus did teach vegetarianism, was a vegetarian, and therefore did not eat flesh food. This is consistent with his teachings of love of all God's creatures, his commitment not to kill any life according to the highest understanding of the Law of Moses that "Thou shalt not kill" (man or animal), the original teachings of vegetarianism in Genesis 1:29, and his stand in the Temple against the sacrifice of animals. Jesus taught that compassion should extend to all of God's creatures. He taught a humane way of life and was a shining example of a fully humane being. To be humane is to be kind, merciful, and a fully humane human being. To be humane is to be kind, merciful, and not to kill any living creature. The slaughter of animals can in no way be considered humane."[552]

Chapter 12

Animal Proteins: Inflammatory
for PD, AD and MS

Saint Augustine also wrote: "The flesh, has been accustomed to restraint in regard to its own satisfaction. Of course, care must be taken to avoid merely changing instead of lessening pleasures; that, in place of meat, they procure food of manifold variety and appeal; that they store up, as opportune for this season, delights which they would be ashamed to indulge in at other times. In this way, the observance of Lent becomes, not the curbing of old passions, but an opportunity for new pleasures. Take measures in advance, my brethren, with as much diligence as possible, to prevent these attitudes from creeping upon you. It is not that certain kinds of food are to be detested, but that bodily pleasure is to be checked."[553]

a. Inflammation: The Brain on Fire!

Inflammation is a problem with Parkinson's, Alzheimer's and other brain diseases. A major cause of this inflammation are animal proteins that become distorted and a meat-based diet, which is high in saturated fats and toxins. It is impossible to get rid of all inflammation unless a person gets rid of all meat and animal products in their diet. Animal products are a major source of inflammation for PD, AD and MS. This elimination of meat and dairy is especially beneficial for older people. In the elderly, the acid in their stomach decreases as they age and they have difficulty digesting and breaking down animal products. Some elderly lose their taste for meat as they age and naturally eat less of it. A protein powder supplement might be a good recommendation for them.

This researcher, Parris Kidd, PhD, has called the inflammation present in these diseases: 'The Brain on Fire.' He believes "that nowhere is damage from runaway inflammation more evident than in the brain, as I learned over the past several years while publishing in-depth reviews on brain diseases. Parkinson's disease is inflammatory, burning away the *substantia nigra* and other brain zones. Multiple Sclerosis is a more sporadic, on and off type of progression, but inflammatory just the same. Alzheimer's involves several overlapping breakdown processes, of which inflammation is definitely a major one. Runaway inflammation causes a stroke. Autism in children features subtle but telltale features of inflammation. The brain is particularly susceptible to runaway inflammation because it [the brain] uses a lot of oxygen and has a lot of flammable material (the fatty nerve insulation). Toxins accelerate the burn, and in Parkinson's, pesticides and mercury are undoubtedly involved. Because the brain lacks pain receptors, the afflicted person does not know his brain is inflamed. There are keys to turning this story around, which lie not in drugs, but in lifestyle, diet, and nontoxic dietary supplements."[554]

Poor nutrition, in general, especially a low dietary intake of B vitamins and a high intake of simple sugars, has been associated with an increased risk of Parkinson's disease and with more rapid progression of the disease in patients who already have it.[555] High dietary intake of meat increases absorption of iron and consumption of animal fats, both of which are associated with an increased risk of Parkinson's. Red meat is rich in iron, yet excessive amounts of iron should be avoided (heavy metals are found in the brains of Parkinson's patients).[556]

b. Decreasing Protein Intake is Useful in PD

Parris Kidd, PhD, a nutrient expert, cites the study: *Decreasing Protein intake is useful in PD* which is a convincing double-blind study that compared low protein intake (50 g/day for men and 40 g/day for women) to high protein intake (80 g/day for men and 70 g/day for women). Total performance scores were significantly improved, along with tremor, hand agility, and mobility in the low protein groups.[557] In another study, modifying meal patterns to eat the majority of protein in the evening also improved symptoms.[558]   Yet, actually 50g/day is not that low of a protein diet compared to a vegan diet which is about 35g/day, which is healthier."

A vegan diet can help bring Parkinson's into remission. The evidence is growing from various studies that a vegan diet, juicing, fasting and supplements can help to prevent and slow down PD, and thus helps to bring PD into remission. Not only is this found to be the case with peer reviewed journal studies, but it is also the findings of non-peer reviewed studies and healthcare practitioners.

"Three case-control studies conclude that diets high in animal fat or cholesterol are associated with a substantial increase in risk for Parkinson's disease (PD). In contrast, fat of plant origin does not appear to increase risk . . . The possibility that vegan diets could be therapeutically beneficial in PD, by slowing the loss of surviving dopaminergic neurons, thus retarding progression of the syndrome, may merit examination. Vegan diets could also be helpful to PD patients by promoting vascular health and aiding blood-brain barrier transport of L-dopa (*Med Hypotheses,* 2001)."[559] The important fact is this major journal is citing three case control studies that have shown animal products are a major problem for people with Parkinson's. Also cited is an early study showed that a low protein diet was beneficial to Parkinson's patients.[560] Therefore, not only are animal proteins a potential problem, but high protein diets are also a real problem according to peer reviewed journal studies. On a high-protein diet, all patients were immobilized by bradykinesia for most of the day."[561]

The Physician's Committee for Responsible Medicine in Washington, D.C. cites studies on protein, "The beneficial effects of a protein–reduced diet, or the redistribution of almost all protein to evening meals on L–dopa availability (and subsequent control of dyskinesis) have been subsequently documented in patients who experience erratic responses to levodopa therapy.[562] In these studies, reducing protein intake resulted in an improved therapeutic response in many (though not all) individuals. Low protein diets resulted in improvements in neurologic scoring. Similarly, redistributing all but 7 grams of protein intake to the evening meal resulted in improvement in the Northwest Disability and AIMS Dyskinesia Scale. Both low protein diets, and diets reserving protein for evening meals, were associated with significant reductions in the need for L–dopa."[563]

A few points here are helpful:
- An early study (*Eur J Clin Nutr*, 1991) showed that a low protein diet was beneficial to Parkinson's patients.[564]
- In a case controlled study of 342 PD patients (*Neurology*, 1996), they found that certain proteins 'may be associated with the development of PD.'[565]
- Another case-control study concluded: 'Although these data support previous findings of no association of past intake with most food groups and PD risk, they confirm an increased risk of PD associated with foods containing animal fat (*Mov Disord.*, 1999).'"[566]

c. Cholesterol, PD and Alzheimer's

Sherry Rogers, MD, in her book, *The Cholesterol Hoax*,[567] gives an overview of the many problems with cholesterol lowering drugs. "Statin drugs work by poisoning a liver enzyme that makes cholesterol. ... Clearly this drug class will bring on a lot more Alzheimer's and senility, which are already soaring to unprecedented levels. And more on the amnesia, depression, nerve, heart and muscle damage and suicide that statins bring on later. ... Cholesterol drugs guarantee an avalanche of new symptoms, especially cancer and more serious heart disease ... they have been proven to slowly deteriorate and shrink the brain and deteriorate the intellect within less than five years (Novasc, Procardia, Calan, Dilacor). ... Cholesterol-lowering drugs cause memory loss, amnesia, Alzheimer's, and mimic strokes."[568]

The *Journal of the American Medical Association*, for example, shows that "death rates actually go up, not down when efforts are made to lower cholesterol with drugs."[569] "Too low of a cholesterol is just as dangerous as too high. Cholesterol is needed for all membrane structure and function, hormones, hormone receptors, and release of cytokines that fight off infection and cancers. And when the cell membrane is cholesterol-starved, it can malfunction and trigger autoimmune diseases, cancers, Alzheimer's and much more. In fact, folks with a cholesterol under 160 mg/dL have double the risk of brain hemorrhage and increased risk of cancers of the liver, lung, pancreas, and leukemia, plus cirrhosis and suicide (Behar)."[570]

In another study, "low cholesterol folks had more than double the death rate from non-cardiac conditions. Besides doubling death, low cholesterol dramatically damages mental-health leading to depression, suicide, mania, and more (Cassidy, Engleberg). One of the fascinating things is that low cholesterol has been well known to be associated with cancer in scores of studies. Most of these studies were published well over 20 years ago, and in the most prestigious journals like *Lancet, Journal of the National Cancer Institute, Journal of the American Medical Association*, and much more."[571]

The book *Selling Sickness* noted, "It is estimated that almost 90 percent of those who write guidelines for their peers have conflicts of interest because of financial ties to the pharmaceutical industry. The ties between guideline-writers and the industry are just one corner of the vast web of interrelationships between doctors and drug companies. The industry's influence over doctors' practices, medical education, and scientific research is as widespread as it is controversial - not just distorting the way physicians prescribe medicines but actually affecting the way conditions like 'high cholesterol' are defined and promoted."[572] If the guidelines are followed, sales of cholesterol-lowering statin drugs will increase by at least from $20 billion to $30 billion per year."[573]

In the journal, *Med Hypotheses* (2001) a major study found that; "Three recent case-control studies conclude that diets high in animal fat or cholesterol are associated with a substantial increase in risk for Parkinson's disease (PD); in contrast, fat of plant origin does not appear to increase risk. ... The possibility that vegan diets could be therapeutically beneficial in PD, by slowing the loss of surviving dopaminergic neurons, thus retarding progression of the syndrome, may merit examination."[574] Another case-control study concluded: "Although these data support previous findings of no association of past intake with most food groups and PD risk, they confirm an increased risk of PD associated with foods containing animal fat (*Mov Disord.*, 1999)."[575]

Recent studies (2002) show that choosing foods that lowered your cholesterol might also cut your risk for Alzheimer's disease. The people who chose these low cholesterol foods had significantly less risk of cognitive impairment as they aged. Furthermore, an amino acid that comes from animal protein, called homocysteine, appears to increase the risk of Alzheimer's disease.[576] Plant-based proteins, rather than animal-based proteins, help to reduce the risk of Alzheimer's disease. As noted, it has been found that the one diet that helps Parkinson's patients to live longer is a vegan diet. In addition, toxic proteins are found in the brains of Alzheimer's patients.

d. Animal Fats/Proteins Unhealthy

A lot of studies have been done on fats and brain degenerative diseases. Unhealthy fats are part of the problem and healthy fats are involved in the healing process of PD. Meat and animal fats contain unhealthy fats and should be avoided by people with PD and MS and all other degenerative diseases:

- 'This population-based case-control study evaluated nutrient intake as a risk factor for Parkinson's disease (PD) . . . Conclusions: These results suggest an association of PD with high intake of total fat, saturated fats, cholesterol, lutein and iron.' (*Int J Epidemiol*, 1999);[577]
- 'Background: Unsaturated fatty acids are important constituents of neuronal cell membranes and have neuroprotective, antioxidant, and anti-inflammatory properties. Objective: To determine if a high intake of unsaturated fatty acids might be associated with a lower risk of Parkinson's disease (PD) . . . Conclusion: These findings suggest that high intake of unsaturated fatty acids might protect against Parkinson's disease.'[578] (*Neurology*, 2005)."

A study showed that certain plant-based diet foods (seedlings, pods, and beans) might have a beneficial effect on PD patients.[579] This is more evidence that confirms why people with PD and MS who eat a vegan diet, or better yet a Living Foods diet with sprouts, live longer and healthier.

A plant-based diet has a positive effect on drug usage whereas a meat-based diet has a negative effect on drug usage. If a person has Parkinson's and takes pharmaceutical drugs, they are better off with a plant-based diet, low protein diet, which the following studies indicate:

- In 1987, a journal (*Arch Neurol*) indicated the benefit of a low protein diet and sensitivity to levodopa.[580]
- In 2004, a journal (*Parkinsonism Relat Disord.*) states, 'A rich protein diet has been shown to impair the clinical effect of levodopa.'[581]
- In 2006, (*Mov Disord.*) 'Protein intake interferes with levodopa therapy. Patients with advanced Parkinson's disease (PD) should restrict daily protein intake and shift protein intake to the evening.'[582]
- Another study (*Mov Disord.* 2006) agrees with the above study.[583]
- In another study shows that: 'There is considerable evidence for the suggestion that the long-term use of levodopa accelerates the progression of PD (*Int J Mol Med.*, 2004).[584]

e. Mutated and Misformed Proteins Aggregate

The pathogenic microorganisms that enter the body through meat-based diets end up in the gut and the liver and can end up in the brain. This is one of the reasons why there is protein aggregation in the brain such as with Lewy bodies. In addition, the mitochondrial damage is a known issue with Parkinson's. A little known fact is that meat-based protein is different on the molecular level than plant-based protein. Meat-based protein has a double-helix bond whereas plant-based protein has a single-helix bond, making it more flexible, and it takes less energy to break down in the ATP cycle in the plants.

The single vs. double helix bonding causing issues with the brain is a hypothesis, but it does fit in with some of the science studies. One raw food scholar David Wolfe, MS pointed out in his book, *Eating for Beauty*, that plant-based proteins have a single helix bond and meat-based proteins have a double helix bond.

The Embden-Meyerhof glycolytic pathway and the Krebs' Cycle both have as their starting point protein which breaks down to amino acids (and to glucose and ketones). This is the final pathway that all nutrient metabolites are involved in for energy production which involves the mitochondria. The studies on Parkinson's have found that: "The concept that mitochondrial dysfunction can cause a Parkinsonian syndrome came into focus with the observation that MPTP induced PD in drug addicts.°"[585] (*J Neurochem* 2001)

Furthermore, research into Parkinson's disease finds that: 'Mutated and misformed proteins tend to aggregate.' (*J Biol Chem*, 1999) The Lewy bodies in the brains of Parkinson's patients, the neurological problems in the brains of MS and the high levels of amyloid plaque found in Alzheimer's in the brain, are or could be also directly related to high animal protein levels in the body.

The average person on a meat-based diet eats two to three times the amount of protein that they actually need (80-120g for the average 150 lb. male). A plant-based diet provides the right amount of protein needed (35-54g for the average 150 lb male).[p] The high protein level in an animal protein based diet causes acidosis. This acidosis starts because of the excess of uric acid that comes from the breakdown of excess amino acids in the body.

This buildup of animal-based proteins not only causes inflammation, it also causes the growth of fungi and causes a buildup of excess protein-based substances that eventually could end up in the Lewy bodies and amyloid plaques of PD, MS and AD patients. The Lewy Bodies and other deformed proteins in the brains of PD, MS and Alzheimer's patients are animal-based proteins (double helix bonds) which are dead foods or misformed proteins

---

° (*Psychiatry Res*, 1979; *Science*, 1983; Vintage Pub., 1996)
Mitochondrial dysfunctions are now recognized to be the major cause of nigral degeneration in experimental models of PD and possibly even in idiopathic PD (*J Neurochem*, 2001; *Bioessays*, 2002).
[p] 35g is ideal and 54 is recommended for the average 150 lb male.

f. Genetic Engineering - Protein Misfolding

The book, *Genetic Roulette - The Documented Health Risks of Genetically Engineered Foods*,[586] states that genetic engineering is a huge multi-billion dollar business and it has a strong influence in the government. It also has become a world-wide health issue, with documented health-risks causing deaths, illnesses, diseases, and genetic engineering creates wide-spread, unpredictable changes in the food chain.

Proteins expressed in a Genetically Modified plant may be processed differently and those changes, which could include misfolding or molecular attachments, can be harmful in unpredicted ways. According to the Centre for Integrated Research on Biosafety (INBI), "proteins derived from natural sources generally regarded as safe can be [toxic to cells] if allowed to re-fold under different conditions. Sometimes, refolding can result in groups of proteins aggregating into shapes with harmful consequences. INBI points out that certain aggregations of 'proteins' that have sustained mutations or have been misfolded (amyloid fibrils) are involved in a variety of medical conditions such as Alzheimer's and Parkinson's diseases. (*Journal of Nature*, 2002)"[587]

g. Kosher has Lower Toxicity Levels

A fascinating study by a researcher, Dr. David Macht of Johns Hopkins University, looked at Leviticus XI and Deuteronomy XIV. He did a study in which he reported "the toxic effects of animal flesh on a controlled growth culture. A substance was classified as toxic if it slowed the culture's growth rate below 75 percent. In each case, the blood, of all the animals Dr. Macht tested showed up more toxic than the flesh."[588] "His results show that the lower the growth percentage of the culture, the more toxic the flesh. Note that the flesh of animals and fish given to us by God for food are all nontoxic, but all forbidden animals lie in the toxic range."[589]

"He was basically comparing those animals classified as kosher to those animals classified as non-kosher in the Bible. All those animals that are kosher or nontoxic were in the safe range for human consumption with low toxicity levels. But the non-kosher animals all had high toxicity levels that would be considered unsafe for human consumption. In other words, all forbidden animals in the bible lie in the toxic range. As it turned out the toxic animals are all meat eaters, while the non-toxic animals are plant-based eaters (vegetarians)! This confirmed the biblical insight concerning meat consumption, when the people rebelled and wanted to eat meat."[590]

Chapter 13

Sprouted Grains versus Dormant Grains

Clement of Alexandria, (b. 150 AD), was a well-educated teacher. His *Paidagogos,* is a handbook of Christian etiquette that discusses the practical needs of life involved with eating, drinking and table manners. Clements' aim throughout the treatise is to inculcate the virtue of temperance. Clement also appeals to medical opinion and cites Antiphanes, "a Delian physician, for the assertion that rich food is one of the causes of diseases."[591] The Law was wise, he stresses, to prohibit rich food, which, in addition to being unhealthy and fattening, engenders greed, is expensive, and absorbs attention and resources that are better spent elsewhere.[592]

a. Grain Products and Raw Fooders

Grains grown in a farm setting have only been around for the last 10,000 years, since the agricultural revolution. A hypothesis is that human gene structure is not designed for grains that is why different grains give us so many health problems. A vegan diet cuts out animal products and a raw vegan diet cuts out grain products, unless they are sprouted. The raw food movement uses minimal grains or no grains at all, unless they are sprouted. This is a big difference between being a vegan and a raw vegan. For those with MS, they need to restrict most grains. Some writers say that it is only certain grains that are damaging to the myelin sheath for those with MS. Grains also have a negative effect for Parkinson's.

Grains are dormant foods and are not living foods until they are soaked and sprouted. Most raw food writers and chefs, in the 1990 to 2008 publications, emphasized no grains for the raw vegan diet, unless sprouted, including:

Gabriel Cousens,[593] Doug Graham,[594] David Wolfe,[595] Victoria Boutenko,[596] Rhio,[597] Chad Sarno,[598] Juliano,[599] Nomi Shannon,[600] Elizabeth Baker,[601] Frederic Patenaude,[602] Brenda Cobb,[603] Charlie Trotter and Roxanne Klein,[604] Shazzie,[605] Alex Ferrara,[606] Elaine Love,[607] Matthew Kenney,[608] Igor Boutenko,[609] Sergei and Valya Boutenko.[610] Julie Wandling.[611] Paul Nison,[612] Fred Bisci[613] Stephen Arlin,[614] Robert Young,[615] Brian Clement,[616] Anna Maria Clement,[617] Cherie Soria,[618] James Tibbetts, Anne Marie Tibbetts [619] Brigitte Mars,[620] James Levin, Natalie Cederquist,[621] Jeremy Safron & Renee Underkoffler,[622] Rita Romano,[623] Annie Padden Jubb and David Jubb,[624] Jeremy Safron,[625] Rose Lee Calabro,[626] Elysa Markowitz,[627] Johann Schnitzer[628] Charlotte Gerson[629] Jameth Dina,[630] George Malkmus,[631] Ronda Malkmus,[632] Dorit,[633] Jordan Maerin,[634] Alissa Cohen, Roe Gallo, Harvey Diamond, Marilyn Diamond.[635]

Melissa Diane Smith, RD, a nutritionist, who has a book on the ill effects of grains in a diet.[636] The problem rising up is that, some of the new raw vegan's books, after 2008, are emphasizing the use of grains (not sprouted).

Some believe that too much food from grains (starches, cereals) burden the digestion, cause acidosis and impure blood, arthritis, cancer, other metabolic problems, and are considered to be the chief factors in skin disorders. One author cites, "Some doctors, who had spent their entire careers in the study of degenerative diseases, were specifically opposed to the use of cereals as suitable foods in the human diet."[637]

b. Grain Damage and Health Problems

One raw food author Doug Graham, D.C. has a booklet called *Grain Damage*, he writes; "Optimum nutrition can only come from foods to which we are biologically adapted, such as fruits and vegetables. Anatomically, humans are classed as anthropoid primates, along with gibbons, chimpanzees, bonobos, gorillas, and orangutans. There is not one example in nature of an animal with anatomy and physiology similar to ours that consumes grains. All of the anthropoid primates thrive on a diet consisting solely of fruits, vegetables, nuts, and seeds."

"Grains contain a substance known as phytic acid. During the process of digestion, the body binds phytic acid with calcium, a powerful alkaline, in order to neutralize its acidity. Grains contain very little calcium, and are also low in sodium, chlorine, iodine, sulfur and other base minerals. Fruits and vegetables contain from ten to one hundred times as much calcium and other base minerals, per calorie as do grains. Grains also contain abundant quantities of acid forming minerals. The body must yield up calcium from the bones to neutralize the acidity in grains. Eventually, we run low on calcium, resulting in a common condition known as osteoporosis."[638]

Dr. Graham continues, "Foods that require cooking to be consumed are not only nutritionally deficient; they must be suspect in terms of their health value. This is because the vitamins, minerals, enzymes, co-enzymes, proteins and fats are damaged, deranged or destroyed by the heat of cooking. This results in foods that will not sustain us. What does remain after cooking, however, are calories. Therefore, when we eat starches, we consume the maximum number of calories with the minimum amount of nutrients." "Because they must be cooked to be consumed, grains cannot, by definition, be considered a 'natural' food for mankind."[639]

"Heating foods generates the creation of substances known to be harmful to humans. Free radicals, created by the heating of fats, are proven to be carcinogenic. Heated fats lower the blood's ability to carry oxygen, and also block capillaries with fat globules. Additional, fatty deposits build up on the vascular walls, a major contribution to atherosclerosis and other forms of heart disease." "Heated fats not only cloud one's thinking, hasten cancers, and foster heart disease; they are fattening."[640]

"The fiber in grains must be considered a health destroyer. Humans have delicate digestive systems; look at the number of people with digestive problems - nine out of ten in the U.S. Our system requires the soft, soluble fiber found in fruits and tender vegetables. Grain's fiber, however, is coarse and sharp, like finely ground glass. Nutritionists refer to it as non-soluble fiber. It acts as an irritant in our system. Irritation of the mucosa of the intestine is considered a risk factor in many different diseases including ulcers, diverticulosis, spastic colon, Crohn's, colitis, irritable bowel, and colon cancer."[641]

"The presence of non-soluble fiber in the intestines causes food to move through the bowels more rapidly than normal, reducing nutrient absorption. Coupled with the irritating quality of non-soluble fiber, this rapid movement of foods leads to mal-absorption syndromes, nutritional deficiencies, and overall loss of health. In the production of refined flour, bran is left over. This waste product is sold, at an inflated price, as if it were a health food."[642]

"Since animal proteins contain no fiber, they pass through the digestive system more slowly than other foods. At one hundred degrees, in a dark, wet environment, undigested meat will go bad (rot) rather rapidly. The partial digestion of meat that occurs when it is eaten with grains very often accounts for the putrefaction so obvious when feces are expelled. The gas formed during fermentation is eventually released visa the anus."

"Grains, fortunately, do not tend to putrefy. They do, however, ferment. Fermentation results from the mixture of sugar and starch found, for example, in a raisin bagel, a fruit pie, or dessert after a starchy meal. There are two products that result from the fermentation of grin: alcohol and gas. Alcohol quickly penetrates the gut lining and becomes blood alcohol. Alcohol is a protoplasmic poison, meaning that it destroys every cell with which it comes in contact. The production of alcohol within the gut is never a good thing. "[643]

"The list of health problems associated with eating grains is quite long. Asthma, allergies, gluten intolerance, digestive disturbances, yeast infections, various mucus and congestive conditions, several types of arthritis, and even chronic overeating are all linked with the consumption of grains. This is not to say that grains are all bad, for they are a far better choice than their animal alternative. However, the healthiest choices are fruits and vegetables. Many sufferers of nasal congestion, asthma, and allergies are pleased to discover that their symptoms are relieved once they embark upon a starch-free diet."[644]

"Gluten, a protein found in many grain products, has been named as a causative factor in several psychoses and neurological disorders. It has been proven to chemically contain fifteen different opioid sequences, or morphine-like molecules. Opioids that come from outside the body are called 'exorphins.' Exorphins are labeled by scientists as addictive and neurotoxic. They have psychoactive properties and cause related behavioral problems such as addictive eating patterns. Gluten consumption has repeatedly been liked to learning disorders and schizophrenia by scientists since the mid 1960's."[645]

Dr. Graham continues, "Central nervous system disorders such as nausea, sedation, truncal ridgidity, euphoria, dysphoria, and meiosis (papillary contraction) are linked to opioid consumption. Opioids are known to interfere with our neurotransmitter chemistry, cause various types of epilepsy and result in digestive disturbances such as constipation, urinary retention, reduced production of ADH (an anti-diuretic hormone that results in reduced urine production,) biliary spasm, slowed gastric emptying and slowed digestion."[646]

"The following is a partial list of the toxic chemicals used in the processing of grain: mercury, cyanide, ammonium salts, chlorine, (each causes insanity and death) fluorine, mineral oil, alum (high intensity toxins) and aspartine (a known neurotoxin that causes birth defects). Daily consumption of such powerful drugs takes its toll and negatively affects health, fitness, performance, sanity, and beauty. Could we all have gone a little crazy?"[647]

c. Grain Allergies, Acidity and Neurotoxicity

Dr. Cousens writes, "A high percentage of my clients have grain allergies and get much better when they stop eating grains. Grain allergies not only cause the typical mucus membrane irritation, congestion, asthma, and sinusitis, but can have an effect on the mental state as well. Gluten, an ingredient in many grain products, has been associated with several forms of mental and neurological disorders. Some research has found that gluten contains fifteen different opioid sequences (morphine-like molecules). These can add to the addictiveness and neurotoxin effect of the grains. I believe that these opioids are in some way connected to the addictive eating patterns associated with grains, as well as to some learning disorders and to schizophrenic reactions in some people. Not only do grains on their own create problems, but many toxic chemicals are used in the processing of grains. These include mercury, cyanide, ammonium, salt, chlorine, fluorine, mineral oil, alum, and aspartame."[648]

Dr. Cousens points out, "Most grains create acidity except for buckwheat and millet. Grains contain very little calcium and are also low in sodium, chlorine, iodine, sulfur, and other minerals. In fact, vegetables as well as fruits contain from ten to a hundred times more calcium and other base minerals per calorie then grains. But grains do contain high amounts of acid-forming minerals. Grains are primarily acid-forming. We must remember that acidity is one of the main things that push the recycle or rotting button. In order to neutralize some of the uric acid from grins, our bodies use up available calcium and must bull calcium from our bones to replace the loss."[649]

Dr. Vivian Virginia Vetrano, a Natural Hygiene raw vegan since the early 70's, answered the question on grains: "We all know that people can live on them, but the question is, can people actually be superbly healthy by partaking of grains, especially a lot of them? The answer is no. A diet of pure grains is acid-forming, and it does not supply the proper proportion of the alkaline minerals to balance the acidic ones."[650]

In the work, *Going Against the Grain*, the author, Melissa Smith, a nutritionist, notes: "Many nutritionists recommend whole grains in place of refined grains, and at first thought, this sounds like good dietary advice. On paper, at least, whole grains contain more nutrients. They also have more blood sugar-regulating fiber. Because of that fiber, they generally rank lower on the glycemic index and offer more protection against Type 2 diabetes and heart disease than refined grains.[651] [652] (citing[q]) However, whole grains have numerous nutritional shortcomings that make these foods far less beneficial to health than they've been made out to be. Their key nutritional downfalls include high carbohydrate content, anti-nutrients that impair the

---

[q] *(Journal of the American Medical Association; American Journal of Clinical Nutrition)*

absorption of minerals such as calcium, iron, and zinc, and lectins that wreak havoc with intestinal and immune function. The more that whole grains are eaten, the more their nutritional shortcomings aggravate body function and lead to serious mental problems. Ironically, many people switch from a high-refined grain diet to a high whole-grain diet in search of better health but actually set themselves up for conditions such as bone problems, iron-deficiency anemia, and autoimmune conditions.'"[653]

Norman Walker, D.Sc., a respected health advocate and author, in discussing Multiple Sclerosis writes. "MS is a degenerative state of the nervous system due to starvation of nerve and cerebrospinal cells. This disease is the most conclusive evidence of the destructive effect of starches and grains used as food for humans. No permanent improvement has ever been achieved, in my 50 years of observation, while the patient was allowed to eat bread, cereals and other starchy foods. Many people however have been helped slowly to recover, by omitting these, and meat, from the diet, eating instead mostly raw fruits and vegetables, drinking at least 3 quarts of fresh raw juices daily, and with frequent colonic irrigations (or colon therapy). The greatest danger in this disease comes from neglecting to follow this program consistently, and so develop secondary complications."[654]

d. Candida and its Neurotoxins

One theory which is used by some doctors is that one of the problems with Parkinson's and MS is *Candida*, (*Candida albicans*) overgrowth and its by-products (mycotoxins). This yeast/fungus is harmless yeast, residing in the gastrointestinal tract on the mucous membranes, and on the skin. Antibiotics kill both the good and bad bacteria in the gastrointestinal tract but do not affect *Candida*. This causes an overgrowth of *Candida* which puts out its own mycotoxins, and this weakens the immune system and attacks the myelin sheath in those with MS. Some of these toxic by-products of mycotoxins can damage neurons, disrupt RNA and DNA synthesis, are carcinogenic, and thus upset the communication of cell interactions. *Candida* leaks through the gut and gets into the rest of the body.

One study notes: "Candida overgrowth and its mycotoxins can attack any organ or system in your body. The attack is relentless, twenty-four hours a day until treated. If not arrested, yeast overgrowth will change form into a pathogenic fungus with roots that cause myriad symptoms. This fungus burrows its roots into the intestinal lining and creates leaky gut - porous openings in the gut lining- that allows the yeast/fungus and its by-products to escape into the blood stream. This systemic yeast/fungal infection is called *candidiasis*, and *Candida albicans* is the most common human systemic pathogen, causing both mucosal and systemic infections, particularly in immune-compromised people."[655] (*Science* Journal, 2000)

Ann Boroch, ND, states, "Once *Candida* is in an overgrowth state, the body has to deal not only with the overgrowth but also with the fact that *Candida albicans* puts out its own toxic by-products or 'mycotoxins - 79 at latest count,' according to one expert, Orian C. Truss, MD, all of which weaken your immune system and attack the myelin sheath in those with MS."[656]

Ann Boroch, ND continues, "Mycotoxins are neurotoxins that destroy and decompose tissues and organs. Mycotoxins are so powerful that they upset the very communication of cell interactions, disrupt RNA and DNA synthesis, damage and destroy neurons, are carcinogenic, produce ataxia (lack of coordination), and even convulsions. These pernicious yeast toxins confuse body system, which accounts for the cross-wiring problems of your immune system once you have MS."[657]

"*Candida* toxins commonly get through the gut lining when it becomes leaky. They then enter the bloodstream, where the liver can detoxify them. However, if the liver's detoxification ability is impaired due to inadequate nutrition and toxic overload, these toxins will settle in other organs and tissues such as the brain, nervous system, joints, skin, and so forth. Over time, chronic disease will occur."[658]

This yeast/fungus overgrowth thrives on diets that have dairy, refined carbohydrates, processed foods, refined sugars, alcohol, and refined grains and meats.

The world-renowned neurologist, David Perlmutter, MD, writes in an article, *The Powerful Therapy for Challenging Brain Disorders*: "The frequency of focal white matter lesions in patients with inflammatory bowel disease is almost as high as that in patients with Multiple Sclerosis. These findings provide convincing evidence supporting that relationship between gut abnormalities and brain pathology. New research clearly reveals a very important relationship between MS and problems in the digestive system like inflammatory bowel disease, yeast overgrowth, and low levels of healthful bacteria. This organism (*Candida albicans*) has been associated with hyper-immune diseases and specifically MS."[659] "*Candida albicans* and its mycotoxins accumulate in the central nervous system, where they attack and create lesions on the myelin sheath."[660]

Dr. Perlmutter is saying that this chronic toxicity over-taxes the immune system, which then loses its ability to function and starts attacking itself. He routinely screens for yeast overgrowth, and when working with MS patients, he integrates an anti-yeast treatment. In another article, he states that the possible link between various autoimmune diseases and infection with the yeast *Candida albicans* has been described by well-respected researchers over the past two decades. He believes that these data provide compelling evidence that candidiasis may, at the very least, be a frequent occurrence in patients with Multiple Sclerosis. In addition, these data seem to indicate that intestinal dysbiosis may be common in MS patients. He now routinely performs serum analysis for *Candida* immune complexes and *Candida* antibodies (IgG, IgM, and IgA) as well as a comprehensive digestive stool analysis on his MS patients. His success in reducing fatigue in MS with treatments designed specifically to reduce *Candida* activity lends further support for the suggested relationship between MS-related fatigue and *Candida* activity. Further, he suggests that intestinal dysbiosis may play a pivotal role with respect to the actual pathogenesis of MS as an autoimmune disease entity.[661]

Dr. Perlmutter also points out a study that 90% of MS patients show large amounts of IgG, manifesting as oligoclonal bands, in brain and cerebrospinal fluid (CSF). Oligoclonal bands are typically a response to infectious pathogens. A decade ago, Vanderbilt researchers found IgG specific to C. pneumonia in CSF from 16 of 17 MS patients but none of 14 controls.[662] (*Neurology*, 2001). The clinical significance of these findings was largely ignored. More recently in 2009, Italian investigators found similar results."[663] (*Neurovirol*, 2009)

There are some strong similarities between candidiasis and MS:
- MS affects more women than it does men, as does candidiasis.
- MS symptoms are ones that impair the nervous system (numbness, tingling, fatigue, poor coordination, urinary frequency, depression, and erratic vision). These are also the symptoms of chronic candidiasis.
- In both conditions, Intestinal dysbiosis, an imbalance between the good and bad bacteria in the gut, is common.
- Both MS and candidiasis suppress the immune system and cause the body to be in an inflammatory state.
- Fatigue is the most common symptom in both conditions.
- Both people with Candidiasis and MS patients have vitamin and mineral deficiencies.

- Food allergies and gluten intolerance are common in both conditions.
- Epstein-Barr virus has been linked with MS and candidiasis.
- Both conditions will respond with dietary changes and an antifungal regime.

A strict Live Plant-based nutrition approach will do this automatically over time. *Candida* exists because a person is eating too much of the wrong carbohydrates. Pharmaceutical drugs only mask this condition and make the candidiasis worse. A faulty diet and taking medications for AD, MS and PD is a major part of the problem and only masks *Candida*.

This would explain the reason why if a person eats this Live Plant-based diet, the fungus stays in remission. If a person goes back to the standard American meat-based diet, the diseases usually comes back within a month, because the fungus starts feeding again. This has been the experience of people who have these diseases.

In the 1950's, there was a drug developed for Parkinson's that was an antifungal that was found to be somewhat successful in Asia and it was written up in a book, but then the use of it faded away. When it was tried in other countries, apparently it didn't work with Parkinson's for some reason, and the results were not consistent in Asia either. A reason it probably worked in Asia is that people are more likely to be vegetarian, and most Asian diets are more natural. The typical Asian diet has a lot of greens, and is healthier than the standard American diet.

Dana Flavin, MD, an expert in toxicity, was asked what she thought was a primary cause or influence in Parkinson's. She mentioned several things, one of them was fungus. She was asked if she thought that a person could have fungus in the brain. She replied, "Of course, it is all over the body even in the brain. It would be one of the main reasons for the inflammation in the brain in people with Parkinson's."[664]

e. Sprouting Brings Grains Alive

Sprouting is not a new development. Not only did the Essenes, during the time of Jesus, use this technique, but the history of sprouting goes as far back as 3000 B.C. in China with the recorded use of bean sprouts.

Learning to sprout regular seeds like alfalfa seeds is an easy way to learn how to sprout. Sprouting is considered a superfood and is a part of a Living Foods lifestyle. Steve Meyerowitz is known as The Sproutman. He has written a book entitled *Sprouts the Miracle Food*.[665] He travels around giving talks on it, and has a sprouting machine he sells, which waters the sprouts automatically. They are great in salads.

If the grains cannot be sprouted, a small amount of cooked grains can be part of the diet. The paradigm of 80 percent live-foods to 20% cooked foods is adequate for supporting general health, and is widely accepted, even though experts like Paavo Airola, Viktoras Kulvinskas, and Gabriel Cousens, MD believe that 100% is the ideal and will provide maximum health and healing. Dr. Cousens states, "For those with major degenerative diseases it is best that the more Live-Foods, eaten the better, the more biogenic and bioactive foods consumed the better."[666]

Gabriel Cousens, MD, a leading raw food expert, gives a good insight into the scientific basis for soaking and sprouting: "In the Conscious Eating Kitchen, (his facilities kitchen), all of the nuts, seeds and grains we use are sprouted and/or soaked. Soaking and sprouting serve several important functions. First, nutrients begin to be broken down into their simplified form. For example, proteins start to break down into amino acids, carbohydrates into simple sugars, fats into fatty acids, while minerals chelate or combine with proteins. This significantly improves digestion and assimilation, and it is why soaked or sprouted foods are considered predigested."[667]

Dr. Cousens continues: "Second, the actual content of nutrients dramatically increases during soaking and sprouting process. Proteins, vitamins, enzymes, and minerals increase 300 to 1200%. For example, zinc present in alfalfa sprouts increases from approximately 6.8 mg per 100 grams of seed to 18 mg per 100 grams dried weight in the sprout. One cup of alfalfa sprouts provides twice the US RDA for zinc. Enzyme inhibitors, phytic and oxalic acids, and mineral chelates are washed away during the soaking and sprouting process. These chemicals function as natural defenses against bacterial, fungal, insect and animal predators in the growing process of the plant, but many interfere with digestion and assimilation when consumed. Finally, chlorophyll develops in the sprouts as they turn green."[668]

"Grains constitute the next class of yeast/fungi/mold-stimulating foods after the high-sugar foods and fruits in particular. Research shows that stored grains ferment in ninety days. Within that time many mycotoxins are produced. In essence, stored grains are a mycotoxic hazard. A correlation was found between 112 patients with esophageal cancer and consumption of stored grains (*Cancer, 1987*). There was a particular risk factor for stomach cancer among Scandinavian and German men eating stored grains reported in *The Fungal/Mycotoxin Etiology of Human Disease*, vol. 2. Stored potatoes also represent a mycotoxic risk. The black spots on them are caused by the fungi aspergillums and fusarium, which produce the mycotoxins aflatoxin and fumosium. Some grains are not stored and therefore are not a mycotoxin hazard. These include pelt, amaranth, quinoa, millet, buckwheat, and wild rice. Buckwheat is often thought of as a seed, but it is actually classified as a grain."[669]

Dr. Cousens concludes, "Grains do not rot like fruit, but they do ferment. This fermentation is the mixture of starch, sugar, and sometimes yeast. The result of these products is alcohol and gas. The alcohol is a mycotoxic by-product and can create what we refer to by the phrase 'food drunk.' Alcohol is a protoplasmic poison, which means that it has a negative effect on any cell in the body. Grains generally have been associated with a series of problems: allergies, asthma, gluten and gliadin intolerance, digestive disturbances, yeast infections, various mucous and congestive conditions, and several types of arthritis. These are, of course, linked with mycosis [process of making mycotoxins], either directly by eating grains, or indirectly through eating the animals that feed on them and drinking the animals milk."[670]

Sprouting helps to create biogenic foods, which means that these foods have more life energy in general or specifically: live foods have more enzymes, bioelectrical energy, bioluminescence, bioactive electrons, bio-photons, phytonutrients, and higher SOEF energy patterns.

Dr. Cousens explains in his book, *Spiritual Nutrition*: "Sprouts are alkaline-producing and energy-charged. They are high in enzymes, predigested complete proteins, chelated minerals, nucleic acids, vitamins, RNA, and DNA, and B12. The process of soaking is used because it activates the proteases, which neutralize the enzyme inhibitors that keep the seeds, legumes, and grains from germinating at the wrong time. Germinating and sprouting increase the enzyme content by six to twenty times. Plant hormones are also activated and phytates are split off, and there is a tremendous increase in metabolic activity. Starches are broken down into simple sugars, proteins are predigested into easily assimilated free amino acids, and fats are broken down into soluble fatty acids. Vitamin and mineral content increase with sprouting; this was one of the clues of the phenomenon of biological transmutation."[671]

"They are the highest class of foods because they are *biogenic*, in other words a cell-renewing and life-generating food. These are the most life-generating, high-energy type of foods. These biogenic foods have the capacity to generate a totally new organism. It is the life force of these foods that is transferred to people and aids their healing and regeneration."[672]

"The second category is *bioactive* foods. These are foods that are capable of sustaining and slightly enhancing an already healthy life force. Bioactive foods include fresh, unprocessed, raw fruits and vegetables."

"The third category is *biostatic* foods. These foods are neither life-sustaining nor life-generating; they diminish the quality of body functioning. They are life-slowing foods that slowly increase the process of aging. These are cooked foods and foods that, although raw, are no longer fresh."

"The fourth category is called *bioacidic*, or life-destroying foods. These are foods that have gone through many processes and refinements and are full of additives and preservatives. They rapidly break down life function."

"In their whole state, live foods have more enzymes, bioelectrical energy, bioluminescence, bioactive electrons, bio-photons, phytonutrients, higher SOEF energy patterns, and life force energy in general. When we eat live foods, we are consuming the living energy of the planet and fully immersing ourselves in the full energy of food as a Love note from God."[673]

i. Make Bread of Them

Grains are spoken of as good in the bible, yet remember everything back in biblical times was organic, free of pesticides, heavy metals and other contaminants. Sprouting grains is superior to dormant grains.

"For the Lord thy God brings thee into a good land, a land of brooks, of water, of fountains with depths that spring out of valleys and hills; a land of wheat, and barley, and vines, and fig trees, and pomegranates; a land of oil, of olives, and honey."   (Deuteronomy 8.7, 8)

"Take wheat and barley, beans and lentils, millet and spelt, and put them into a single vessel and make bread of them."   (Ezekiel 4.9)   Bread made of this combination is a complete protein source.

Chapter 14

Living Foods versus Dead Foods

With the rise of monasticism in the fourth century, the question of a suitable diet for a Christian monk was answered by Saint Pachomius (292-348) a founder of Christian monasticism. He stipulated two meals a day, one during the day and one in the evening. The main meal was in the day and consisted of bread and cooked vegetables and a dessert of some kind, possible dried fruit or some other morsel.[674] The monks lived on a diet of herbs, olives, and cheese.[675] Another reference states "almost all the brothers practice abstinence and do not eat cooked food. The cooks had taken it upon themselves to decide that it was right to encourage every member of the community to eat raw food."[676] "Basil of Caesarea (d. 379) suggests one meal a day, vegetables, and fruits." "The fifth-century historian Sozomen mentions a group of Syrian ascetics called 'grazers' who lived on grass cut with a sickle."[677] These are very important quotes because they show one of the first recorded raw food or Live-Food emphasis was found in a community, a monastery in the fourth century.

a. Living Plant-based Foods

A Living Foods approach versus a dead foods approach, is all about life and living to the full, which can only be fully achieved on Living Foods. The nutritional approach is a raw vegan diet that ranges from 80/20 to 100% raw. The 80/20 means 80% raw and 20% cooked foods, on average. There are thousands of choices of dishes that can be simply made from raw fruits and vegetables, nuts and seeds. These can easily supply all of one's nutritional needs. This leads a person into living foods, or Live-Food. Living foods are foods that are alive and have all the enzymes, nutrients and cellular structures still alive and not dead or dying. The body grows and matures optimally on living foods not dead foods.

The body uses a Live-Food program for curing diseases like PD, AD or MS, it is a therapeutic program. A karate master was at a tournament and was asked about how he would fight for points in China and he replied: "I never fought for points, I only fought for life, either I win and kill my opponent or he kills me." This is what happens with these degenerative diseases like Parkinson's or Alzheimer's or MS you must fight for life and not for points. Either you fight and kill the disease or it will kill you.

A 2009 book cites a news report stated that: Raw food is one of the seven most popular diets in the world. Google.com has 1.7 million sites devoted to this style of eating. Most raw foodists prepare most of their food at home, but raw food restaurants are opening everywhere.[678]

Live-Foods Nutrition is a new paradigm. It is another level of nutrition that is above the level of nutrition medical science currently works with. Nutrition today is still very much linear and Newtonian, where A influences B which influences C in a linear fashion. Living Foods is holistic and has multiple things happening on several different levels, which are not linear in fashion - it is another paradigm shift. The linear nature of interactions between matter and energy in the Newtonian biology school of thought has changed to complex holistic pathways today in the Quantum biology school of thought.

What is the difference between raw foods and Living Foods? A leading Live-Food promoter Brenda Cobb explains it this way: "Let's talk about the difference between raw and Living Foods. Raw foods are those picked off trees or vines, such as apples, berries, cucumbers, avocados, squash, tomatoes and bananas, etc. Living Foods are beans, grains, nuts, and seeds that have been soaked and sprouted. When the sprout comes out of the grain, seed or berry, it becomes a 'Living Food,' full of life and increased nutritional value. Ann Wigmore made the distinction between raw and Living Foods, and promoted the Living Foods Lifestyle."[679]

b. PD Olfactory Dysfunction

"Cooking can be a problem for people with degenerative diseases. One neurodegenerative symptom that makes a nutritional program hard for Parkinson's, Alzheimer's and others, is the problem with the sense of smell. This is also reported in the book, *Geriatric Nutrition*. 'Olfactory dysfunction is reported in a wide range of neurodegenerative disorders, including Alzheimer's disease (AD), Parkinson's disease (PD) (and variants), Huntington's disease and Down's syndrome,[680] as shown through a meta-analysis of 43 studies.[681] Olfactory dysfunction appears to be an early marker in those at risk for developing AD,[682] and most patients with AD have, but are unaware of, olfactory dysfunction.[683] Olfactory dysfunction is seen in 9 of 10 individuals with PD (a rate that exceeds the presence of tremors, a hallmark sign of PD), and they are unaware of the dysfunction.[684] The severity of PD does not correspond with the degree of olfactory dysfunction. Medications used to treat PD do not improve olfactory functioning.'[685] 'Olfactory dysfunction can disrupt dietary behaviors[686] and cause loss of appetite and weight[687] in animals. In humans, the relationship between appetite and olfactory dysfunction is not consistent. Up to 48% of individuals seen for a chemosensory disturbance report a decreased appetite with the onset of the disorder.[688]""

A person should go 100% raw vegan for long periods of time, then you can have a little bit of cooked vegan foods as long as your diet is above 80% raw. Living plant-based nutrition is   superior to cooked foods. Fresh, Ripe, Raw Living foods contain all the nutrients necessary for good health, growth, maintenance and repair.

c. Living Foods versus dead foods

Living Foods avoid the stimulant highs and depressant lows (Sugar, coffee, caffeinated tea, soda, rich foods, overeating, alcohol, etc.)
Living Foods are easier to prepare and digest.
Living Foods are much easier to clean up after.
Living Foods help the body to achieve a normal weight.
Living Foods restore the natural *appestat* (appetite control).
Living Foods do not cause or support degenerative diseases.
Living Foods help a person feel better and have more energy.
Living Foods provide the highest nutrient count per calorie.
Living Foods allow a person to spend less time sleeping.
Living Foods minimizes bad breath, body odor and gas.
Living Foods cost less when it becomes a lifestyle.

A well-known study on natural foods-vs-cooked foods was a 10 year research project conducted by Dr. Francis M. Pottenger using 900 cats. "His study was published in 1946 in the *American Journal of Orthodontics and Oral Surgery*. Dr. Pottenger fed all 900 cats the same food, with the only difference being that one group received it raw, while the others received it cooked. The results dramatically revealed the advantages of raw foods over a cooked diet. Cats that were fed raw, living food produced healthy kittens, year after year, with no ill health or premature deaths. But cats fed the same food, only cooked, developed heart disease, cancer, kidney and thyroid disease, pneumonia, paralysis, loss of teeth, arthritis, birthing difficulties, diminished sexual interest, diarrhea, irritability, liver problems and osteoporosis (the same diseases common in our human cooked-food culture). The first generations of kittens from cats fed cooked food were sick and abnormal, the second generation was often born diseased or dead, and by the third generation, the mothers were sterile."[689]

"Cooking, baking roasting, broiling, boiling and steaming destroy from 30% to 90% of the nutrition in the food, resulting in a nutrient-deficient diet, the main cause of degenerative diseases. 97-100% of the enzymes are destroyed in cooking. Minerals are leached into the cooking water when cooking; and liquids (broth) are often poured out.

Cooked foods become so devitalized they take more energy to digest than they give and are difficult to digest.

Cooked foods shorten our life span.

Cooked foods cause far more build-up of toxins, a factor suppressing the immune system and making the body more susceptible to disease of all kinds.

Cooked foods encourage over eating, resulting in weight gain. Since they are nutrient-deficient, they leave the system still hungering for and craving food.

The natural fiber is broken down, increasing transit time of food through the gastrointestinal tract. Increased transit time means sugars ferment, proteins putrefy, and fats turn rancid, loosening toxins for absorption.

The carcinogenic substances are formed from foods-cooked or grilled over charcoal forms during some cooking procedures. The meat drippings drop onto the charcoal and carcinogenic substances are transmitted by steam onto the cooked meats.

Leucocytosis (an increase in white blood cell count and associated with a pathological condition) increases upon ingestion of cooked food.

There is poor mastication resulting in decreased saliva and enzyme flow; food is, therefore, poorly prepared for digestion.

Cooked food is most often fragmented/refined/deficient.

Cooked food is most often highly chemicalized.

Cooked food is prepared in utensils that give off toxic metal/plastic/paint particles.

Cooked food is most often addicting and promotes overeating.

Finally cooked foods falsely satisfy the taste and appetite but cause abnormal cravings for sugary foods (candy, cakes, pies, ice creams, cookies, etc.) Heavy meats, richly-seasoned starches, such as breads with spreads, deep fat-fried potato and corn chips, French fries, spicy, rich grain and legume dishes also cause abnormal cravings. After such a meal, the coffee drinker craves coffee for the caffeine fix, which over-stimulates the pancreas to produce more enzymes to digest all the heavy food."[690]

On grocery shelves, there sit more than 5,000 items processed from whole natural foods into empty edibles. Some 65% of the American adults and 25% of children under 17 now live with chronic diseases which are fed by cooked foods and commercially prepared foods.

d. Cooking to Brown: Millard Reaction

When certain foods are roasted or baked, they turn brown or golden and their taste and aroma are enhanced. This is from the Maillard reaction, which occurs when amino acids are cooked in the presence of carbohydrates (particularly reducing sugars such as glucose). This reaction can produce compounds called advanced glyco-oxidation end products (AGEs), which are of significant concern. This negative or bad effect on a macro-molecular level can be the cause or feed degenerative diseases in the future.

AGEs are linked to cancer and "enhanced cancer progression,"[691] diabetes, kidney disease, aging,[692] and neurodegenerative diseases such as Alzheimer's.[693] AGEs are also implicated in slower healing of wounds in diabetics[694] as well as diabetes-related autoimmunity.[695] AGEs may reduce nutritive value,[696] as well as increase protein stability, and therefore allergenicity. Higher levels of AGEs are also detected in patients with Creuzfeld-Jacob Disease (CJD or mad cow disease), but it is not clear if they contribute to the disease.[697]

e. Sodium-potassium balance

Another issue is that we need sodium. Table salt is heated to over a thousand degrees, it is not organic, and it's dead. Natural organic salts are found in fruits and vegetables. Even though this is basic nutrition the real emphasis is the sodium-potassium balance.

We still need a certain amount of sodium every day and a person can easily get that through your daily vegetables and greens. A little sea salt in items can give some additional sodium. Most Americans have too much sodium in their systems and not enough potassium, so their sodium-potassium pumps are unbalanced. The sodium-potassium pumps exist in every cell in the body.

The Gerson therapeutic diet and the Natural Hygiene diets are very strong about a "no salt" diet and they even tell people "no salt in the water system." Even if people don't drink the water, they shower in the water and that water will get into the skin through the pores. A person needs to detox themselves of salt to re-establish the proper sodium-potassium balance in the cells.

f. Healthy, Life-Giving Bread

Life and living are rooted in our physical being, our body, which is the Temple of the Holy Spirit. As scripture points out, "If anybody should destroy the temple of God, God will destroy him, because the temple of God is sacred, and you are that temple." Or another place, "Your body, you know, is the temple of the Holy Spirit, who is in you since you received him from God." Also it states, "A man never hates his own body, but he feeds it and looks after it; and that is the way Christ treats the Church, because it is his body - and we are its living parts." (1 Cor 3:17; 1 Cor 6:19; Eph 5:29) Even the Jesus Christ who is the new Adam refers to himself as "the Bread of Life." In Aramaic it means the healthy, life-giving bread. Jesus said; "Give us each day our daily life-giving bread." Lk 11.2

Chapter 15

Salads, Smoothies & Juices

St. Thomas Aquinas[r] (d. 1274) writes about how our "Health of body" needs to become a habit in our life. As St. Thomas writes, "Habits are concerned with human action. They can be related to the human action directly or indirectly. Some habits then can be found in the essential parts of his nature - his body and soul. Health of body or beauty of body, are habits that affect man's nature directly and his actions indirectly. Health makes a man's body well-disposed in itself and a fit instrument of the soul and the powers of the soul in search of happiness. A healthy man [or woman] can work better than a sick one."[698]

"Health of body enables man [or woman] to live and act efficiently in the natural order. Since most habits are acquired by human activity, it follows that they can be increased or lessened. They can grow or diminish. The more frequently a man acts honestly, the stronger becomes the habit of honesty."[699]

St. Thomas Aquinas states, "There are seven capital sins or vices: pride, covetousness, gluttony, lust, envy, anger and sloth. They are disordered inclinations. Our survey of the causes of sin in human life shows clearly that the chief cause of sin is the human will. Every man is free to choose good or evil. Reason may be ignorant; the sense appetite may be strong. But in the last analysis it is the will which chooses evil. It is the will which sins."[700] Americans often live a comfortable armchair spirituality and also dietary practices involving these sins.

---

[r] St. Thomas Aquinas in his *Summa*, II.5, "Happiness and Habit".

a. The basic Diet for PD, AD and MS

When dealing with PD, AD and MS the recommended nutritional approach promotes salads, smoothies and juices. A simplified format for this Live-Food Nutrition approach has been noted earlier.

- A 100%/95% Live-Food diet is the ideal.
- An 85/15% raw vegan diet, usually one meal is a large salad; this is a 100% vegan, 85% raw plant-based foods which have less than 15% cooked foods.
- Six, 8 oz glasses of freshly-juiced carrot or apple or cucumber juice daily.
- Six teaspoons of a green powder like barley grass powder (or green powders like: barley, wheat and/or alfalfa grass combinations) daily.
- Breakfast should be juice, a smoothie, some fruit, or a light meal
- Lunch and Dinner consists of two large raw vegan meals (one meal is a large salad and fermented foods)
- Vigorous walking or other aerobic exercise like flow yoga, at least ½ to 1 hour a day to help digestion;
- Sunshine, fresh air, prayer, and meditation daily.
- Finally, a weekly meeting with a mental health professional or counselor is needed to work through the issues, both past and present.

In summary we could say:
1. Two raw vegan meals; lunch and dinner (one meal is a large salad with some fermented foods or drinks), breakfast is juice, smoothie, fruit or light meal.
2. Six 8 oz glasses of freshly juiced carrot/ apple/ and/or cucumber juice or other veggie juice and a smoothie.
3. Six teaspoons of a green powder; like barley grass powder, 2 to 3 times a day.

This is the nutritional therapy in a nutshell. It has a history of healing MS and Parkinson's from the authors have met and/or researched, as noted in this book. It brings a strong dimension of purification to the physiology for both people with MS and PD and even AD.

b. Salads and Greens

There are a lot of good raw vegan salad books and raw food prep books on the market. The following is a recommended Alleluia salad.

One to two times daily, a person with Parkinson's, AD, or MS needs to have a large salad. This salad is not to be cooked, but raw, and should be primarily vegetables, but some fruits could be added in. The salad should be composed of primarily vegetables such as: cucumbers, carrots, tomatoes, spinach, yellow or orange peppers, green onions, parsley, turnip, broccoli, cauliflower, asparagus, beets, turnips, cabbage, avocado, and nuts (soaked nuts and seeds like walnuts, almonds, or seeds like sunflower seeds), and any other vegetables. It's best to have half a dozen to a dozen different vegetables. It is easiest to cut up a few days to a weeks' worth of vegetables in a food processor, into small pieces and put them into covered containers. Making enough for a week is the easiest way to do this salad. It is best to leave out the cucumbers, tomatoes and any other soft juicy vegetables, which adds liquid to the salad decreasing the shelf life in the refrigerator. Putting these soft vegetables in a separate container and adding them in later.

It is best to leave out the leafy greens such as kale, spinach, or lettuce and add them in separately or use them in a smoothie. When leafy greens are whirled in a blender, cellular structures break open, making the chlorophyll easily digested. That's why smoothies contain so many beneficial nutrients.

c. Green Smoothie's, Juices and Powders

What about green smoothies? There are some good books out on this one recommended is the book by James and Anne Marie Tibbetts on *Living Green with Smoothies and Chlorophyll Rich Foods*. It give a rather complete overview of the literature, the science behind it and is a how to do smoothies book.

The green smoothie is one of the keys for degenerative diseases. Blending breaks open the cellular structure and releases the chlorophyll into the liquid. A liquid, colloidal form is one of the best ways to take nutrients. A smoothie basically contains fresh fruit (such as banana, apple, berries, peaches, mango, pineapple chunks, etc.); 2-3 cups water; 1-2 cups juice; leafy greens (such as kale, spinach, Swiss chard, arugula, mescaline, romaine lettuce, etc.); juicy vegetables like cucumbers or tomatoes; optional a large scoop of protein powder, a teaspoon or two of barley, wheat grass or other green powder, or avocado which adds a smooth texture. Blend it all together; if it is too thick, add more water or juice.

Make up three or four at once since they will keep for several days. There's an old saying an apple a day keeps the doctor away, well now the saying is "a smoothie a day keeps the doctor away!"

What about juices, why carrot juice? There is a long history of juicing using carrot juice with many books discussing it. Primarily because it is an easy vegetable to juice and it yields a lot of juice. There are surely some anti-Parkinson's and Anti-MS Nutrients in carrot juice that will fight both Parkinson's and MS, but there is not enough research to prove this yet. The main proof is in the clinical arena: in the testimonials mentioned earlier.

The Gerson Institute, in San Diego, California promote the use of 6 glasses of carrot juice and 6 glasses of green juices daily for cancer and other degenerative diseases. Other medical experts, like Dr. Bernard Jensen, also recommend carrot juice to clients to promote healing.

Other juices like cucumber and apple can be beneficial if they are freshly juiced, no store bought juices since these are all pasteurized. Cucumber and apple juice can add some more flavor to the carrot juice. At least four glasses daily are needed to promote the cure but six are recommended. This is a lot of juice but a person with a degenerative disease needs to flood the cellular structure with these nutrients and juicing is the easiest way, although the salads and smoothies are still needed and add fiber and many other nutrients.

What if a person has a hard time having fresh juices, smoothies made for him or her, wouldn't store-bought juices work just as well? Yes but to a limited degree. I discourage buying juices in the store because they are not organic, are all pasteurized at high temperatures, which destroys a lot of the nutrients, enzymes and other component in juice, and most have a high sugar content from the way they are processed. Most I (Jim T.) would not recommend for many different reasons.

Are there any you would recommend? There are many good health food type of juices like: R.W. Knudsen, Santa Cruz, Lakewood organic, Bionature, and others. One juice that is bio-culture organic, an advanced growing of produce (since 1957) and has lower pasteurization temperature and has a strong reputation for being a functional food/juice (for curing) is "Biotta". *Biotta Natural* [s] is an excellent organic juice, definitely one of the best, if not the best on the market. Drinking 2 bottles a day (four to 6 cups)

---

[s] On the web (Biottajuices.com) is from Switzerland and sold in some health food stores and but it is expensive, about twice the cost of other juices.

could replace the 6 cups of freshly made juice but as of yet there are no documented results using these juices, whereas with freshly made juices there is a track record of success and they are less expensive.

What about protein powders? These are very good for vegans but not always necessary. A plant-based protein powder is necessary like the companies *Vega* or *Sunwarrior or Garden of Life*. *Vega* has a whole line of vegan supplements and is found in most health food stores. They are the only completely vegan company or one of the few.

What about the green powders? The use of green powders I spoke of earlier are a major means of purification for the body.[t] It is very difficult to eat as many greens as are needed to bring a cure of the disease and making green juices from fresh, ripe, raw, organic plants is difficult and expensive. As I just said, the Gerson Institute promotes 6 glasses of green drinks and 6 glasses of carrot juice a day for their patients, which are mostly cancer patients. You need an expensive juicer and a lot of time to put into all the work of making green juices. Therefore using green powders is the next best option, to colloidal liquid nutrients such as wheat grass juice. Two of the best green powders are wheat grass and barley grass; they are best because a lot of research has been done on them showing their therapeutic value. About three grams or one heaping teaspoon of barley powder is the equivalent of about two handfuls, or 100 grams, of fresh young barley leaves.

But four to six teaspoons of barley grass a day is a lot, isn't it? Yes it is a lot for a healthy person maybe; but not for a person with Parkinson's or MS or any other degenerative disease. This has been the clinical experience for healing these kinds of diseases. The barley grass can be mixed in with the juice or with the smoothie or taken with water.

---

[t] Green powders in chapter on Plant-based Diets are Reconstructive.

The meals should be an 80/20% or 85/15% raw vegan diet, at least one meal is a large salad is daily. It includes as much raw as possible, 95% to 100% would be ideal but at least 80-85% raw foods. It would be best to have the smoothie in the morning and the large salad at lunch or dinner. It is a very simple nutritional therapy but discipline and determination are needed.

d. Low Stomach Acidity

This is a problem with a lot of older people with or without diseases and this diet is very helpful with it. Hydrochloric acid in the stomach is important for human health. This impacts the digestion and absorption of many nutrients and a shortage of Hydrochloric acid can lead to nutritional deficiencies and this could develop into diseases. Professor W. A. Walker from the Department of Nutrition at Harvard School of Public Health, states that, "Medical researchers since the 1930's have been concerned about the consequences of hypochlorhydria. While all the health consequences are still not entirely clear, some have been well documented."[701] Hypochlorhydria is low stomach acidity, when the body is not producing enough stomach acid. This impacts digestion and absorption of nutrients. Stomach acid also destroys all harmful microorganisms, pathogenic bacteria, parasites and their eggs, and fungi that enter the body through the mouth.[702] If the stomach acid is insufficient then there is no barrier against these organisms.

As we get old does HCL decrease? As we age, especially after 40, the level of hydrochloric acid (HCL) decreases. If we abuse our body through excess food and the wrong types of foods it can also causes the hydrochloric acid to decrease. "Overeating, especially over consumption of fats and proteins, wears out the parietal cells of the stomach that secret HCL."[703] "Stomach acid helps to digest large protein molecules. If stomach acid is low, then incompletely digested protein fragments get absorbed into the bloodstream and cause allergies and immunological disorders."[704]

Is there a simple solution for this? Yes, green smoothies, because blending foods is similar to chewing foods. Unfortunately, most people do not chew their foods enough to break them down completely. A high speed blender breaks the foods down for easier assimilation. The food doesn't stay in the stomach as long so less hydrochloric acid is needed. The process of blending aids the body in that it doesn't need to produce more HCL, saves energy, and promotes easier assimilation. Having green smoothies is a good solution to help this situation.

e. Maximize the Colors on your Plate

An easy way to get started is to eat a rainbow colored plant-based diet. A rainbow of colors brings peace to the soul. There is a mosaic of colorful fruits and vegetables and the more colorful your food choices the better. Over the course of a week, you want to maximize the colors on your plate. In the book, *The Color Code: a Revolutionary Eating Plan for Optimum Health* by James Joseph, PhD, Daniel Nadeau, MD, and Anne Underwood, they emphasize the importance of eating a variety of colors every day for prevention and healing. 'Indeed, almost every colorful food – from fresh-picked apples to cool green kiwis, bright red strawberries, and zesty, ripe oranges – is loaded with disease fighters. Many of them are found in the pigments themselves. Consider:

- The natural dye that makes tomatoes red may help ward off prostate cancer. A Harvard study found that 10 servings of tomato products a week reduced the risk of aggressive tumors by nearly half.
- The crimson in sour cherries may alleviate your arthritis pain. Researchers in Michigan found sour cherries to be 10 times stronger than aspirin in relieving pain.

- The yellow in corn could protect your eyesight. Repeated studies have found that it helps prevent macular degeneration, the leading cause of blindness in people over 65.
- The golden pigment in curry powder can reduce inflammation. Researchers are now studying its potential to prevent colon cancer, which is often linked to inflammation.
- The blue in bilberries, a close relative of blueberries, appears to enhance night vision. The indigo pigments in blueberries may starve off the natural mental decline that occurs as we age.'"[705]

"The pigments that give the color fall into two main classes known as carotenoids and anthocyanins. The carotenoids are the yellow-orange-red end of the spectrum. They are also found in leafy green vegetables, but the strong color of green chlorophyll masks these other colors. In the fall, in trees, the cold pushes aside the chlorophyll and the golden hues of yellow, orange and red appear. "There are over 600 carotenoids in nature, but only 50 in the human diet – of which 25 or so get into the bloodstream. The most important of these are alpha- and beta-carotene, beta-cryptoxanthin, lycopene, lutein, and zeaxanthin."[706]

"The other major class of pigments found throughout the plant kingdom, are 'the anthocyanins which have hues ranging from crimson and magenta to violet and indigo. These are widely distributed in the food we eat. Cherries, plums, red currants, and blueberries all owe their beautiful hues to anthocyanins. There are more than 300 of these pigments, 70 of which have been reported in fruits.'[707]

f. Deficient in Phytonutrients

If a person with PD, AD or MS are they low in some of these phytonutrients? Phytochemicals are not considered nutrients like proteins, fats, and carbohydrates and vitamins. Yet the term phytonutrient has started to be used along with phytochemical as scientists are become more aware of their great importance in the body. Our bodies have different uses for the majority of antioxidants and phytochemicals than plants do. "The human body evolved with most of those chemicals," says botanist James Duke, author of *The Green Pharmacy* and compiler of a massive USDA phytochemical database, "that's why you need them in your diet. Cancer, in many cases, is a deficiency of antioxidants, so is heart disease. Scientists are starting to think of these diseases as a shortage of phytochemicals."[708]

Scientists are still learning what all the phytochemicals in foods of these different colors indicate. Researchers are learning how they work in their vast synergistic networks. Even though they can be dehydrated some of the beneficial benefits can be lost. The best way to get all these benefits is by eating living foods in various color combinations. "There are thousands of compounds in plants that are associated with lower disease rates," says Cornell University biochemist T. Colin Campbell, who helped conduct the longest running nutrition study to date of the Chinese diet and disease prevention. The only way to take advantage of them all is by eating a diet rich in brightly-colored fruits and vegetables, not popping supplements every day. Dr. Campbell says, "There are no magic bullets."[709] Try to eat a kaleidoscope of different colored life-giving fruits and vegetables.

g. Healing or Purified in the Gospels

Healing plays a large role in the Gospel, where four different verbs are used to express it. One of the words is *katharizo*, which means 'purify' and this is found in various Gospel texts (Mt 8:2, 3; 11:5; Mk 1:40; Lk 5:12; 17:14). This is a very significant insight since back in Biblical times for a person to be cured meant that they were purified or cleansed and it involved eating and fasting.
- "That penance (or purification) and remission of sins should be preached to all nations." Lk 24.47

- "Purify thyself and believe the Good News." Mk 1:15
- "He shall purify himself." Num 19:12
- "Keep thyself pure ..." 1 Tim 5:22
- "sanctifieth to the purifying of the flesh." Heb 9:13

The four different verbs are used to express healing or being cured are:

- One is *therepeuo*, which is used forty-two times in the New Testament (Mt 16; Mk 6; Lk 13; Jn 1; Ac 4; Apoc 2).

- Another is *iaomai* (*iatros*, 'physician,' is a noun from the same root), which is used twenty-six times in the New Testament, especially by Luke, who was himself a physician (Lk 11; Ac 4; Mt 4; scattered use in other New Testament books).

- A third is *katharizo*, which means 'purify' (Mt 8:2,3; 11:5; Mk 1:40; Lk 5:12; 17:14), (used many times in Old Testament).

- The fourth verb is *sozein*,[u] 'save,' which is often used of 'salvation' in the full and transcendent sense, but is also used in the sense of 'heal' (notably in Mt 9:21-22; 14:36; Mk 5:23, 28; 6:56; Lk 7:3; 8:36, 48 50; 17:19; Jn 11:12; Ac 4:9; 14:9; Jam 5:15)."

---

[u] Examples of *sozein*: "...fringe of his cloak. And all those who touched it were completely cured [saved]." Mt 9:21 "Do come and lay your hands on her to make her better and save [heal] her life." Mk 5:23; "When he (the centurion) heard about Jesus he sent some Jewish elders to him, asking him to come and save [heal] the life of his servant." Lk 7:3; Jesus said to her, 'Daughter, it is your faith that has cured [saved] you. Now go in peace." Lk 8:48; "Fear is useless; what is needed is trust and her life will be spared [healed]." Lk 9:50 He said to the man, 'Stand up and go your way; you faith has been your salvation [healing]. Lk 17.19 "crippled ... restored to health [saved] ... in the name of Jesus." Acts 4:9; "Paul looking directly at him and saw that he had the faith to be saved [healed]." Acts 14:9; "the prayer of faith will save [heal] the sick man." James 5:15.

Chapter 16

Supplements for AD, PD and MS

St. Gregory of Sinai (d. 1360) says: "The partaking of food has three degrees: abstinence, adequacy and satiety. To abstain, means to remain a little hungry after eating; to eat adequately, means neither to be hungry, nor weighed down; to be satiated, means to be slightly weighed down. But eating beyond satiety is the door to belly-madness, through which lust comes in. But you, firm in this knowledge, choose what is best for you, according to your powers, without overstepping the limits: for the perfect, according to the Apostle, ought "both to be full and to be hungry . . . and do all things through Christ which strengthened." (Phil. 4:12, 13)."[710]

a. Helpful but they do not Cure AD, PD or MS

Supplements can be helpful but by themselves, they will not cure AD, PD or MS. They are a short-term solution for nutritional deficiencies. The long-term use of Living Food and fasting as we have been discussing is the method to put into remission or to cure these diseases.

Reviews of the use of vitamins and minerals in journal studies have not found enough consistent evidence to recommend them. This includes: vitamins A, B_{12}, C, and E; selenium, zinc, folic acid, docosahexaenoic acid and Omega 3 fatty acids. The herbals: curcumin, ginkgo and cannabinoids (marijuana) have shown little, to no positive effects in improving the symptoms of AD or dementia. The problem with the journal studies done on all of these is that they are from various countries around the world and mostly with people who eat a meat-based diet. If they were testing a strict vegetarian population, then these vitamins would have a better chance of getting more positive results. Diets have effects on the nutrients that are taken in, especially with the body that has an acidic pH on the cellular level, from a meat-based diet. Whereas, a proper alkaline pH of 7.0 to 7.6 in the body, found in a healthy vegetarian person, could have a positive effect.

Brian Clement, PhD in his book *Killer Fish* points out "A 'meta-analysis' published in the Journal of the American Medical Association (*JAMA*) that purported to show how the consumption of vitamins A, E, C, and beta-carotene – the 'antioxidant' group of nutrients – may 'significantly increase mortality' among supplement users, 'significantly' being defined here as a 5-percent overall increase in the risk of death."[711]

A second critical examination of the JAMA study, cited above, this one done by physicians associated with the Alliance for Natural Health in Britain (2007), pointed out they used synthetic supplements. "It was seriously remiss of [the JAMA study authors] not to emphasize that the studies they used to condemn these vitamins were nearly all performed using synthetic forms of the vitamins that behave in the body in remarkable different ways to the natural forms."[712]

Sherry Rogers, MD, an environmental doctor and author, notes how many people are deficient in certain vitamins or minerals. She points out that basically there's two ways to deal with it: spend several thousand dollars doing tests to find out what they are deficient in, or just have them take mega-vitamins and minerals for two months and that will force the nutrients deep down into the body (which a multivitamin may not reach). This will balance out and fill out their needs for those deficient nutrients. Then she would recommend that they reduce the mega-nutrients to just a multi-vitamin and/or dosages of certain nutrients. It is very important to get enough vitamins and minerals, and concentrated intake can help to ensure this will happen.

Dana Flavin, MD, an American who is living and working in Germany, explained the following to author in 2009. She is an internationally known Neuro-pharmacologist and a physician who says, the key to healing degenerative diseases, like Parkinson's, is the synergistic activity of the detox, diet and nutrients together. Dr. Flavin emphasizes that detox is very important since you need to keep detoxing the body to get the toxins and poisons out and to re-balance the biochemistry, otherwise the nutrients may not be able to work. The same goes for modern drugs, they work much better if the biochemical environment is clean.

Dr. Flavin points out that most people in the US don't want to do the nutritional therapy the way they are supposed to. Overseas in Germany and other European countries they are much more accepting and willing to cooperate with nutritional therapy. Most people in the US just want some vitamins and herbs or other "XYZ natural product" to take. These patients do not want to make lifestyle changes. They have to have the 'will' to make these changes. It is more than just an act of the 'will', it is also involved with their level of peace and low levels of stress. If they are stressed out, then their hormone levels will be all over the place and these simple XYZ products just will not be able to work. The neurotoxicity in Parkinson's disease continues even after treatments. The toxicity is caused by many factors which may be influenced by both diet and nutritional supplements.[713]

b. Probiotics: Gut-brain Connection

Dr. Alan Logan in *The Brain Diet* notes "*Lactobacilli* and *Bifidobacteria* can lower levels of brain-toxic compounds that can otherwise build up through digestive and other metabolic processes. While many mainstream gastroenterologists and neurologists would be quick to dismiss the functioning of *Lactobacilli* and *Bifidobacteria* as being of no relevance to brain function and behavior, emerging research supports a connection. Recently, bacteria belonging to these genera have been shown to lower immune cytokine levels, not only locally in the gut, but also in the body-wide bloodstream when orally administered."[714]

c. Neuronutrients help the brain

Paris Kidd in a journal article (*Nutrition*) relates some categories of brain helping nutrients. Evidence suggests that neuronutrients help the brain in the following ways:

- Building-block nutrients help the brain form new neurons (neurogenesis).[715]
- Neurotransmitter nutrients help the brain synthesize the chemicals that enable nerve transmission.[716]
- Vasodilator nutrients boost blood flow to the brain, bringing abundant oxygen and nutrition.[717]
- Antioxidant nutrients protect the brain from oxidative stress and degeneration.[718]
- Energizing nutrients supercharge the brain so it can fire on all cylinders.[719]

d. Antifungal's for Fungus and Yeast

Dr. Ann Cook's book, *The Yeast Connection,* makes the link between *Candida* and MS. She mentions several cases of patients with MS, who from their medical history, seemed good candidates for anti-Candida treatment. In all of the cases described in her book, the MS symptoms improved as the Candidasis was treated. She also cites, *The Yeast Syndrome*, noting: "Once *Candida albicans* and its by-products have entered the bloodstream, they so severely debilitate the body that victims could become easy prey for far more serious diseases such as acquired immune deficiency syndrome, multiple sclerosis, rheumatoid arthritis, myasthenia gravis, colitis, regional ileitis, schizophrenia, and possibly, death from *Candida* septicemia."[720] "The antifungal supplement is crucial. It can be either herbal or pharmaceutical. Many of the pharmaceutical antifungals are harsh on the liver. Herbal antifungals are easily available and are safer."[721] She recommends: *Candida Cleanse*, (Rainbow Light company); *Primal Defense*, (Garden of Life company); *Pau d'arco* (Lapacho Company)." See section on Candida.

e. Glutathione Therapy is Helpful

In the last five years (from 2008), over 25,000 medical articles about this substance have been published, and the scientific understanding of glutathione is gradually becoming common knowledge. Dr. Perlmutter was involved in a study on Glutathione Therapy for Parkinson's in 2009. It was a randomized double-blind, pilot evaluation of intravenous glutathione in Parkinson's disease involving Dr. Perlmutter and four others in the study. Twenty one subjects were used and it showed that there were no significant differences in the changes in Unified Parkinson's Disease Rating Scale (UPDRS) scores over the three month study. Glutathione was well tolerated and no safety concerns were identified.[722] Even though the study was not shown to be successful with glutathione in the long haul, it looked like it was successful in the short run.

Dr. Robert O. Young, PhD, DSc, a biochemist and raw vegan nutrition expert, has suggested that dairy products are some of the most toxic or acidic foods one can eat and should be eliminated from any diet in order to maintain the alkaline design of the human body. "One of the best protectors of the alkaline body and especially your bowels, blood and brain (especially in the prevention and reversal of Parkinson's), is from a phyto-compound (a tri-peptide) known as Glutathione. Glutathione is a powerful anti-oxidant in buffering the negative effects of glucose, acetylaldehyde (vinegar) and lactic acid from dairy products, over-exercise and/or lack of oxygen."[723]

In one study in *The Lancet* it states, "For Neurological Dis-ease: Low glutathione levels have been associated with neuro-degenerative dis-eases such as MS (Multiple Sclerosis), ALS (Lou Gehrig's Dis-ease), Alzheimer's and Parkinson's."[724] Another study (in *An Neurol*) notes: "Glutathione helps to preserve brain tissue by preventing damage from free radicals (acids) and destructive chemicals formed by the normal processes of metabolism, toxic elements in the environment, and as a normal response of the body to challenges by acidic agents or other stresses. With the understanding that glutathione is important for brain protection and that this protection many be lacking in the brains of Parkinson's clients due to glutathione deficiency, it can be seen as very beneficial."[725]

f. Essential Fatty acids (EFAs) are Needed

Dr. Julian Whitaker, MD, in her newsletter *Health & Healing,* October 2009, writes about the breakthrough discovery that Medium Chain Triglycerides (MCT's), that are found in coconut oil, had a very salutary effect on restoring brain function. Dr. Whitaker now recommends coconut oil for other neuro-degenerative diseases such as Parkinson's disease, Dementia, Multiple Sclerosis and ALS (commonly known as Lou Gehrig's disease). Coconut oil could be used for the millions who currently suffer from Alzheimer's disease, Parkinson's disease, Huntington's Chorea, Multiple Sclerosis, ALS, Type I and Type II diabetes, as well as any number of other conditions that involve a defect in transport of glucose into neurons and other cells. The treatment was pioneered by Dr. Mary Newport, MD, who first initiated the therapy on her husband who had Alzheimer's disease.[726]

In a Parkinson's study on a "hyperketogenic" diet that was adhered to for 28 days, Unified Parkinson's Disease Rating Scale scores improved in all five categories during the use of this hyperketogenic diet.[727] Some other research worth noting was done by Dr. Richard L. Veech, of the NIH, (2001), and others, and they published an article entitled, 'Ketone bodies: Potential therapeutic uses.'[728] In 2003, George F. Cahill, Jr. and Dr. Veech authored, 'Ketoacids? Good Medicine?'[729] In 2004, Dr. Richard Veech published a review of the therapeutic implications of ketone bodies.[730] In Alzheimer's disease, the neurons in certain areas of the brain are unable to take in glucose,[731] [732] due to insulin resistance, and slowly die off, a process that appears to happen one or more decades before the symptoms become apparent. If these cells had access to ketone bodies, they could potentially stay alive and continue to function. It appears that persons with Parkinson's disease,[733] Huntington's disease,[734] Multiple Sclerosis[735] and ALS[736] have a similar defect in utilizing glucose but in different areas of the brain or spinal cord. These and other studies give evidence for the use of coconut oil.

g. Green Powders and Protein Powders

Green powders were discussed earlier.[v] The use of Green powder is essential for the body to cure PD, AD and MS, without them PD, AD and/or MS probably cannot be cured. It just is not possible to get enough greens when we are sick, and perhaps even when we are well. Green powders such as Barley Grass powder, Wheat Grass powder or other green powders are needed.

Protein powders can be used if there is a need for more protein, even though most people do not realize that eating this much greens in salads and a living foods diet will probably give enough protein. There are a lot of different protein powders on the market. The only ones that should be used are vegan, 100% plant-based, with no whey products. The nutrition therapy for curing PD, AD and MS should only include plant-based food powders.

h. Biblical Purification vs. uncleanness

Biblical Kosher means purity or cleanness, and goes back to the extensive texts on the clean and the unclean in the Bible. There is a theology behind purity or cleanness which relates directly to unhealthy, impure and sin. The words "clean" and "unclean" and similar words occur hundreds of times in the Bible, it was a major concern to Biblical writers. There is a close relationship between the terms, "uncleanness" and "sin."   And it was usually the priests job

---

[v] See chapter 12, Plant-based diets.

to "separate the sacred from the profane, the unclean from the clean." (Lev 10:10; 11:47; 20:25; Ezek 22:26)

The term has numerous forms such as cleanness;[w] cleanness; to cleanse; to cleanse oneself; purifying; cleansing; clean. Also to cleanse; to cleanse oneself; purifying; cleansing; clean; in the purifying rituals "to sin" is normally translated as "to cleanse," and to cleanse oneself; and to cleanse oneself; morally clean.

The unclean is prohibited or repulsive to God, or it belongs to the realm of the demonic which is opposed to God, and uncleanness is described as an abomination to Yahweh, or is... opposed to God.[x] Since Yahweh was a moral God he demanded ethical purity 'clean hands and a pure heart' (Ps 24:4). There is a close connection between holiness and cleanliness, but they are not the same. The Day of Atonement (a day of fasting) was specifically for the purification of the person that may be in sin or unclean. It is a day in which they were to afflict their souls (Lev 23:27, 32) by fasting (cf. Ezra 8:21) and repenting of one's sins (Ezek 18:30-31).

---

[w] Cleanness (Lev 15:13; 22:4); to cleanse (Lev 16:30; Num 8:6); to cleanse oneself (Num 8:7; Josh 22:17); purifying (Lev 12:4); cleansing (Lev 13:7: Num 6:9); clean (Gen 7:2; Lev 11:47). Also to cleanse; to cleanse oneself; purifying; cleansing; clean; in the purifying rituals 'to sin' is normally translated as 'to cleanse', (Lev 14:52; Num 19:19; Ezek 43:20), and to cleanse oneself (Num 19:12-13, 20); and to cleanse oneself; morally clean. (Job 15:14; 25:4; 33:9; Ps 73; 13; Isa 1:16).

[x] An abomination to Yahweh (Is 35:8; 52:1; Ezek 39:24; Rev 21:27; Lev 7:21; 11:10; Deut 17:1), or is... opposed to God (Zech 13:2; Mk 1:23; Lk 4:33; Ac 5:16).

Part IV
Counseling, Exercise and Prayer

Chapter 17
Counseling is Needed as Part of the Cure

St. Jerome (347-420) writes: "During the whole time of Lent, they have been free for prayer and fasting, they have slept in sackcloth and ashes, seeking future life in the confession of their sins. Because they have poured forth tears in sorrow and lament, it is said to them: 'Those that sow in tears shall reap rejoicing' (Ps 125.5); 'Blessed are they who mourn, for they shall be comforted.' (Matt 5.5) 'What does Christ say to you?'"[737]

a. Depression for PD and MS

Handbook of Parkinson's Disease (3rd Edition),[y] points out three areas that are directly affected by nutrition. The first is Depression. "Depression affects up to 50% of patients [with Parkinson's] and may be present at any stage of the illness or even precede the onset of motor symptoms.[738] [739] Although depression correlates poorly with the severity of motor symptoms,[740] it is probably the single most important contributor to poor quality of life in Parkinson's."[741] [742]

The second area directly affected by nutrition is Dementia. "Reported frequency of Dementia in PS ranges from 2% to 81%, although most were minimally affected in these studies.[743] [744] Some cognitive impairment has been

---

[y] Peer review journals cited: *Am J Psychiatry; BMJ; Arch Neurol; Mov Disord; J Neurol Neurosurg; Psychiatry Neurology; Am J Psychiatry.*

reported even in mild early Parkinsonian patients,[745] [746] and is more likely in depressed patients."[747] [748]

The third area directly affected by nutrition is Anxiety. "Anxiety is common in PD, occurring about as frequently as depression. One researcher found that 9 of 24 patients (38%) with PD suffered from a significant anxiety disorder and that anxiety did not correlate with the severity of Parkinsonism or with anti-Parkinsonian drug exposure."[749] [750]

David Healy, in his book: *Let Them Eat Prozac: The Unhealthy Relationship between the Pharmaceutical Industry and Depression*, gives a detailed account of the antidepressant drugs which have a long involved history. The antidepressant Prozac was released in 1988 and by the mid 1990's there were over 200 civil suits and various crimes associated with it.[751]

A good approach is found in the book by the psychiatrist, Gabriel Cousens, MD, *Depression-Free for Life, A Physician's All-Natural, 5-Step Plan*. The table of contents gives the Five Steps which are:

Step One: Take Mood-Boosting Amino Acids
Step Two: Optimize Your Supplements
Step Three: Make the Fatty Acids Essential
Step Four: Diet for Mental Health
Step Five: Eight Lifestyle Choices You can make to
            Help Beat Depression.

The eight lifestyle choices a person can make to beat depression include:
1. exercise or stay physically active
2. stay connected to close friends and family
3. have a creative outlet
4. cultivate a sense of humor
5. breathe right
6. sleep well

7. relax in a mindful manner
8. touch and be touched in a nurturing way

b. Compliance is the Number One Problem

It is hard to believe but the author's experience over the years is that most people would rather keep their disease than change their diets, especially if they have to give up meat and dairy products and go vegan! For example, there is the story related earlier of Darlene who had advanced MS in the 1970's; she was getting close to death. She started changing her diet, influenced by the teachings of Ann Wigmore, one of the pioneers of Living Foods, and slowly turned her condition around in about five years. To this day, she's living a healthy plant-based lifestyle. When she was completely cured, her doctor was so amazed he had her write up her story and the doctor gave it to all his MS clients. Not one of his clients chose to change their diet in order to be cured. Darlene said, "I don't get it, these people would rather suffer this awful disease with all its symptoms than change their diet!"

Did she ever go back to her old meat-based diet? Once she decided to go back to her old dietary lifestyle, and within thirty days the MS disease came back with a vengeance! This has been found true with others who were cured, when they left the raw vegan diet for more than a month, the disease comes back. So Darlene and the others all returned to the Live-Foods Nutrition approach and the disease went away again, back into remission.

Compliance is the number one problem with nutritional therapy: people don't want to make the lifestyle changes in their diets to cure these awful diseases. Obviously with non-compliant people there are a lot of psychological and social issues in the background. Educating a person about nutrition is necessary, but it is not enough, because it doesn't deal with the human emotions, motivations, fears and addictions. Someone trained in this field like a counselor or health coach is needed to help them succeed. Very few can be healed without a counselor. In order to successfully conquer Parkinson's, AD, MS or any neurological disorder, a professional counselor or psychologist is usually needed.

c. These Diseases are Psychogenic

There is a psychological element. If a person with PD, AD or MS is extremely angry, then they will not be healed no matter what nutritional therapy or drug they use. Anger and other negative emotions affect the nervous system and these diseases are mediated through the nervous system. These negative emotions will affect the nervous system, which will continue to feed the disease biochemically.

For example, a counselor, Bill Irwin, had a client who had MS who was doing the therapeutic diet perfectly and progressing. Then she got angry about having the disease and her progress stopped. Bill Irwin said that she will not continue to improve until she can let go of her anger. Her anger was reinforcing the disease. It was feeding the disease, because these diseases are psychogenic. This means the disease is tied into the psychic and the nervous system.

Robert Young, PhD, an expert on acid and alkaline balance in the body, gives some good insights into the energies in the soul. Our thoughts and emotions require energy and energy metabolized can create an acid in the body. "Your alkaline or healthy thoughts create less acid than your acidic or negative thoughts. We either have an alkaline lifestyle and diet, and we enjoy a fit and healthy body, or we have an acidic lifestyle and diet, and experience the aches, pains and suffering from metabolic acids."[752]

Dr. Young relates that, "When you are constantly having negative thoughts, they give rise to feelings like hatred, revenge, anger or fear. These thoughts provoke negative feelings can lower the pH of your urine (the urine pH indicates tissue pH) by over 100 times. This can cause the body to go into preservation mode 24/7, using up your alkaline buffering reserves. Once the alkaline reserves are used up the body goes into body wasting from all the acids." "If the acidic waste products from your thoughts are not eliminated through urination, perspiration, respiration or defecation, they will be absorbed into your tissues to protect and maintain the delicate pH of the blood at 7.365. Acids absorbed into the tissues will burn, ferment, spoil and even rot any cells and tissues they come into contact with.'[753] This is part of the psychogenic component when trying to cure PD, AD and MS. Good coaching and counseling is needed.

d. Emotions and Happiness

From the book of Genesis, through the latter prophets, history developed and matured with the Jewish people. Emotions are a strong motivation in the area of diet. Emotions have been connected to the development of the Jewish culture over time in the Bible. This is found in a study by James Tibbetts (Mayer; Tibbetts, fall 1994, *Journal of Psychohistory*). The study analyzed the emotional content of the Old Testament over a twelve century period with the Jewish people's evolution. Word frequency correlations were run and it was discovered that the basic emotion of "happiness" was statistically significant. "Our procedures led to the clear conclusion that happiness increased with time in the Hebrew Bible."[754] A key emotional term in the New Testament is "Joy" or "Happiness," this became a way of life for the early Jewish people.

Cell biologist, Bruce Lipton, PhD relates that because of chronically-elevated stress hormones: "Almost every major illness that people acquire has been linked to chronic stress. (Segerstom and Miller 2004;[755] Kopp and Rethelyi 2004;[756] McEwen and Lasky 2002;[757] McEwen and Seeman 1999[758]) Between 75 and 90 percent of primary-care physician visits have stress as a major contributing factor. (Atkinson 2000[759])."[760]

Bruce Lipton, PhD states, "Our positive and negative beliefs not only impact our health but also every aspect of our life. Learning how to harness your mind to promote growth is the secret of life, which is why I called this book *The Biology of Belief.* Of course, the secret of life is not a secret at all. Teachers like Buddha and Jesus have been telling us the same story for millennia. Now science is pointing in the same direction. It is not our genes but our beliefs that control our lives. 'Oh ye of little belief!'"[761]

e. Rule of Life - a Way of Life

Nutrition needs to become a way of life, a rule of life. "My brothers, be united in following my rule of life." And with this rule of life we need to "Persevere under disciple." (Phil 3:17; Heb 7.7) As Paul the Apostle wrote: "And be not conformed to this world; but be ye transformed by the renewing of your mind, that ye may prove what is that good and acceptable and the perfect Will of God." (Romans 12:2)

"Listen to advice; accept correction, to be the wiser in the time to come. Many are the plans in the human heart, but the purpose of Yahweh - stands firm.'" Prov. 19:20, 21

Chapter 18

Exercise is needed as Part of the Cure

A brother asked <u>Abba Agathon</u>, a 4th century monk: "Tell me, Abba, which is greater, physical work or guarding what lies within?" The Abba replied: "Man is like a tree, physical work is the leaves and guarding what lies within is the fruit. Now it says in the Gospel, 'Every tree which bringeth not forth good fruit is hewn down and cast into the fire (Mt 3:10).' Clearly, then, all our care should be about the fruit, that is, about guarding the mind. But we also need the protection and adornment of leaves, that is, physical work."[762]

a. Brain Cell Growth through Exercise

Physical activity is associated with a reduced risk of AD.[763] The three things that are helpful are mental stimulation, exercise, and a balanced diet which have been found to delay cognitive symptoms but not the brain pathology.[764]

To a limited degree, exercise can help and will slow the disease process down, but the disease marches on. From our review of the literature, only the type of plant-based nutritional remedies as found in this book put PD, AD and MS into remission.

Yoga is one of the most advanced systems of physical exercise and therapeutic methods of healing. In India's public schools yoga is taught as an exercise system and not as a religion. In America, public schools teach push-ups, sit-ups, jumping jacks and other exercises. Yoga, Pilates and other therapeutic exercises can be beneficial for those with AD, PD and MS.

Elevating the feet above the head is one of the most important exercises or postures to do for these diseases since it increases the circulation of blood in the brain and enables it to carry away more toxins and poisons. Inversion exercises do this very well. Increased oxygen to the brain is very important. The inversion postures in yoga, where you bring the feet over the head, are great exercises for brain diseases like Parkinson's, MS and Alzheimer's.

A keynote presentation, "Feeding Your Brain" at an American College of Nutrition conference in New York City was presented by neurologist David Perlmutter, MD. He pointed out that that exercise is free for us all to take advantage of now for the plasticity of our brains. He noted that scientists[765] found that walking increases functional connectivity in the aging brain and attenuates age-related brain dysfunction. Physical exercise is a key that is better than any pharmaceutical drug for enhancing brain activity.[766]

In a journal article, Dr. Perlmutter writes: "The important role of physical exercise in treatment protocols for various diseases, including coronary artery disease, diabetes, depression, and obesity is well established. Research clearly indicates that exercise reduces not only the risk for development of these and other conditions, but limits their progression and serves to enhance clinical improvement as well. Each of these conditions shares several important features with Alzheimer's disease. All are characterized by higher levels of inflammatory markers including C-reactive protein, as well as increased markers for oxidative stress. All are more common in individuals with higher caloric intake as well as those maintaining a sedentary lifestyle. Both inflammation and oxidative stress are key players in the pathophysiology of these conditions and both of these processes are ameliorated by physical exercise. Like calorie restriction, physical exercise enhances neurogenesis."[767] Multiple animal studies have validated the role of physical exercise in reducing memory deficits. Human studies are now confirming the same relationship.[768]

Perhaps one of the reasons that people with Parkinson's have tremors is because the body intuitively knows that it needs to get rid of the poisons, pesticides or whatever else is in the brain and body and the shaking could help to do this. Exercise like shaking helps to dislodge and get rid of things. This is a hypothesis of the author.

b. Brain Exercises for Dementia

A study published in the *New England Journal of Medicine* (2003) monitoring 470 older Americans for five years, found that different types of brain exercises done by the people in the study promoted a lower risk for developing dementia. (124 subjects with dementia, 61 of them with Alzheimer's) Scientists believe such leisure activities involving the brain help maintain mental fitness by stimulating connections between brain cells -- and building up new brain cells that replace those that die.[769]

The authors of *Keep Your Brain Alive*, "Researchers are finding that brain circuits for emotions are just as tangible as circuits for the senses, and advanced imaging techniques can now observe this. It is also clear from a number of studies that one's ability to remember something is largely dependent on its emotional context. As studies on aging have clearly demonstrated, social interactions they have positive effects on overall brain health. Interestingly, in the brains of individuals afflicted with Alzheimer's disease, this growth did not occur."[770]

c. Exercise and Oxygen

In the book: *Exercises for Multiple Sclerosis* by Brad Hamler, a fitness professional, he states: "A 1996 study done at the University of Utah by Jack Petajan, MD, PhD, found that regular aerobic exercise, vigorous enough to raise the pulse and respiration rate, increased fitness, muscle strength, and workout capacity and improved bowel and bladder control in people with Multiple Sclerosis. Participants in the study also reported reduced depression, fatigue, anxiety, and anger. Other studies have shown that exercise eases spasticity and poor balance in people with MS while increasing cardiovascular capacity.[771]"

There are three main types of exercise that are good for MS, PD and AD patients. Brad Hamler states, "Exercise is important and necessary no matter what level of MS a person has. Resistance, aerobic, and stretching, is the three main types of exercise beneficial to MS patients:

- Resistance training makes use of weights, springs, and bands. They increase the muscle power and ability and help large muscles burn fat . . .
- Aerobic exercise works the heart and lungs and increases stamina. Stair climbing, walking, jogging, dancing, swimming, and bicycling are all examples of aerobic activities. MS patients are recommended not to push too hard, though . . .
- Stretching is especially helpful for muscles that will be exercised, and it helps prevent injuries caused by sudden muscle elongation. It also fights the spasticity, increases the range of motion in joints, and prevents muscle contracture."[772]

Ozone or Oxidation Therapy is a new use of an old treatment discovered almost 70 years ago. One of the main benefits of exercise is oxygen. Getting more oxygen into the body will help fight the disease. A clinical way of doing this is ozone therapy that is widely used in Germany and other countries. Parkinson's is often treated with ozone therapy. Some of the various specialty areas in which ozone therapy is used include: Proctology, Gastroenterology, Urology Gerontology, Internal Medicine, Neurology, Surgery, Gerontology, Dermatology, General Medicine, Gynecology, Neurology, Orthopedics, Radiology and Dental Medicine.[773]

There are different types of oxygen therapies. What we breathe normally is O_2 but in oxygen therapy what is usually used is active oxygen or O_1 for it to be most effective. There's a big difference between active oxygen (O_1) and the 18 to 21 percent of oxygen in the air we breathe, it is regular stable oxygen (O_2). The emphasis for therapy here is O_1 (or O_3) active oxygen, but stable oxygen O_2 can be helpful too. Ozone therapy is widely used in Germany (by most physicians) and other countries and it is used for Parkinson's as an adjunct therapy, or perhaps as the main therapy.[774]

A Bedroom Greenhouse - A second way to get more oxygen naturally is through a greenhouse. Have you ever walked through an enclosed greenhouse and taken a deep breath? Plants give off oxygen, which is noticeable whether the plants are in a greenhouse or your bedroom. If you put many big leafy plants in your bedroom and living room, they give off oxygen and clean the air in the room. This higher level of oxygen in the air increases the quality of oxygen you breathe into your body. This would help to build your immune system and fight degenerative diseases.

Juices and Smoothies - Another way to get more oxygen into the body is through drinking many freshly made juices. At the Gerson clinic, they emphasis 13- 8 oz. glasses of freshly made raw juice every day, one glass every hour. Of course, there are several reasons for this, one reason being that many nutrients and phytonutrients are entering the body through the juice. A second reason that is often overlooked is the amount of extra oxygen that is taken in. When juice is freshly made, many oxygen molecules end up being attached to the molecules in the juice. These are transported to the cells in the body. These added oxygen molecules in the cellular structure of the freshly made juice are incorporated into the body, raising the level of oxygen in the body naturally. This extra oxygen is an influence in helping the body to cure degenerative diseases.

Protein Powders and Green Powders - Are good for exercise routines but they have to be vegan. *Vega* has a great line of vegan performance protein powders. Avoid "whey" (from milk) and any kind of animal-based powders; it must be plant-based.

d. Sunshine Needs

In an abstract by the Vitamin D Council (2010),[z] they propose that vitamin D plays a role in mental illness based on the following five reasons:

1. Epidemiological evidence shows an association between reduced sun exposure and mental illness.
2. Mental illness is associated with low 25-hydroxyvitamin D [25(OH)D] levels.
3. Mental illness shows significant co morbidity with illnesses thought to be associated with vitamin D deficiency.
4. Theoretical models (*in vitro* or animal evidence) exist to explain how vitamin D deficiency may play a causative role in mental illness.
5. Studies indicate vitamin D improves mental illness.

Sunshine on the skin is an essential component of beauty and health. Denser bones, stronger muscles, richer blood, healthier nerves, and greater endurance are created by regular exposure to sunshine. Understand that over-sunning, like over-eating, is harmful. Over-sunning causes free-radical collagen damage to the skin.[775]

The raw food speaker, David Wolfe, writes, "Some unique facts about sunshine exposure:
- Vitamin D, which assists in mineralizing the bones, is actively formed when the skin is exposed to sunshine.

---

[z] www.vitamindcouncil.org

- Sunshine increases the amount of iron in the blood. This creates a more 'magnetic' presence as is evident in the 'well-tanned' look.
- US cancer rates are highest in the northern states with the least sunshine.
- Rates of breast, prostate, ovarian, and colon cancer are lower in people with more sunshine exposure.
- Sunshine exposure may reduce breast cancer up to 30-40% and ovarian cancer by 80%.
- There are 2,200 sunlight-associated cancer deaths yearly versus 138,000 for the above-mentioned cancers in the US.
- Sunshine-associated cancers (non-melanoma) increase most where sunscreens are most heavily promoted.
- Sunshine raises positive moods in persons with SAD (seasonal affective disorder).
- Psoriatic skin lesions are reduced by sunshine.
- Direct sun exposure kills most forms of mold, fungus, and yeast (athlete's foot, Candida, etc.)
- Daily sunshine exposure normalizes hormone levels in women and men."[776]

There are some real benefits to sunshine for people with AD, MS and Parkinson's and other diseases. Twenty minutes a day would be fine; half an hour or more and may promote sunburn, depending on the person's skin type. Sunshine several times a week would be very helpful. For otherwise healthy persons, the FNB reports adequate intake (AI) for vitamin D is 200, 400, or 600 IU a day, depending on your age. But Dr. Robert Heaney, et al, writing in the *American Journal of Clinical Nutrition* in 2003 said: "The recommendations of the Food and Nutrition Board with respect to oral vitamin D input fall into a curious zone between irrelevance and inadequacy. For those persons with extensive solar exposure, the recommended inputs add little to their usual daily production, and for those with no exposure, the recommended doses are insufficient to ensure desired 25(OH)D concentration."[777] (*N Engl J Med*)

Michael Holick's, MD, PhD (1995), demonstration "that a brief dose of noontime summer sun is comparable to taking between 10,000–25,000 IU of vitamin D. Four earlier papers all found similar amounts of natural vitamin D production. Adam *et al,* found that up to 50,000 IU of vitamin D was released into the circulation of Caucasians after 30 minutes of noontime summer sun."[778] "A minimum of 5,000 IU of vitamin D a day is needed (from all sources, diet, sun and supplements) as recognized by various studies."[779]

Dr. Michael Holick (Boston University, an expert on sunlight) now believes "that a full body minimal erythemal dose of summer sunlight at noontime produces 20,000 IU of vitamin D. The high amount of natural human production of vitamin D is the single most important fact every physician should know about vitamin D because it has such profound implications for the natural human condition. Furthermore, there has never been a reported case of vitamin D intoxication due to excessive sun-exposure such as lifeguards, sun-worshippers, etc. The reason is that once the skin makes enough vitamin D, the sun destroys the excess. Some rather technical benefits in other studies can be cited, but the end result is that yes, there is a connection between brain health and having enough sunlight."[780]

e. Focus on the Finish Line

Concerning sunshine keep in mind that God created man to be outdoors and in the beginning God placed them naked in the Garden of Eden so that the sun would shine upon the entire body and their body soaked in a lot of sun. "And they were both naked, the man and his wife, and were not ashamed." (Gen 2:25) A second teaching from this verse is that it is healthy to be naked with your spouse and to not be ashamed, but to be comfortable with ones' nakedness.

In the book of Genesis God created man to be physically active, and God gave the command to work. "The Lord God took the man, and put him into the Garden of Eden to cultivate it and to keep it." And "Therefore the Lord God sent him forth from the Garden of Eden, to till [to work by plowing, sowing, and raising crops] the ground from whence he was taken." (Genesis 2:15, 3:23; Exodus 20:9; 2)

Paul encourages us onward saying, "That is how I run, intent on winning; that is how I fight, not beating the air. I treat my body hard and make it obey me." (1 Cor 9.26, 27) "Brothers, I do not think of myself as having reached the finish line. I give no thought to what lies behind but push on to what is ahead. My entire attention is on the finish line as I run toward the prize to which God calls me - life on high in Christ Jesus. All of us who are spiritually mature must have this attitude." (Phil 3.13-15)

Chapter 19

Prayer and Meditation are Needed

The bishop <u>St. Gregory of Nyssa</u> (c. 335-395) writes: "Since it has been shown what the scope of reverence is which must be prescribed for those choosing to live the God-loving life which is purity of soul and abiding spiritual progress, give yourselves over to prayer and fasting according to His will, remembering the one who advises us to: 'Pray without ceasing' and 'Be persevering in prayer.'" (1 Thess 5.17; Rom 12.12).[781]

a. Prayer Dimensions

In a brief overview about healing, we find these elements or dimensions in prayer for healing.
1. Levels: three levels of healing; body, soul, spirit
2. Approach: Healing services vs. retreats vs. personal or group prayer
3. Experience: Experience in prayer makes a difference
4. Power to Heal: Through a healer vs. group prayer
5. Time element: Healings take time; hours, days, months
6. Distance element: By laying on of hands or by people praying at a distance
7. Natural healing: Involves healing diets like a Live-Food diet, fasting, juicing and using supplements
8. Human choice: Intensity and openness to being healed
9. Teachings: Openness, knowledge and belief in healing

b. Sister Marie – A Cure from PD

The author (Jim) wrote John Paul II a letter in 2004 and explained to him that Parkinson's could be put into remission through a nutritional approach. He received a letter back from a Cardinal thanking him and that the Pope had physicians who were looking after his condition.

Pope John Paul II had Parkinson's disease, and even with this disease, he gave his life fully to preaching the Gospel. The Vatican confirmed the diagnosis in 2003, after keeping it quiet for about 12 years. Sister Marie Simon-Pierre (age 46) worked in Paris at a maternity hospital run by her order. She was diagnosed with Parkinson's disease in June 2005. She prayed to the late John Paul II (1920 - 2005). One morning after getting up, her Parkinson's had vanished, a mystery confirmed by a local medical team. She recounted her story to Vatican officials. A Vatican-appointed panel of doctors, a psychiatrist, theologians and church officials declared that the French nun was cured of Parkinson's, and said they cannot explain her miraculous recovery.

Sister Marie's claim is called a miracle, which occurred two months after John Paul II died. The panel of doctors determined the French nun's cure had no scientific explanation. She was deemed cured of her Parkinson's because of the intercession by Pope John Paul II. The Vatican has many reports of healings and miracles attributed to the intercession of the late Pope John Paul II. This was one that was investigated and declared a miracle. She prayed to the late Pope John Paul II and she was healed. The testimony, written in 2006, formed part of John Paul II's cause for beatification, in which a miracle is needed.[782]

c. Science, Meditation and Prayer

Dana Flavin, MD, says the more often you pray and meditate, the more positive effect it will have in the body. Changes in the brain wave patterns from alpha state to gamma state occur during meditation. The monks, she says, in meditation, achieve a state of neuroplasticity in their nervous system, and this is good. She notes that meditation lowers the cortisone levels in the body and contributes to other biochemical changes that are beneficial. Studies have shown that there's a 30% improvement in the biochemistry for those who have a prayer life.[783]

Dr. Paavo Airola sums up the basic factors for longevity as: a low-calorie, simple, primarily vegan diet; exercise; fresh air; water; a loving atmosphere and a positive state of mind. Li Chung Yun, the Chinese man documented to be 256 years old, (196 years old by other reports) calls it "inward calm."[784]

Meditation is an activity that can affect the brain and can calm the nervous system, making it valuable for any disease. Meditation over a long period of time will have positive physiological effects on the brain, including those with conditions like Alzheimer's, Parkinson's and MS.

The Harvard Crimson (2005)[785] reported a 2005 study by Harvard instructor, Dr. Sara W. Lazar, which showed that meditation can help to increase brain function, reduce the effects of aging on the brain, and improve concentration and memory.[786]

A study published in the *New England Journal of Medicine* on developing a lower risk for developing dementia stated, "Scientists believe such leisure activities (like meditation) involving the brain help maintain mental fitness by stimulating connections between brain cells -- and building up new brain cells that replace those that die."[787]

A Harvard Health Publication, "Can Prayer Heal the Sick?"[788] by Robert Shmerling, MD (2009) found positive results in reviewing the literature.

A recent survey of more than 1,100 US physicians found that 85 percent believed religion and spirituality (including prayer), had a positive influence on health and recovery. But, only 6 percent of these doctors believed it had any effect on the 'hard' medical endpoints, such as speed of recovery or death. About three-fourths of these doctors thought religion and spirituality helped people cope and maintain a positive outlook.[789]

Other studies have linked meditation with reduced stress, better sleep, pain management, heart protection, and even increased immunity. For example, one recent study found that those who meditate produced more antibodies -- an indicator of robust immune function -- in response to a flu vaccine compared to non-meditators. Other research shows improvement in productivity, job performance and job satisfaction with regular meditation practice.[790]

d. Meditation in the Bible

The word "meditation" occurs over twenty-five times in the Old Testament.[aa] The root in Hebrew of the word 'meditation' means to ponder, to murmur, to reflect, to pray, a murmuring sound, to meditate. The Greek would add to this to revolve in the mind, to imagine, pre-meditate (Lk 21:14), to take care of (1 Ti 4:15). The first instance of meditation in the N.T. is Luke 2:51, where Mary "pondered these things in her heart."[791]

Jesus finds strength in meditating and praying before dawn (Mk 1.35) and He went up onto the mountain to pray, and continued all night in prayer to God (Lk 6.12). He prays regularly in the Synagogue (Lk 4.16). He prays and meditates in solitude (Mk 6.46); He prays twice a day[bb] the basic Jewish Creed of faith: 'and you shall love the Lord, your God, with all your heart, and with all your soul and with all your might.' Deut 6.5-7 Jesus thanks His Father, God; (Mt 11.25-30; Jn 11.41) he praises His Father, God (Lk 10.21; Jn 17), he is transfigured, while he was praying before the Father (Lk 9.28), he prays for his disciples (Jn 17), he acts as an intercessor (Heb 4.14-16), and he teaches his followers to 'Ask.... Seek.... Knock,' (Lk 11.9-13) and to 'pray always and never lose heart.' Lk 18.1

[aa] (Gen 24:63, Jos 1:8, 1 Kgs 18:27, Is 33:18, Sir 6:37, 14:20, 39:7, 50:28, Job 15:4, Ps 1:2, 5:1, 19:14, 49:2, 63:6, 77:3, 77:6, 77:12, 104:34; 119:12, 119:15, 119:23, 119:27, 119:48, 119:78, 119:97, 119:99; 119:148, 119:78, 119.97, 119:99, 119:148, 143:5, 145:5)
[bb] (Mt 14.23; Lk 3.21, 5.16, 6.12, 9.18,28f)

Meditation on the name of Jesus is the oldest and most widely used form of Christian meditation.[cc] The invocation of the name of Jesus may be used alone, "Jesus," or used in a phrase. In the Eastern Church the most common form is: "Lord Jesus Christ, Son of God, have mercy upon me, a sinner." (Mk 10:48) Other invocations may be used: Jesus Thank you, Jesus I love you, Praise you Lord Jesus, Jesus have mercy, etc. A basic way to start is to take one of these four invocations and start saying it. From your mind go down into your heart and meditate on this invocation for at least 10 to 20 minutes, when finished come back up from your heart and let it go.

The author, in his book, T*he Jesus Prayer, Meditation and Praise*, explains Christian meditation and praise as noted above. Prayer is a relationship with God, a communication with the Communion of Saints. Meditation is a spiritual journey within and sometimes it becomes a prayer. Praise is a spiritual journey and usually becomes an act of worship. Charismatic prayer groups are known for their practice of praise. These meditation activities can be helpful in the process of being cured of minor or major degenerative diseases or any personal issue.

The charismatic renewal is a prayer movement that has many healing testimonials. There are charismatic prayer meetings all around the US and even overseas. These groups that use the 9 charismatic gifts, as found in 1 Corinthians 12 in the Bible: the gift of tongues, the interpretation of tongues, prophecy, the word of knowledge, the word of

---

[cc] Citing: Mt 1:21; 1:23; 1:24,25; 10:22; 12:18,21; 18:5; 18:19,20; 19:29; 28:19; Mk 9:38-41; 16:17,18; Lk 10:17; 24:46,47; Jn 1:12; 2:23; 3:18; 14:13,14; 14:26; 15:16; 15:20,21; 16:23, 24, 26; 20:31; Acts 2:21; 2:38; 3:6; 3:16; 4:7, 8, 10, 12, 17,18; 4:29,30; 5:28,40-42; 8:12; 9:14-16; 9:21,27,29; 10:43; 10:48; 15:25,26; 16:18; 19:5; Rom 1:5; 10:13; 1 Cor 1:2; 1 Cor 1:10; 1 Cor 6:11; Eph 5:20; Phil 2:9,10,11; Col 3:17; 2 Thess 1:12; 2 Tim 2:19; Heb 1:4; Heb 6:10; Heb 13:15; Ja 5:14; 1 Pt 4:14; 1 Jn 2:12; 1 Jn 3:23; 1 Jn 5:13; Rev 19:12,13,16; Rev 22:3,4.

wisdom, the discernment of spirit, the gift of healing, the gift of miracles and the gift of faith. The author has been involved in these prayer groups and highly recommends them, especially for people who want prayer for healing.

e. Healing Our Body and the Earth

In the 1800's the world's population reached a billion people and the industrial revolution happened and two major problems of overpopulation and global warming started. In the fall of 2012 there are now 7 billion people on earth. NASA's consensus is that 97% of climate scientists agree about Global Warming. Global warming has many factors but they can be summarized into three main categories:
1. Industrial pollution
2. Car pollution
3. Animal pollution

There are about 70 billion animals of various kinds that are raised and eaten as food every single year. This huge number of animals creates a huge carbon footprint. Growing and eating animals for food is at least 30% of the problem and can be as much as 50% of the carbon footprint, when all the factors are taken in. This problem involves more than just food. It involves land usage; water usage; temperature changes; seawater levels rising; hurricanes and weather becoming more destructive and all the expenses involved with these.

Rabbi Gabriel Cousens, MD gives a Torah Teaching on preserving the earth and says, "The earth is the Lord's and the fullness thereof." (Psalms 24:1) "This is the Torah teaching: that we are to help, as God's co-workers, preserve and improve the world. It is essential to the teaching of *Tikkun*, in which the Torah instructs that it is part of one's role in life to help heal the substance and soul of the planet. This means that we are to protect the resources of the Earth as well as the animal and human inhabitants."[792]

"By cycling our plant protein through the beef, the conversion to beef protein is between one-tenth and one-twentieth of the plant protein yield. This is a 100% loss of complex carbohydrates and a 95% loss of calories when plant protein is cycled through livestock. This is a significant waste of protein, complex carbohydrates, and calorie resources when so many people in the world suffer from malnutrition. It is an ecological shame to realize that meat-eaters, according to the book, *Diet for a New America*, use three and one-half acres per year to supply their meat and dairy consumption lifestyle, whereas vegans require one-quarter of an acre of land. In other words, approximately 14 vegans can live off the same land and water supply that it takes for one meat-eater. A nondairy and nonmeat diet saves one acre of trees per year because of how few resources the diet demands. On our planet, with ever-increasing shortages of land and water, this is a tremendously significant amount of resources wasted."[793]

Eating a plant-based diet will help heal both the human body and the body of the earth. It supports global ecology as well as our personal ecology.

f. Parable of the Sower and the Seed

As the Bible states, "One day a farmer went out sowing. Part of what he sowed landed on a footpath, where birds came and ate it up. Part of it fell on rocky ground, where it had little soil. It sprouted at once since the soil had no depth, but when the sun rose and scorched it, it began to wither for lack of roots. Again part of the seed fell among thorns, which grew up and choked it. Part of it finally landed on good soil and yielded grain a hundred- or sixty- or thirty-fold. Let everyone heed what he hears." Matthew 13:4-9 "Purify thyself and believe the Good News." (Mk 1:15)

Notice

If this book is a significant help to your Parkinson's or Alzheimer's or MS, or other degenerative disease, please let us know and write us about your testimony. We are collecting testimonials and case studies of people who have been helped or cured with this approach. The testimonials and case studies presented in this book are examples of people that were healed. Please contact us; we are always interested when this book is helpful. Thanks and God bless.

Jim Tibbetts
Live- Foods Technology, LLC
P.O. Box 2533
Glenville, New York 12325
www.jimtibbetts.com

Chapter 20
Appendix
a. Bios

James C. Tibbetts, MBA, STL

Academic degrees:
MBA 2009, Salve Regina University, Newport, RI.
STL   1995, Licentiate in Sacred Theology, Marian
              Studies, International Marian Research Institute
              (IMRI), at the University of Dayton, Ohio.
MA   1983, Christian Ministry and Renewal, The
              Franciscan University of Steubenville, Ohio.
BA   1976, Psychology, University of Buffalo,
              Buffalo, New York.

Associations
   ❖ A member of the SFO - Secular Franciscan Order.
   ❖ A member of the American Mariological Society,
           University of Dayton, Ohio.

Businessman
   James is a businessman. He has worked in the mentally
disabled health field, ran several family owned businesses,
including, a national manufacturing business and other
ventures. He promoted a feature film for a Marian
organization, World Apostolate of Fatima in NJ.

Theologian and Retreat Leader
   Jim is an historian and theologian (MA, STL), speaker; his
writings give theological teachings, emphasizing the
historical and scientific evidence. He gives talks and retreats
on Spirituality and Marian topics. He has given retreats and
talks on plant-based diets, fasting, healing and meditation
from the 1990's to the present. He was a speaker at The
International Raw and Living Foods Festival, Portland,
Oregon (2002, 2003) and other events.

Author and Scholar - <u>Books on Nutrition</u>: (books in print)
1. Plant-based Live-Food Nutrition, Alleluia!
2. Live-Food Standards Blueprint, a review of the literature
3. The Bioethics of Drug Intervention
4. Starving Cancer to Death, Nutritional Integrative Cancer Therapies, with Joseph Spaziani, MD
5. Impacting Parkinson's, Alzheimer's and MS to Permanent Remission, Paradigms and Data
6. The Sower's Seeds of Remission and Curing: Alzheimer's, Parkinson's and MS! A Nutrition Therapy Novel with Anne Marie Tibbetts, MS, RD
7. Remission towards Curing: Alzheimer's, Parkinson's and Multiple Sclerosis Nutritional Integrative Therapies with Anne Marie Tibbetts, MS, RD
8. Juice Fasting Simplified, a Practical Approach with Anne Marie Tibbetts, MS, RD
9. Living Green with Juices, Smoothies and Salads with Anne Marie Tibbetts, MS, RD
10. Superior Health for Astronauts as Raw Vegans
11. A Diary on Juice Fasting

<u>Books on Spirituality</u>: (Some books in print)
12. Jesus and Mary were Kosher Vegetarian, the Evidence from the Bible, the Early Church and Nutrition
13. Biblical Nutrition Meditations
14. The Jesus Prayer, Christian Meditation, Praise
15. Biblical Titles of the Virgin Mary - 30 Day Meditation
16. A Ballad of Mary's Biblical Heritage - Meditations
17. Mary the Ark of the Covenant with Fr. Bill McCarthy
18. Guadalupe the Tilma's Conquest - a historical novel, a factual booklet, a CD and a musical.
19. Why Oh God do you not Answer my Prayer to be Cured? with Fr. Richard Carlino
20. Why Oh God . . . Society   - booklet

Video and Audio Production
Several documentaries (*):
*DVD: *Saint Faustina Life and Mission* – award winning
*DVD: *Fr. Ed McDonough the Healing Priest in Boston*
 DVD: The Mime Adventures of Mr. Tibb, James Tibbetts

Scholarship Originals
Article: "Emotion over Time within a Religious Culture: A Lexical Analysis of the Old Testament." *Journal of Psychohistory*, fall 1994, with John Mayer PhD
Received two small grants (2003 travel, 2004 publication) from: Maine Space Grant Consortium. 1. Gave a talk at NASA in Houston, TX (February, 2003), "A vegetarian diet for space travel". 2. Wrote a book (2004) for the Maine Space Grant: *Superior Health for Astronauts as Raw Vegans, the Scientific Evidence.* Gave a talk at the Kennedy Space Center, FL (January 2006).
Jim has written articles such as: "The Early Christian Vegetarian Communities" in *Healing Our World*, Hippocrates Health Institute, (January 2010); and published the magazine: "Just Eat an Apple" raw vegan health magazine - (2004) editor, owner, and writer.

Performer and Mime
From 1978 to 2003, Jim was a professional mime and has performed around the US and in England; solo, duet and with the group "Christsong." From 1991 to 2001, Jim was a Founding Member of "Christsong" and performed as a mime: Jesus, Joseph, other characters; in a 2-hour performance on the life of Christ which included a dancer, mime, singers, and a 5-piece band. They performed around 100 shows in the US, twice-toured England (1994-1995) and appeared on television shows.
"Tibbetts has studied his art under technique-oriented Marcel Marceau and personality-oriented Tony Montanaro. The result has been a critically acclaimed combination of the two." *Arts & Entertainment*, Evening Express, Portland, ME.

Why Oh God ... Society

The question of this Society: "Why Oh God ...?" is asked concerning important questions and issues facing the Church and Society today. The first and primary question for this ministry is that involving health and healing of the individual. For more infor: www.jimtibbetts.com

Personal

Jim is married to Anne Marie Tibbetts. They co-authored several books. He is certified as a Pilates Instructor (2011). He has been a vegetarian since college (1975) and into raw, living foods since about 2000.

James C. Tibbetts
www.jimtibbetts.com

Anne Marie Tibbetts, MS, RD, CSG, CDN

Academic Degrees:

MS   1998, Master of Science, College of St. Rose,
         Albany, NY
BS   1987, Nutrition, Cornell University, Ithaca, NY

Credentials

RD   - Registered Dietitian, Academy of Nutrition and
         Dietetics (formerly American Dietetic Association)
CDN - Certified Dietitian - Nutritionist in New York State
CSG - Certification in Gerontological Nutrition (Certified
         Specialist in Geriatric Nutrition) from the Academy
         Nutrition and Dietetics, Spring 2009, Spring 2014.

Presently: She is a Clinical Dietitian at a large nursing home in New York. She has worked in the nutrition field for over 25 years, at various hospitals, nursing homes and community agencies. She has worked extensively with the Geriatric population, including those with Parkinson's, Alzheimer's, MS, Diabetes and other diseases.

Anne Marie is Certified as a Pilate's Instructor (2010) through Pilates Academy International (PAI), *Pilates on 5th* in New York City. She has practiced yoga for over 15 years and developed the Beads Pilates, Yoga (Rosary Yoga) with her husband, Jim Tibbetts.

Anne Marie enjoys singing in a choir, speed walking, yoga, Pilates and raw food preparation. She has been eating plant-based diets since 2008. She is a member of the Vegetarian Practice Group, as well as the Healthy Aging Practice Group of the Academy of Nutrition and Dietetics. She is a Dominican Associate with the Sisters of Peace in Schenectady, NY.

Some co-authored works by Anne Marie Tibbetts
and James Tibbetts include:
1. Juice Fasting Simplified, a Practical Approach
2. Living Green with Juices, Smoothies and Salads
3. The Sower's Seeds of Remission and Curing:
    Alzheimer's, Parkinson's and MS!
        A Nutrition Therapy Novel
4. Remission towards Curing: Alzheimer's, Parkinson's
    and Multiple Sclerosis Nutritional Integrative Therapies

Anne Marie Tibbetts website:
    www.jimtibbetts.com

b. Endnotes

[1] Dionysius the Areopagite, *The Divine Names and Mystical Theology*, trans by C.E. Rolt, (SPCK, Holy Trinity Church, London, 1979), p. 55.
[2] *Geriatric Nutrition the Health Professionals Handbook*, Chernoff, Ronni, (Jones & Bartlett Pub. Inc., Boston, 2006), p. 433, citing: Faxen-Irving G, Basun H, Cederholm T. Nutritional and cognitive relationships and long-term mortality in patients with various dementia disorders. *J Am Geriatr Soc* 2005;34:136-141.
[3] *Geriatric Nutrition*, Chernoff, Ronni, citing: Lee L, Kang A, Lee HO, Lee B-H, Park JS, Kim J-H, Jung IK, Park YJ, Lee JE. Relationships between dietary intake and cognitive function level in Korean elderly people. *Public Health* 2001;115:133-138.
[4] *Geriatric Nutrition*, Chernoff, Ronni, p. 433, citing: O'Hanlon P, Kohrs MB, Hilderbrand E, et al. Socioeconomic factors and dietary intake of elderly Missourians. *J Am Diet Assoc* 1983;82:646-653.
[5] *Geriatric Nutrition*, Chernoff, Ronni, p. 433, citing: Baker H, Frank O, Thind IS, et al. Vitamin profiles in elderly persons living at home on in nursing homes, versus profile in healthy young subjects. *J Am Geriatr Soc* 1979;27:444-450.
[6] Lieberman, Abraham, MD, *Shaking Up Parkinson Disease*, (Jones and Bartlett Publishers, Sudbury, Massachusetts, 2002), p. 126.
[7] Waldemar G. Recommendations for the Diagnosis and Management of Alzheimer's Disease and Other Disorders Associated with Dementia: EFNS Guideline. *Eur J Neurol*. 2007: 14(1):e1-26.
[8] Brookmeyer R, Johnson E, Ziegler-Graham K, MH Arrighi, Forecasting the global burden of Alzheimer's disease, *Alzheimer's and Dementia*, 2007.
[9] World Health Organization (2006). Neurological Disorders: Public Health Challenges. Switzerland: World Health Organization. pp. 204-207.
[10] Bermejo-Pareja F, Benito-Leion J, Vega S, Medrano MJ, Roman GC. Incidence and subtypes of dementia in three elderly population of central Spain. *J. Neurol. Sci.* 2008; 264(1-2):63-72.
[11] Di carlo A. Incidence of dementia, Alzheimer's disease, and vascular dementia in Italy. The ILSA Study. *J Am Geriatr Soc*. 2002;50(1):41-8.
[12] Kelleher, Colm, A., *Brain Trust*, p. 181, citing: Herbert, L.E. Screrr P.A., Bienais J.L., et al, "Alzheimer's Disease in the U.S. Population: Prevalence Estimates Using the 2000 Census," *Archives of Neurology* 60 no. (8) (August 2003): 1119-1122.
[13] Kelleher, Colm, A., *Brain Trust*, p. 183.
[14] Thompson CA, Spilsbury K, Hall J, Birks Y, Barnes C, Admson J., Systematic Review of Information and Support Interventions for Caregivers of People with Dementia. *BMC Geriatr*. 2007;7:18.

[15] Schneider J. Murray J, Banerjee S, Mann A. EUROCARE: a cross-national study of co-resident spouse cares for people with Alzheimer's disease: I- Factors associated with carer burden. (part II – A Qualitative Analysis of the Experience of Caregiving.) *International Journal of Geriatric Psychiatry.* 1999;14 (8):651-662 (II: 662-667).

[16] Bonin-Guillaume S, Zekry D, Giacobini E, Gold G. Michel JP. Impact economique de la demence (English: The Economical Impact of Dementia). *Presse Med.* 2005;34(1):35-441. French.

[17] Meek PD, McKeithan K, Schumock GT. Economic Considerations in Alzheimer's Disease. *Pharmacotherapy.* 1998; 18(2 Pt2):68-73; discussion 79-82.

[18] Meek PD, McKeithan K, Schumock GT. Economic Considerations in Alzheimer's Disease. *Pharmacotherapy.* 1998; 18(2 Pt2):68-73; discussion 79-82.

[19] Jonsson L. Determinants of Costs of Care for Patients with Alzheimer's Disease. *Int J. Geriatr Psychiatry.* 2006;21(5):449-59.

[20] Meek PD, McKeithan K, Schumock GT. Economic Considerations in Alzheimer's Disease. *Pharmacotherapy.* 1998; 18(2 Pt2):68-73; discussion 79-82.

[21] Findley LJ (September 2007). "The economic impact of Parkinson's disease". *Parkinsonism Relat. Disord* 13 (Suppl):S8-S12.

[22] Alzheimer's Disease International website (ww.alz.co.uk) Dementia statistics, March 2014.

[23] Forsti H, Kurz A. Clinical Features of Alzheimer's Disease. *European Archives of Psychiatry and Clinical Neuroscience.* 1999;249(6):288-290.

[24] World Health Organization (2008) Atlas: Multiple Sclerosis Resources in the World 2008, Geneva: World Health Organization, pp. 15-16.

[25] Miller DH, Leary SM (October 2007). "Primary-progressive multiple sclerosis". *Lancet Neurol* 6(10):903-12.

[26] Forsti H, Kurz A. Clinical Features of Alzheimer's Disease. *European Archives of Psychiatry and Clinical Neuroscience.* 1999;249(6):288-290.

[27] Carlesimo GA, Oscar-Berman M., Memory Deficits in Alzheimer's Patients: A Comprehensive Review. *Neuropsychol Rev.* 1992;3(2): 119-69.

[28] Hauser, Robert, and Zesiewicz, Theresa, *Parkinson's Disease Questions and Answers – Third Edition*, (Merit Publishing International, Coral Springs, Florida), 2000, p. 32.

[29] Hauser and Zesiewicz, *Parkinson's Disease Questions and Answers*, p. 32, citing: Hoehn M. Commentary: Parkinsonism: onset, progression, and mortality. *Neurology* 1998; 50(8):38. Poewe WH, Wenning GD. The natural history of Parkinson's dise. Ann *Neurol* 1998;44(Supp 1):S1-S9.

[30] US National Institutes of Health. Retrieved 2011-01-10 (found 1012 trials for AD)

[31] US National Institutes of Health. Retrieved 2011-01-10 (found 1012 trials for AD)

[32] Francis PT, Palmer AM, Snape M, Wilcock GD. The Cholinergic

Hypothesis of Alzheimer's Disease: a Review of Progress, *J. Neuro. Neurosurg. Psychiatr.*, 1999;66(2):137-47.

[33] Galpern WR, Lang AE (March 2006). "Interface between tauopathies and synucleinopathies: a tale of two proteins". *Anals of Neurology* 59(3):449-58.

[34] Galpern WR, Lang AE (March 2006). "Interface between tauopathies and synucleinopathies: a tale of two proteins". *Anals of Neurology* 59(3):449-58.

[35] Alzheimer's Association. Retried 1 October 2011.

[36] Francis PT, Palmer AM, Snape M, Wilcock GD. The Cholinergic Hypothesis of Alzheimer's Disease: a Review of Progress, *J. Neuro. Neurosurg. Psychiatr.*, 1999;66(2):137-47.

[37] Shen ZX Brain Cholinesterases: II. The Molecular and Cellular Basis of Alzheimer's Disease. *Med Hypotheses*. 2004;63(2):308-21.

[38] Wenk GL. Neuropathologic Changes in Alzheimer's Disease. *Clin Psychiatry*. 2003;64 Suppl 9:7-10.

[39] Hardy J, Allsop D. Amyloid Deposition as the Central Event in the Aetiology of Alzheimer's Disease. *Trends Pharmacol. Sci.* 1991;12(10):383-88.

[40] Mudher A, Lovestone S. Alzheimer's disease-do tauists and Baptists finally shake hands? *Trends Neurosci.*, 2002;25(1):22-26.

[41] Su B, Wang X, Nunomura A, et al. (December 2008). "Oxidative Stress Signaling in Alzheimer's Disease" *Curr Alzheimer Res* 5(6):525-32.

[42] Pohanka, M. "Alzheimer's Disease and Oxidative Stress: A Review". *Curr. Med Chem (Review)* 2013; 21(3):356-64.

[43] Bartzokis G (August 2011). "Alzheimer's Disease as Homeostatic Responses to Age-related Myelin Breakdown". *Neurobiol Aging* 32(8): 1341-71.

[44] Bartzokis G, Lu PH, Mintz J (April 2007). "Human Brain Myelination and Beta-amyloid Deposition in Alzheimer's Disease". *Alzheimers Dement* 3(2):122-5.

[45] Brewer, George J. (March 2012). "Copper excess, zinc deficiency, and cognition loss in Alzheimer's disease" *BioFactors (Review)* 38(2):107-113.

[46] Shcherbatych I, Carpenter DO. The Role of Metals in the Etiology of Alzheimer's Disease. *J Alzheimers Dis*. 2007;11(2):191-205.

[47] Hashimoto M, Rockenstein E, Crews L, Masliah E. Role of Protein Aggregation in Mitochondrial Dysfunction and Neurodegeneration in Alzheimer's and Parkinson's Diseases. *Neuromolecular Med*. 2003;4(1-2)21-36.

[48] Huang Y, Mucke L Alzheimer Mechanisms and Therapeutic strategies. *Cell*. 2012;148(6)1204-22.

[49] Greig NH. New Therapeutic Strategies and Drug Candidates for Neurodegenerative Diseases: p53 and TNF-alpha Inhibitors, and GLP-1 Receptor Agonists. *Annals of the New York Academy of Sciences*,

2004;1035:290-315.

[50] Perlmutter, David, Colman, Carol, *The Better Brain Book*, p. 219.

[51] Hatherill, Robert J., *The Brain Gate*, (Life Line Press, Washington, D.C., 2003), p. 8.

[52] Cook, Michelle Schoffro, *The Brain Wash*, (Toronto, ON: John Wiley & Sons CAN, Ltd., 2007), p. 23.

[53] Compston A, Coles A (April 2002). "Multiple sclerosis". *Lancet* 359(9313):1221-31

[54] Hoffer, Abram, *Healing Schizophrenia Complementary Vitamin and Drug Treatments*, (CCNM Press Inc., Toronto, Canada, Third Printing 2008), p. 154.

[55] Hoffer, Abram, *Healing Schizophrenia*, p. 155.

[56] Wikipedia online encyclopedia, citing CJD.

[57] Colm A. Kelleher, *Brain Trust the Hidden Connections between Mad Cow and Misdiagnosed Alzheimer's Disease*, (Paraview, New York, N.Y., 2004).

[58] National Institutes of Health (NIH) Office of Rare Diseases, 2013, online citation.

[59] Kelleher, Colm, A., *Brain Trust*, p. 180, citing: Manuelidis, E.E. and L. Manuelidis, "Suggested Links between Different Types of Dementias: Creutzfeldt-Jakob disease, Alzheimer Disease, and retroviral CNS infections," *Alzheimer Disease and Associated Disorders* 3 no. (1-2)(1989): 100-109.

[60] Kelleher, Colm, A., *Brain Trust*, p. 181, citing: Boller, F., Lopez O.L., and Mossy J. et al, "Diagnosis of Dementia: Clinicopatholic Correlations," *Neurology* 39 no. (1) (1989): 76-79.

[61] Kidd, Parris, PhD, Parkinson's Disease as Multifactorial Oxidative Neurodegeneration: Implications for Integrative Management, *Alternative Medicine Review*, (El Cerrito, CA, 2000), vol.5,no.6, p. 518.

[62] Carley, Rececca, MD, website, www.drcarley.com, 1/09.

[63] Carley, Rececca, MD, website, www.drcarley.com, 1/09.

[64] *Healthc Demand Dis Manag.* 1998 Aug; 4(8):122-6.

[65] Whitmer RA, et al. *Neurology.* 2008;71(14):1057-64. Epub 2008 Mar 26.

[66] Sofi, F; Macchi, C; Abbate, R; Gensini, GF; Casini, A (2010). "Effectiveness of the Mediterranean diet: can it help delay or prevent Alzheimer's disase?". *Journal of Alzheimer's disease: JAD (Review)* 20(3):795-801.

[67] Solfrizzi V. Lifestyle-related Factors in Predementia and Dementia Syndromes. *Expert Rev Neurother.* 2008;8(1):135-58.

[68] Solfrizzi, V; Panza, F; Frisardi, V; Seripa, D: Logroscino; G; Imbinbo, kBP; Pilotto, A (May2011). "Diet and Alzheimer's disease risk factors or prevention: the current evidence." *Expert Review of Neurotherapeutics* 11(5):667-708.

[69] Kanoski, SE; Davidson, TL (18 April 2011). "Western diet consumption and cognitive impairment: links to hippocampal dysfunction

and obesity". *Physiology & behavior (Review)* 103(1):59-68.

[70] Tejada-Vera, B. (2013). Mortality from Alzheimer 's disease in the United States: Data for 2000 and 2010. Hyattsville, MD: U. S. Department of Health and Human Services, Centers for Disease Control and Prevention, National Center for Health Statistics.

[71] National Institute on Aging. 2006-08-29. Retrieved 2008-02-29.

[72] Katz, Lawrence, Rubin, Manning, *Keep Your Brain Alive*, (Workman Publishing Company, NY, New York, 1999), p. 140.

[73] Katz, Rubin, *Keep Your Brain Alive*, p. 140-141.

[74] Shelton, Herbert; Oswald, Jean, *Fasting for the Health of It*, (Nationwide Press, Pueblo, Colorado, 1983), p. 172.

[75] Hamer and Collinson, *Achieving Evidence-based Practice*, p. 36, Klein R 1996. The NHS and the new scientism: solution or delusion? *Quarterly Journal of Medicine* 89:85-87.

[76] Krimsky, Sheldom, *Science in the Private Interest*, (Rowman and Littlefield Publishers, Inc., Lanham, Maryland, 2003, 2004).

[77] Krimsky, *Science in the Private Interest*, p. 146, citing: Richard A. Davidson, "Source of Funding and Outcome of Clinical Trials," *Journal of General Internal Medicine* 1 (May-June 1986): 155-158.

[78] Krimsky, *Science in the Private Interest*, p. 147, citing: Lise L. Kjaergard and Bodil Als-Nielsen, "Association between Competing Interests and Authors' Conclusions: Epidemiological Study of Randomized Clinical Trials Published in BMJ," *British Medical Journal* 325 (Aug. 3, 2002):249-252.

[79] Krimsky, *Science in the Private Interest*, p. 148, citing: H.T. Stelfox, G. Chua, G.K. O'Rourke, A.S. Detsky, "Conflict of Interest in the Debate over Calcium-Channel Antagonists," *New England Journal of Medicine* 338 (January 8, 1998): 101-106.

[80] Krimsky, *Science in the Private Interest*, p. 158, citing: Department of Health and Human Services, National Institutes of Health Conference on Human Subject Protection and Financial Conflicts of Interest, Bethesda, MD, August 15-16, 2000.

[81] Hamer and Collinson, *Achieving Evidence-based Practice*, p. 19, citing: Brooks M 1997, "Let's hear it for failure." *New Scientist* 15, March 4:6.

[82] Hamer and Collinson, *Achieving Evidence-based Practice*, p. 40, citing: Dyer C 1997, Consultant struck off over research fraud. *British Medical Journal* 315:205. Smith R 1997, Misconduct in research: editors respond. *British Medical Journal* 315:201-202. Wilkie T 1997, Sources in science: who can we trust? *Lancet* 347:1308-1311.

[83] Uffe, Ravnskov, *The Cholesterol Myths, Exposing the Fallacy that Saturated Fat and Cholesterol cause Heart Disease*, (New Trends Publishing, Inc., Washington, DC, 2003), p. 52-53, citing: Kannel WB. The role of cholesterol in coronary artherogenesis. *Medical Clinics of North America* 58, 363-379, 1974.

[84] *Early Fathers from the Philokalia*, edited by E. Kadloubovsky and

G.E.H. Palmer (Faber and Faber Limited, London, 1976), p. 40, 41.

[85]   *Circulation* 1954;9:335.

[86]   *Am J Med* 1959;26:68.

[87]   *Lancet* 1974;2:1061.

[88]   *Lancet* 1963;1:26.

[89]   Graham, Judy, *Multiple Sclerosis A Self-Help Guide to Its Management*, (Healing Arts Press, VT, 1989), p. 40, citing: Millar, J.H.D., Zilkha, K.J., Longman, M.J.S., et al. *British Medical Journal* 1:765, 1973.

[90]   Graham, Judy, *Multiple Sclerosis*, p. 41, citing: Bates, D., Fawcett, P.R.W. Shaw, D.A.,Weightman, D. British *Medical Journal* 2:765, 1973.

[91]   Graham, Judy, *Multiple Sclerosis*, p. 40, citing: "Long term studies on the effect of diet on the red blood cell membranes of patients with multiple sclerosis." By Dr. R. Jones and Dr. A. Preece (Bristol Royal Infirmary); Mr. L. Harbige and Proffessor M. Crawford … International Symposium on Multiple Sclerosis at Charing Cross and Westminster Medical School, London, Sept. 24-26, 1986. Published by ARMS in *Symposium Summaries*.

[92]   *Arch Neurol* 1970;23:460.

[93]   McDougall, John A., MD, writing (website) article for Physicians Committee for Responsible, Medicine, Washington, DC.

[94]   Swank R. Effect of low saturated fat diet in early and late cases of multiple sclerosis. *Lancet*. 1990 Jul 7;336(8706):37-9.

[95]   Swank R. Multiple sclerosis: fat-oil relationship. *Nutrition.* 1991 Sep-Oct;7(5):368-76.

[96]   Swank R. Multiple sclerosis: the lipid relationship. *Am J Clin Nutr. 1988* Dec;48(6):1387-93.

[97]   Swank R. Multiple sclerosis: twenty years on low fat diet. *Arch Neurol.* 1970, Nov;23(5):460-74.

[98]   John A. McDougall website 2012: www.drmcdougall.com

[99]   John A. McDougall website 2012: www.drmcdougall.com

[100]   Hurst, Judi, *Back to the Garden magazine*, (Hallelujah Acres, Shelby, NC, Fall 1999/Winter 2000), Issue no. 19.

[101]   Malkmus, George, Dye, Michael, *God's Way to Ultimate Health* (Hallelujah Acres Publishing, Shelby, NC, 1995), p. 188.

[102]   Hallelujah Diet website: www.hacres.com (2012)

[103]   Hallelujah Diet website: www.hacres.com (2012)

[104]   Hallelujah Diet website: www.hacres.com (2012)

[105]   Hallelujah Diet website: www.hacres.com (2012)

[106]   Hallelujah Diet website: www.hacres.com (2012)

[107]   Hallelujah Diet website: www.hacres.com (2012)

[108]   Hallelujah Diet website: www.hacres.com (2012)

[109]   Hallelujah Diet website: www.hacres.com (2012)

[110]   Hallelujah Diet website: www.hacres.com (2012)

[111]   Hallelujah Diet website: www.hacres.com (2012)

[112]   Hallelujah Diet website: www.hacres.com (2012)

[113] Hallelujah Diet website: www.hacres.com (2012)
[114] Hallelujah Diet website: www.hacres.com (2012)
[115] Hallelujah Diet website: www.hacres.com (2012)
[116] Hallelujah Diet website: www.hacres.com (2012)
[117] Graham, Judy, *Multiple Sclerosis*, p. 117.
[118] Graham, Judy, *Multiple Sclerosis*, p. 121-122.
[119] Sawyer, Ann D., and Judith E. Bachrach, Judith, *The MS Recovery Diet*, (Avery Books, The Penguin Group, New York, NY, 2007).
[120] Sawyer, Ann D., Judith E. Bachrach, *The MS Recovery Diet*, p. 184.
[121] Sawyer, and Bachrach, *The MS Recovery Diet*, p. 188.
[122] Sawyer, Ann and Bachrach, Judith, *The MS Recovery Diet*, (Avery Books, New York, NY, 2007).
[123] Sawyer, Ann; Bachrach, Judith, *The MS Recovery Diet*, p. 141.
[124] Sawyer, Ann; Bachrach, Judith, *The MS Recovery Diet*, p. 145-147.
[125] Sawyer, Ann; Bachrach, Judith, *The MS Recovery Diet*, p. 145-147.
[126] Joseph Malfara article, Never Give Up, *Healing Our World*, Hippocrates Health Institute, (Vol. 34, issue 1), p. 25.
[127] Matt Goodman, Interview via. email with him (2014) and also the article, "Can Raw Foods Help Reverse Multiple Sclerosis?" Interview by Tom Fisher, RN, BA. *Healing Our World*, (Hippocrates mag. Issue 32-1; 2012) and from Matt's website.
[128] Matt Goodman, Interview via. email with him. (2014)
[129] Matt Goodman, Interview via. email with him. (2014)
[130] *The Art of Prayer an Orthodox Anthology*, compiled by Igumen Chariton of Valamo, (Faber and Faber Limited, London and Boston, 1978), p. 208.
[131] Perlmutter, David, Colman, Carol, *The Better Brain Book*, (Riverhead Books, New York, 2004), p. 62.
[132] Kidd, Parris, PhD, Parkinson's Disease as Multifactorial Oxidative Neurodegeneration: Implications for Integrative Management, *Alternative Medicine Review*, (El Cerrito, CA, 2000), vol.5, no.6, p. 518.
[133] Shelton, Herbert; Oswald, Jean, *Fasting for the Health of It*, (Nationwide Press, Pueblo, Colorado, 1983), p. 172.
[134] Haag, Tosca, (in a letter August 2009) Rest of Your Life Retreat (ROYL), La Vernia, TX.
[135] Bisci, Fred, *Your Healthy Journey, Discovering Your Body's Full Potential*, (Bisci Lifestyle Books, N.J., 2008), p. 105.
[136] Nisson, Paul, *The Raw Life becoming Natural in an Unnatural World*, (343 Publishing, West Palm Beach, FL, after 2002), p. 31.
[137] Kent, Ray communication via. Email with Jim Tibbetts, June 2011.
[138] Ellioit Gallin interview with Maria Krajnak, Killing Giants, *Healing Our World*, Hippocrates Health Institute, (Vol. 34, issue 1), p. 28.
[139] Testimonials, hacres.com section.
[140] *The Fathers of the Church a New Translation*, Volume 16, (The Fathers of the Church, New York, 1952), Saint Augustine, Treatises on Various Subjects: The Usefulness of Fasting, p. 89-92.

[141] Biser, Sam, *Curing with Cayenne*, p. 31-32.

[142] Biser, Sam, *Curing with Cayenne,* p. 32-33.

[143] Hildenbrand, G., and S. Gavin. "Five-Year Survival Rates of Melanoma Patients Treated by Diet Therapy after the Manner of Gerson: A Retrospective Review." *Alternative Therapies in Health and Medicine* 1:4 (1995), 29-37.

[144] Hildenbrand, Gar, J., *Natuopath Med.*, 1996; 6(1):49-56.

[145] *St. Benedict's Rule for Monasteries*, (Liturgical Press, Collegeville, Minnesota, 1948), citing Chapter 1, p. 6.

[146] *Geriatric Nutrition the Health Professionals Handbook*, Chernoff, Ronni, (Jones & Bartlett Pub. Inc., Boston, 2006), p. 433, citing: O'Hanlon P, Kohrs MB, Hilderbrand E, et al. Socioeconomic factors and dietary intake of elderly Missourians. *J Am Diet Assoc* 1983; 82:646-653.

[147] *Geriatric Nutrition*, Chernoff, Ronni, p. 433, citing: Singer JD, Granahan P, Goodrich NH, et al. Diet and iron status, a study of relationships: United States 1974. *Vital Health Stat* 1982; 229(11).

[148] *Geriatric Nutrition*, Chernoff, Ronni, p. 433, citing: McGrandy RB, Russell RM, Hartz SC, et al. Nutritional status survey of healthy non-institutionalized elderly: energy and nutrient intakes from three day records and nutrient supplements. *Nutr Res* 1986; 6:785-798.

[149] Sawyer, Ann; Bachrach, Judith, *The MS Recovery Diet*, p. 147-150.

[150] Johann G. Roten, Marian Devotion for the New Millennium, *Marian Studies*, (University of Dayton, 2000) p. 54.

[151] *Early Fathers from the Philokalia*, edited by E. Kadloubovsky and G.E.H. Palmer, p. 132, 144.

[152] Campbell, Colin, T., *The China Study*, (Benbella books, Dallas, TX, 2004), p.

[153] Newsweek article on CEO with Parkinson's around 2008.

[154] Hunot S, Hirsch EC. Neuroinflammatory Processes in Parkinson's Disease. *Annals of Neurology* 2003;53S3:S49-S60.

[155] C. Holmes et al., "Long-term effects of $A\beta_{42}$ immunisation in Alzheimer's disease: follow-up of a randomised, placebo-controlled phase I trial," *Lancet*, 372:216-23, 2008.

[156] Griffin, W. Sue T., "What Causes Alzheimer's? Researchers and pharma companies have tried to attack this disease by reducing amyloid plaques, but inflammation may be the real culprit." *The Scientist, Magazine of the Life Sciences*, Sept. 2011.

[157] W.S. Griffin et al., "Interleukin-1 expression in different plaque types in Alzheimer's disease: significance in plaque evolution," *J Neuropathol Exp Neurol*, 54:276-81, 1995.

[158] D. Goldgaber et al., "Interleukin 1 regulates synthesis of amyloid beta-protein precursor mRNA in human endothelial cells," *PNAS*, 86:7606-10, 1989.

[159] W.S. Griffin et al., "Brain interleukin 1 and S-100 immunoreactivity are elevated in Down syndrome and Alzheimer disease," *PNAS*, 86:7611-15, 1989.

[160] J.C. Breitner et al., "Inverse association of anti-inflammatory treatments and Alzheimer's disease: initial results of a co-twin control study," *Neurology*, 44:227-32, 1994.

[161] S.C. Vlad et al., "Protective effects of NSAIDs on the development of Alzheimer disease," *Neurology*, 70:1672-77, 2008.

[162] J.C. Breitner et al., "Extended results of the Alzheimer's disease anti-inflammatory prevention trial," *Alzheimers Dement*, 7:402-11, 2011.

[163] Y.Li et al., "Neuronal-glial interactions mediated by interleukin-1 enhance neuronal acetylcholinesterase activity and mRNA expression," *J Neurosci*, 20:149-55, 2000.

[164] Griffin, W. Sue T., "What Causes Alzheimer's? Researchers and pharma companies have tried to attack this disease by reducing amyloid plaques, but inflammation may be the real culprit." *The Scientist, Magazine of the Life Sciences*, Sept. 2011.

[165] Griffin WST, Stanley LC, Ling C, White L, Macleod V, Perrot LJ, White CL, III, Araoz C. Brain interleukin 1 and S-100 immunoreactivity are elevated in Down syndrome and Alzheimer disease. Proc Natl Acad Sci USA. 1989;86:7611–7615.

[166] Rogers J, Luber-Narod J, Styren SD, Civin WH. Expression of immune system-associated antigens by cells of the human central nervous system: relationship to the pathology of Alzheimer's disease. *Neurobiol Aging*. 1988;9:339–349.

[167] Akiyama H, Barger S, Barnum S, Bradt B, Bauer J, Cole GM, Cooper NR, Eikelenboom P, Emmerling M, Fiebich BL, Finch CE, Frautschy S, Griffin WST, Hampel H, Hull M, Landreth G, Lue L-F, Mrak R, Mackenzie IR, O'Banion MK, Pachter J, Pasinetti G, Plata-Salaman C, Rogers J, Rydel R, Shen Y, Streit W, Strohmeyer R, Tooyoma I, Van Muiswinkel FL, Veerhuis R, Walker D, Webster S, Wegrzyniak B, Wenk G, Wyss-Coray A. Inflammation and Alzheimer's disease. *Neurobiol Aging*. 2000;21:383–421.

[168] Eikelenboom P, Bate C, Van Gool WA, Hoozemans JJ, Rozemuller JM, Veerhuis R, Williams A. Neuroinflammation in Alzheimer's disease and prion disease. GLIA. 2002;40:232–239. doi: 10.1002/glia.10146.

[169] Orr CF, Rowe DB, Halliday GM. An inflammatory review of Parkinson's disease. *Progr Neurobiol*. 2002;68:325–340. doi: 10.1016/S0301-0082(02)00127-2.

[170] Ishizawa K, Dickson DW. Microglial activation parallels system degeneration in progressive supranuclear palsy and corticobasal degeneration. *J Neuropathol Exp Neurol*. 2001;60:647–657.

[171] Gehrmann J, Banati RB, Wiessner C, Hossmann KA, Kreutzberg GW. Reactive microglia in cerebral ischaemia: an early mediator of tissue damage? *Neuropathol Appl Neurobiol*. 1995;21:277–289.

[172] Touzani O, Boutin H, Chuquet J, Rothwell N. Potential mechanisms of interleukin-1 involvement in cerebral ischaemia. *J Neuroimmunol*. 1999;100:203–215. doi: 10.1016/S0165-5728(99)00202-7.

[173] Graeber MB, Scheithauer BW, Kreutzberg GW. Microglia in brain tumors. GLIA. 2002;40:252–259. doi: 10.1002/glia.10147.
[174] Griffin, W. Sue T., "What Causes Alzheimer's?" *The Scientist,* Sept. 2011.
[175] Griffin, W. Sue T., *ScienceBlog*, September 2002, from University of Arkansas for Medical Sciences, Little Rock, Arkansas, Archives 202C.
[176] Victoria BidWell, www.naturecurerawfoodhealthretreat.com, The Bedrock Teachings and other material.
[177] Fields, R. Douglas, *The Other Brain*, (Simon & Schuster, New York, 2010).
[178] Fields, R. Douglas, *The Other Brain*, p. 17.
[179] Fields, R. Douglas, *The Other Brain*, p. 17.
[180] Fields, R. Douglas, *The Other Brain*, p. 18, 4-7.
[181] Fields, R. Douglas, *The Other Brain*, p. 180.
[182] Fields, R. Douglas, *The Other Brain*, p. 179.
[183] Fields, R. Douglas, *The Other Brain*, p. 181-182.
[184] Eriksson PS, Perfileva E, Bjork-Eriksson T, Aborn AM, Nordbord C, Peterson DA, Gage FH. Neurogenesis in the adult human hippocampus. *Nat Med* 4(11):1313-1317, 1998. Cited in Phosphatidyserine (PS): Mental Clarity at Any Age by Parris M. Kidd, PhD (Natraceutical Publishing, Bohemia, NY, 2007).
[185] Kidd, Parris, PhD, Parkinson 's disease as Multifactorial Oxidative Neurodegeneration: Implications for Integrative Management, *Alternative Medicine Review*, (El Cerrito, CA, 2000), vol.5, no.6, p. 518.
[186] Brian Clement, *Food is Medicine, the Scientific Evidence*, Vol. One, (Hippocrates Pub., FL, 2012), p. 22/
[187] Victoria BidWell, w.naturecurerawfoodhealthretreat.com, Bedrock Teachings website.
[188] Victoria BidWell, Ibid., website section: Bedrock Teachings.
[189] Cousens, Gabriel, *Rainbow Green Live-Food Cuisine*, (North Atlantic Books, Berkely, CA, 2003), p. 120; Also Essene Vision Books, Patagonia, Arizonia, 2003.
[190] Cousens, Gabriel, *Rainbow Green Live-Food Cuisine,* p. 113-114.
[191] Cousens, Gabriel, *Rainbow Green Live-Food Cuisine*, p. 116.
[192] Cousens, Gabriel, *Rainbow Green Live-Food Cuisine*, (North Atlantic Books, Berkely, CA, 2003), p. 120-21; Also Essene Vision Books, Patagonia, Arizonia, 2003.
[193] Cousens, Gabriel, *Rainbow Green Live-Food Cuisine*, (North Atlantic Books, Berkely, CA, 2003), p. 120-21; Also Essene Vision Books, Patagonia, Arizonia, 2003.
[194] Cousens, Gabriel, *Rainbow Green Live-Food Cuisine*, (North Atlantic Books, Berkely, CA, 2003), p. 107; Also Essene Vision Books, Patagonia, Arizonia, 2003.
[195] Lipton, Bruce, *The Biology of Belief*, p. 74, citing: Li, S., C.M. Armstrong, et al. (2004). "A Map of the Interactome Network of the Metazoan C. Elegans." *Science* 303:540+.

[196] Lipton, Bruce, *The Biology of Belief*, p. 74, citing: Giot, L., J.S. Bader, Et al. (2003). "A Protein Interaction Map of Drosophila melanogaster." *Science* 302:1727+.

[197] Lipton, Bruce, *The Biology of Belief*, p. 74, citing: Jansen, R., H. Yu, et al. (2003). "A Bayesian Networks Approach for Predicting Protein-Protein Interactions from Genomic Data." *Science* 302:449-453.

[198] Lipton, Bruce, *The Biology of Belief*, p. 74, citing: Barry, Patrick (2008). "It's the Network, Stupid." *Science News* 173.

[199] Lipton, Bruce, *The Biology of Belief*, p. 74-74.

[200] Lipton, Bruce, *The Biology of Belief*, p. 81.

[201] Lipton, Bruce, *The Biology of Belief*, p. 81, citing: Liboff, A.R. (2004). "Toward an Electromagnetic Paradigm for Biology and Medicine." *Journal of Alternative and Complementary Medicine* 10(1):41-47.

[202] Lipton, Bruce, *The Biology of Belief*, p. 81, citing: Goodman, R. and M. Blank (2002). "Insights Into Electromagnetic Interaction Mechanisms." *Journal of Cellular Physiology* 192:16-22.

[203] Lipton, Bruce, *The Biology of Belief*, p. 81, citing: Sivitz, L. (2000). "Cells proliferate in magnetic fields." Science News 158:195

[204] Lipton, Bruce, *The Biology of Belief*, p. 81, citing: Jin, M., M. Blank, et al. (2000). "ERK1/2 Phosphorylation, Induced by Electromagnetic Fields, Diminishes During Neoplastic Transformation." Journal of Cell Biology 78:371-379.

[205] Lipton, Bruce, *The Biology of Belief*, p. 81, citing: Blackman, C.F., S.G. Benane, et al. (1993). "Evidence for direct effect of magnetic fields on neurite outgrowth." Federation of American Societies for Experimental Biology 7:801-806.

[206] Lipton, Bruce, *The Biology of Belief*, p. 81, citing: Rosen, A.D. (1992). "Magnetic field influence on acetylcholine release at the neuromuscular junction." *American Journal of Physiology-Cell Physiology* 262:C1418-C1422.

[207] Lipton, Bruce, *The Biology of Belief*, p. 81, citing: Blank, M. (1992). Na, K-ATPase function in alternating electric fields. 75th Annual Meeting of the Federation of American Societies for Experimental Biology, April 23, Atlanta, Georgia.

[208] Lipton, Bruce, *The Biology of Belief*, p. 81, citing: Tsong, T.Y. (1989). "Deciphering the language of cells." *Trends in Biochemical Sciences* 14:89-92.

[209] Lipton, Bruce, *The Biology of Belief*, p. 81, citing: Yen-Patton, G.P.A., W.F. Patton, et al. (1988). "Endothelial Cell Response to Pulsed Electromagnetic Fields: Stimulation of Growth Rate and Angiogenesis in Vitro." *Journal of Cellular Physiology* 134:37-46.

[210] The following leaders attended and support these principles: (listed in alphabetical order) Solveig Almqvist – Sweden; Tommy Axelsson – Sweden; Fred Bisci, PhD – USA; Tamara Campbell – Vision,

USA; Rajaa Chbani – Pharmacie L'Unite – Morocco; Anna Maria
Clement, CN, NMD, PhD – Hippocrates Health Institute – USA; Brian
Clement, CN, NMD, PhD – Hippocrates Health Institute – USA; Brenda
Cobb – Living Foods Institute – USA; Michael Cousens, MD, MD(H) –
USA; Carole Dougoud – Institute Haute Vitalite – Switzerland; Kare
Engstrom – Dietician – Sweden; Viktoras Kulvinskas – "Grandfather" of
the Living Foods Movement – USA; Marie Christine L'hermitte –
Chemin du mas Magnuel – France; George Malkmus – Hallelujah Acres
– USA; Rhonda Malkmus – Hallelujah Acres – USA; Paul Nisson – The
Raw Life – USA; Claudine Richard – Naturopath – France; Jameth
Sheridan, ND – HealthForce Nutritionals – USA; Michael Saiber –
Vision – USA; Diana Store – Raw Superfoods – UK/Holland; Jill Swyers
– Living Foods for Health – UK/Portugal; Jim Tibbetts – USA; Walter J.
Urban – USA – Costa Rica.

211 Tibbetts, James, Tibbetts, Anne Marie, *Live-Foods Nutrition
Blueprint, A Review of the Literature's Principles*, (LF Tech books,
Schenectady, NY, 2008).
212 *Killer Clothes*, Anna Maria Clement, Brian Clement, (Hippocrates
Publications, 2011), p. 87-88.
213 *Killer Clothes*, Anna Maria Clement, Brian Clement, (Hippocrates
Publications, 2011), p. 87-88.
214 Buby, Bertrand, SM, *Mary of Galilee, The Marian Heritage of the
Early Church*, Alba House, New York, NY, 1995, (New York:
Scribner=s, 1926), 249. Citing: Irenaeus *Against Heresies*, XXII, 4;
Roberts and Donaldson, op. cit., vol. 1, 449, p. 20.
215 Kalchofsky, Roberta, *Vegetarian Judaism*, (Micah Publications, Inc.,
N.H. 1998), p. 168.
216 *The Fathers of the Church a New Translation*, Volume 16, (The
Fathers of the Church, New York, 1952), Saint Augustine, *Treatises on
Various Subjects: The Usefulness of Fasting*, p.114, 160.
217 *The Fathers of the Church a New Translation*, Volume 16, St.
Augustine, *Treatises on Various Subjects: The Usefulness of Fasting*, p.
201, 336, 395-6, p. 114, 160.
218 Cousens, Gabriel, *Conscious Eating*, p. 415-416.
219 Page, Linda, N.D., Ph.D., *Detoxification*, p. 18.
220 Airola, Paavo N.D., PhD., *Juice Fasting*, (Health Publishers,
Phoenix, Arizona), 1971), p. 39.
221 Airola, *Juice Fasting*, p. 40.
222 Airola, *Juice Fasting*, p. 38.
223 Airola, *Juice Fasting*, p. 34.
224 Breuss, Rudolf, *The Breuss Cancer Cure*, Forward, p. ix-x.
225 Airola, Paavo N.D., PhD., *Juice Fasting*, (Health Publishers,
Phoenix, Arizona), 1971), p. 42.
226 Bragg, Paul, *The Miracle of Fasting*, p. 84.
227 Shelton, Herbert; Oswald, Jean, *Fasting for the Health of It*, (1983).
228 Shelton, Herbert; Oswald, Jean, *Fasting for the Health of It*.

[229] Lawlor, T., M.B.,B.S., and D. G. Wells, M.B., B.S., "Metabolic Hazards of Fasting", *The American Journal of Clinical Nutrition.*, Vol. 22, No. 8, August 1969, p. 1148.

[230] Shelton, and Oswald, *Fasting for the Health of It*, p. 212, citing: Dr. Benesh and Dr. McEachen.

[231] Shelton, and Oswald, *Fasting for the Health of It*, p. 211, citing: Dr. William Esser.

[232] Shelton, and Oswald, *Fasting for the Health of It*, p. 213, citing: Dr. Robert Gross.

[233] Lawlor, and D. G. Wells, "Metabolic Hazards of Fasting," p. 1145; (1.) Bloom, W.L., "Fasting as an Introduction to the treatment of obesity," *Metab. Clin. Exptl.* 8:214, 1959. (2.) Drenick, E.J., M.E. Swendseid, W.H. Bland and S.G. Tuttle, "Prolonged starvation as treatment for severe obesity". *J. Am. Med. Assoc.* 187: 100, 1964. (3.) Thomson, T. J., J. Runcie and V. Miller, "Treatment of Obesity by total fasting for up to 249 days."
Lancet 2:992, 1966.

[234] Shelton, Herbert; Oswald, Jean, *Fasting for the Health of It*, (Nationwide Press, Pueblo, Colorado, 1983), p. 172.

[235] Shelton, and Oswald, *Fasting for the Health of It*, p. 212, citing: Dr. Benesh and Dr. McEachen.

[236] Shelton, and Oswald, *Fasting for the Health of It*, p. 211, citing: Dr. William Esser.

[237] Shelton, and Oswald, *Fasting for the Health of It*, p. 213, citing: Dr. Robert Gross.

[238] Shelton, Herbert; Oswald, Jean, *Fasting for the Health of It*, p. 184.

[239] Shelton, Herbert; Oswald, Jean, *Fasting for the Health of It*, p. 171.

[240] Shelton, Herbert; Oswald, Jean, *Fasting for the Health of It*, p. 186.

[241] Shelton, Herbert; *Fasting Can Save Your Life*, (Natural Hygiene Press, CT, 1964, to 1981).

[242] Shelton, Herbert; Oswald, Jean, *Fasting for the Health of It*, p. 173.

[243] Shelton, Herbert, *Fasting Can Save Your Life*, p. 99.

[244] Shelton, Herbert, *Fasting Can Save Your Life*, p. 102.

[245] Shelton, Herbert, *Fasting Can Save Your Life*, p. 102.

[246] Shelton, Herbert, *Fasting Can Save Your Life*, p. 102.

[247] Shelton, Herbert, *Fasting Can Save Your Life*, p. 102.

[248] Cott, Allan, *Fasting: the Ultimate Diet*, (Bantam Books, New York, 1975, 16th printing 1981).

[249] Cott, Allan, *Fasting: the Ultimate Diet*, p. 34-35.

[250] Cott, Allan, *Fasting: the Ultimate Diet*, p. 34-35.

[251] Cott, Allan, *Fasting: the Ultimate Diet*, p. 36.

[252] Hoffer, Abram, *Healing Schizophrenia Complementary Vitamin and Drug Treatments*, (CCNM Press Inc., Toronto, Canada, Third Printing 2008), p. 79.

[253] Hoffer, Abram, *Healing Schizophrenia*, p. 154.

[254] Hoffer, Abram, *Healing Schizophrenia*, p. 154.

255 Hoffer, Abram, *Healing Schizophrenia*, p. 155.
256 Dr. Scott's website: fastingbydesign.org (outside Cleveland, Ohio).
257 Airola, Paavo, PhD, ND, *Cancer Causes, Prevention and Treatment, the Total Approach*, (Health Plus, Publishers, Sherwood, Oregon, 97140, 1972), pp. 9, 28, 34.
258 Airola, Paavo, PhD, ND, *Cancer Causes, Prevention and Treatment, the Total Approach*, pp. 9, 28, 34. Airola, Paavo O., *How to Get Well*, (Health Plus Publishers, P.O. Box 1027, Sherwood, Oregon, 97140).
259 Red Beet Juice therapy for cancer and leukemia, as recommended by Dr. Siegmund Schmidt and Dr. A.
Ferenezi - *March of Truth on Cancer*, (Arlin Brown Inf. Center, P.O. Box 251, Fort Belvoir, Virgina, 22060).
260 "Modified Grape Cure" and "Grape Cure". (Arlin Brown Inf. Center, P.O. Box 251, Fort Belvoir, Virginia, 22060).
261 Airola, Paavo O., *Are You Confused?*, (Health Plus Pub., P.O. Box 1027, Sherwood, Oregon, 97140).
262 Breuss, Rudolf, *The Breuss Cancer Cure*, (Alive Books, Burnaby BC Canada, 1995), p. 28-29.
263 Breuss, Rudolf, *The Breuss Cancer Cure*, (Alive Books, Burnaby BC Canada, 1995), p. 28-29.
264 Breuss, Rudolf, *The Breuss Cancer Cure*, p. 33.
265 Tibbetts Jim and Anne Marie, *Juice Fasting Simplified a Practical Approach,* (www.jimtibbetts.com, 2011).
266 Airola, Paavo, N.D., PhD., *Rejuvenation Secrets from around the World,* (Health Publishers, Phoenix, Arizona, 1971), p. 61-62.
267 Lee, C., et al. ☐Age Associated Alterations of the Mitochondrial Genome,☐ *Free Rad Bio Med* 22, 7 (1977): 1259-69. Quoted from Peter Bennett, N.D., Stephen Barrie, N.D., *7-Day Detox Miracle,* (Prima Health, Roseville, CA.), 1999, p. 255.
268 *Ann Neurol.* 1999 Jan; 45(1):8-15.
269 Perlmutter, David "Integrative Medicine Approaches for Early Alzheimer's Disease", *Swedish Medical Journal*, (November 22, 2010). Dr. Perlmutter's site, Citing: www.vanguardneurologist.com
270 Dr. Perlmutter's site, Citing: article, for endnotes see: wwww.vanguardneurologist.com
271 *Encyclopedia of the Early Church*, citing: Cels. 5, 49 and 8, 30.
272 *Encyclopedia of the Early Church*, citing: In *Lev.* 10, 1-2; cf. Ambr., *In Ps.* 40, 1: Greg. Nyss.,
Beat. IV; Util. ieiun. 1,1.
273 *Encyclopedia of the Early Church*, citing: Basil, Ieiun. Hom. 2, 5; cf. Chrom., Serm. 35.4 and In Mt. 29.
274 *Encyclopedia of the Early Church*, citing: Ambr., Hel. 3,4; 4,7; Ep 63, 17).
275 *Encyclopedia of the Early Church*, citing: Jov. 2,6; Ep 54, 105.
276. *Encyclopedia of the Early Church*, citing: Basil, *Ieiun.* 1 and 2; Cass., *Coll* 21.13ff, and Inst. *coen.* 5,5 ff; cf. Hipp., *Trad.* ap. 25; Epiph., *Haer.*

330

3; Exp. *fid.* 23; Theodor., *Haer. fab.* 5,29.

[277] *Encyclopedia of the Early Church*, citing: Rule 4,39-41, 49.

[278] *Encyclopedia of the Early Church*, citing: 12-20; 39-50; 86-94, *Serm.* 13,1.

[279] *Writings from the Philokalia on Prayer of the Heart*, translated by E. Kadloubovsky and G.E.H. Palmer (Faber and Faber Limited, London, 1977), p. 294.

[280] Levin, Buck, *Environmental Nutrition*, p. 215, citing: Stehr-Green PA. (1989). Demographic and seasonal influences on human serum pesticide residue levels. *J Toxicol Environ Heal* 27(4):405-421.

[281] Levin, Buck, *Environmental Nutrition*, p. 181, citing: Henriksen GL, Ketchum NS, Michalek JE it al. (1997). Serum dioxin and diabetes mellitus in veterans of Operation Ranch Hand. *Epidem* 8(3):252-258.

[282] Levin, Buck, *Environmental Nutrition*, p. 181, citing: Hill RH Jr, Ashley DL, Head Sl et al. (1995). P-dichlorobenzene exposure among 1,000 adults in the United States. *Arch Environ Health* 50(4):277-280.

[283] Levin, Buck, *Environmental Nutrition*, p. 181, citing: Hammand TA, Sexton M, and Langenberg P. (1996). Relationship between blood lead and dietary iron intake in preschool children. *Ann Epidemiol* 6(1):30-33. Also: Kim R, Landrigan c, Mossmann P et al. (1997). Age and secular trends in bone lead levels in middle-aged and elderly men: three-year longitudinal follow-up in the Normative Aging Study. *Am J Epidemiol* 146(7):586-591.

[284] Levin, Buck, *Environmental Nutrition*, p. 181, citing: Yamamura Y, Yoshinaga Y, Arai F et al. (1994). Background levels of total mercury concentrations in blood and urine. *Sangyo Igaku* 36(2):66-69.

[285] Levin, Buck, *Environmental Nutrition*, p. 181, citing: Chia SE, chan OY, Sam CT et al. (1994). Blood cadmium levels in nonoccupationally exposed adult subjects in Singapore. *Sci Total Environ* 145 (1-2): 119-123.

[286] Levin, Buck, *Environmental Nutrition*, p. 181, citing: Wolff MS, Anderson HA, and selikoff IJ. (1982). Human tissue burdens of halogenated aromatic chemicals in Michigan. *JAMA* 247(15):2112-2116.

[287] Levin, Buck, *Environmental Nutrition*, p. 181, citing: Hill RH Jr, Head SL, Baker S et al. (1995). Pesticide residues in urine of adults living in the United States: reference range concentrations. *Environ Res* 71(2): 99-108.

[288] Levin, Buck, *Environmental Nutrition*, p. 215, citing: Guengerich FP and Shimada T, *op. cit.*

[289] Levin, Buck, *Environmental Nutrition*, p. 215, citing: Nakajima T and Wang RS. (1994). Induction of cytochrome P450 by toluene. Int J Biochem 26(12):133301340.

[290] Levin, Buck, *Environmental Nutrition*, p. 215, citing: Ungv-rg G. (1990). The effect of xylene exposure on the liver. *Acta Morphol Hungar* 38:245-258.

[291] Levin, Buck, *Environmental*, p. 215, citing: Casazza JP, Felver ME,

and Veech RL. (1984). The metabolism of acetone in the rat. *J Biol Chem* 259:231-236.

[292] Levin, Buck, *Environmental Nutrition,* p. 215, citing: Albores A, Sinal CJ, Cherian MG et al. (1995). Selective increase of rat lung cytochrome P450 1A1 dependent monooxygenase activity after acute sodium arsenite administration. *Can J Physiol Pharmocol* 73(1):153-158.

[293] Levin, Buck, *Environmental Nutrition,* p. 215, citing: Keyon EM, Kraichely RE, Hudson KT, it al. (1996). Differences in rates of benzene metabolism correlate with observed genotoxicity. *Toxicol Appl Pharmacol* 136(1):49-56.

[294] Levin, Buck, *Environmental Nutrition,* p. 215, citing: Zheng J and Hanzlik RP. (1992). Bromo(monohydroxyl)phenyl mercapturic acids: a new class of merapturic acids from bromobenzene-treated rats. *Drug Metabol Dispos* 20:688-694.

[295] Levin, Buck, *Environmental Nutrition,* p. 215, citing: Guengerich FP and Shimada T. (1992). Human cytochrome P450 enzymes and chemical carcinogenesis. Chapter 2. In: Jeffrey EH. (Ed). Human drug metabolism from molecular biology to man. *CRC Press,* Boca Raton, pp. 5-12.

[296] Levin, Buck, *Environmental Nutrition,* p. 215, citing: Guengerich FP. (1994). Metabolism and genotoxicity of dihaloalkanes. *Adv Pharmacol* 27:211-236.

[297] Levin, Buck, *Environmental Nutrition,* p. 215, citing: Cheever KL, Cholkis JM, et-Hawari AM et al. (1990). Ethlyene dichloride: the influence of disulfiram or ethanol on oncogenicity, metabolism and DNA covalent binding in rats. *Fund Appl Toxicol* 14(2):243-261.

[298] Levin, Buck, *Environmental Nutrition,* p. 215, citing: Lapadula DM. (1991). Induction of cytochrome P450 isozymes by simultaneous inhalation exposure of hens to n-hexane and methyl iso-butyl ketone (MiBK). *Biochem Pharmacol* 41(6-7):877-883.

[299] Levin, Buck, *Environmental Nutrition,* p. 215, citing: Kocarek TA. (1991). Selective induction of cytochrome P450e by kepone (chlordecone) in primary clutures of adult rat hepatocytes, *Mol Pharmacol* 40(2):203-210.

[300] Levin, Buck, *Environmental Nutrition,* p. 215, citing: Stresser DM and Kupfer D. (1997). Catalytic characteristics of CYP3A4: requirement for a phenolic fuction in ortho hydroxylation of estradiol and mono-O-demethylated methoxychlor. *Biochem* 36(8):2203-2210.

[301] Levin, Buck, *Environmental Nutrition,* p. 215, citing: Vezina M, Kobusch AB, du Souich P et al. (1990). Potentiation of chloroform induced hepatotoxicity by metyl isobuty ketone and two metabolites. *Can J Physiol Pharmacol* 68(8):1055-1061.

[302] Levin, Buck, *Environmental Nutrition,* p. 215, citing: Hogan GK, Smith RG, and Cornish HH. (1976). Studies on the microsomal conversion of dichloromethane to carbon monoxide. *Toxicol App Pharmacol* 37:112-119.

[303] Levin, Buck, *Environmental Nutrition*, p. 214, citing: Levin W et al. (1982). Oxidative metabolism of polycyclic aromatic hydrocarbons to ultimate carcinogens. *Drug Metab Rev* 13:555-580.

[304] Winter, *Poisons in Your Food*, p. 5, citing: Howard J. Sanders, "Food Additives," *Chemical and Engineering News,* October 17, 1966. James L. Goddard, M.S., FDA Commissioner, tape-recorded interview with author, May, 1968.

[305] Winter, *Poisons in Your Food*, p. 5, citing: Pharmaceutical Manufacturers Association, Washington, D.C., fact booklet, 1967.

[306] Winter, *Poisons in Your Food*, p. 67, citing: *Medical Tribune,* August 8, 1968.

[307] Levin, Buck, *Environmental Nutrition...*, p. 179, citing: Murphy R. and Harvey C. (1985). Residues and metabolites of selected persistent halogenated hydrocarbons in blood from a general population survey. *Environ Health Perspect* 60:115-120.

[308] Levin, Buck, *Environmental Nutrition*, p. 179, citing: Lordo RA, Dinh KT, and Schwemberger JG. (1996). Semivolatile organic compounds in adipose tissue: estimated averages for the US population and selected subpopulations. *Am J Pub Heal* 86(9):1253-1259.

[309] Hatherhill, J. Robert, PhD, *The BrainGate:...,* p. 32. Cited by: Cook, *The Brain Wash*, p. 31.

[310] Finefrock, Anne E. MD; Bush, Ashley, MD, PhD, Doraiswamy, Muralim MD; "Current Status of Metals as Therapeutic Targets in Alzheimer's Disease;" *J Am Geriatr Soc* 51:1143–1148, 2003.

[311] Finefrock, Anne E. MD; Bush, Ashley, MD, PhD, Doraiswamy, Muralim MD; "Current Status of Metals as Therapeutic Targets in Alzheimer's Disease;" *J Am Geriatr Soc* 51:1143–1148, 2003.

[312] Cook, Michelle Schoffro, ND, *The Brain Wash*, (Toronto, ON: John Wiley & Sons Canada, Ltd., 2007), p. 23.

[313] Cook, *Brain Wash*, p. 225.

[314] Pro-Lab Inc., "Lead in Water." www.prolabinc.com, Cited by: Cook, *The Brain Wash*, p. 36.

[315] Mercola, MD and Klinghardt, MD, "Mercury Toxicity and Systemic Elimination Agents," *Journal of Nutritional and Environmental Medicine*, March 2001. Also citing Taggart, by Cited by: Cook, *The Brain Wash*, p. 36.

[316] Perlmutter, David, MD, FANC and Carol Colman, *The Better Brain Book*, p. 146. Cited by, Cook, *The Brain Wash*, p. 36.

[317] Rachael Moeller Gorman, "Food for Thought: Can healthy eating help your brain stay sharp?" *Eating Well*, April/May 2006. Cited by Cook, *The Brain Wash*, p. 29.

[318] Philpott, William H. MD and Kalita, Dwight K., *Brain Allergies: The Psychonutrient and Magnetic Connections* (Los Angeles, CA: Keats Publishing, 2000), 68-69. Cited by Cook, *The Brain Wash*, p. 29.

[319] Perlmutter, David, MD, FANC and Carol Colman, *The Better Brain Book* (New York, NY: Riverhead Books, 2004), 28. Cited by, Cook, *The*

Brain Wash, p. 29.

[320] Hatherhill, J. Robert, PhD, *The BrainGate: the Little-Known Doorway that Lets Nutrients In...,* p. 133. Cited by: Cook, *The Brain Wash*, p. 81.

[321] Perlmutter, David, MD..., *The Better Brain Book*, p. 56. Cited by, Cook, *The Brain Wash*, p. 27.

[322] Hatherhill, J. Robert, PhD, *The BrainGate:...,* p. 149. Cited by: Cook, *The Brain Wash*, p. 27.

[323] Martyn, C.N., Barker, D.J.P., Osmond, C., Harris, E.C., Edwardson, J.A., Lacey, R.F. "Geographical Relation Between Alzheimer's Disease and Aluminum in Drinking Water." *The Lancet*. January 14, 1989, pp. 59-62.

[324] Piccardo, P., Yanagihara, R., Garruto, R.M., Gibbs, C.J. Jr., Gajdusek, D.C. "Histochemical and X-ray Microanalytical Localization of Aluminum in Amyotrophic Lateral Sclerosis and Parkinsonism-Dementia of Guam." *Acta Neuropathologica*. 1988, 77(1) pp. 1-4.

[325] Domingo, J., et al. "Citric, Malic and Succinic Acids as Possible Alternatives to Deferoxamine in Aluminum Toxicity." *Journal of Toxicology - Clinical Toxicology*. 1988. 26 (1-2), pp. 67-79.

[326] Dean, Ward, M.D., Morgenthaler, John, *Smart Drugs and Nutrients*, (Health Freedom Publications, Menlo Park, CA., 1991), p. 172-73.

[327] Hatherhill, J. Robert, PhD, *The BrainGate:..,* p. 36. Cited by: Cook, *The Brain Wash*, p. 30.

[328] *Geriatric Nutrition the Health Professionals Handbook*, Chernoff, Ronni, (Jones & Bartlett Pub. Inc., Boston, 2006), p. 107, citing: Chadwick, D, Whelan J, eds. *Aluminum in Biology and Medicine*. Chichester, England: Wiley and Sons, Ltd; 1992.

[329] *Geriatric Nutrition*, Chernoff, Ronni, citing: Flaten T, Aluminum as a risk factor in Alzheimer's disease, with emphasis on drinking water. *Brain Res Bull* 2001;55:187-196.

[330] *Geriatric Nutrition*, Chernoff, Ronni, citing: Flaten T, Alfrey A, Birchall J, et al. Status and future concerns of clinical and environmental aluminum toxicology. *J Toxicol Environ Healt* 1996:12:152-167.

[331] *Geriatric Nutrition*, Chernoff, Ronni, citing: Perl D. Aluminum and Alzheimer's disease, methodologic approaches. In: Sigel H, ed. *Metal Ions in Biological Systems*. New York, NY: Marcel Dekker; 1988.

[332] *Geriatric Nutrition*, Chernoff, Ronni, citing: Kruck R, McLachlan D. Mechanisms of aluminum neurotoxicity: relevance to human disease. In: Sigel H, ed. *Metal Ions in Biological Systems*. N.Y., NY: Marcel Dekker; 1988.

[333] *Mov Disord*. 1993;8(1):87-92.

[334] *J Neural Transm*. 1997;104(6-7):649-60.

[335] *Mov Disord*. 1998;13 Suppl 1:13-6.

[336] *Neurology*. 2003 Jun 10;60(11):1761-6.

[337] *Lancet Neurol*. 2004 Jul;3(7):431-4.

[338] *Behav Pharmacol*. 2006 Sep;17(5-6):425-30.

[339] Hatherill, Robert J., *The Brain Gate*, (Life Line Press, Washington,

D.C., 2003), p. 8.

[340] Hatherill, Robert J., *The Brain Gate*, p. 129, 130.

[341] Cook, *The Brain Wash*, p. 50.

[342] Gerlach M, Koutsilieri E, Riederer P. N-methyl-(R)-salsolinol and its relevance to Parkinson's disease. Lancet 1998;351(9106):850-1.

[343] Fleming L, Mann J.B, Bean J, Briggle T, Sanchez-Ramos JR. Parkinson's disease and brain level of organochlorine pesticides. Ann Neurol 1994;36(1):100-3.

[344] Source: *BioMedCentral-Neurology* 2008, on their website.

[345] Fleming L, Mann J.B, Bean J, Briggle T, Sanchez-Ramos JR. Parkinson's disease and brain level of organochlorine pesticides. *Ann Neurol* 1994;36(1):100-3.

[346] Rapp, Doris J., MD, *Our Toxic World: A Wake Up Call: Chemicals Damage Your Body Brain, Behaviour and Sex* (Buffalo, NY: Environmental Medical Research Foundation, 2004) p. 319, Cited by: Cook, *The Brain Wash*, p. 51-52.

[347] Cook, *Brain Wash*, p. 225.

[348] Colgan, Michael, *Save Your Brain* (Vancouver: Science Books 2007).

[349] Organic Consumers Association, "Pesticides causing brain damage," *Organic Bytes*, April 14, 2003. Cited by: Cook, *The Brain Wash*, p. 51-52.

[350] Rockoff, Jonathan D., "New life seen for vaccine industry," Baltimore Sun, June 6, 2006. Cited by: Cook, *The Brain Wash*, p. 64.

[351] Verrealut, Rene, et al., Past exposure to vaccines and subsequent risk of Alzheimer's disease, *CMAJ: Canadian Medical Association Journal*; 11/27/2001, Vol.165 Issue 11.

[352] Verrealut, Rene, et al., Past exposure to vaccines and subsequent risk of Alzheimer's disease, *CMAJ: Canadian Medical Association Journal*; 11/27/2001, Vol.165 Issue 11.

[353] Cook, *The Brain Wash*, p. 63-64, citing Dan Olmsted, "The Age of Autism".

[354] Carley, Rececca, MD, website, www.drcarley.com, 1/09.

[355] Williams, Rose Marie. "Fragrance Alters Mood and Brain Chemistry – Health Risks and Environmental Issues." The Townsend Letter for Doctors and Patients, 2004. Cited by: Cook, *The Brain Wash*, p. 65.

[356] Winter, *Poisons in Your Food*, p. 5, citing: Howard J. Sanders, "Food Additives," *Chemical and Engineering News,* October 17, 1966. James L. Goddard, M.S., FDA Commissioner, tape-recorded interview with author, May, 1968.

[357] Cook, *The Brain Wash*, citing: Fitzgerald, p. 70. Krohn, Jacqueline, MD and Taylor, Francis, MA, *Natural Detoxification: A Practical Encyclopedia* (Port Roberts, WA: Hartley and Marks Publishers, Inc. 2000), 115.

[358] Cook, *The Brain Wash,* p. 82-83.

[359] Hatherill, Robert J., *The Brain Gate*, (Life Line Press, Washington, D.C., 2003), p. 50.

[360] Hatherill, Robert J., *The Brain Gate*, p. 51.

[361] Hatherill, Robert J., *The Brain Gate*, p. 51.

[362] Olney, J.W. *Prog. Brain Res.* 73(1988):283-294. Also Olney, J.W. *J. Child. Neurol.* 4(1989):218-226.

[363] Blaylock, Russel L., *Excitotoxins the Taste that Kills*, (Health Press, Santa Fe, New Mexico, 1997), p. 117.

[364] Blaylock, Russel L., *Excitotoxins the Taste that Kills*, p. 34.

[365] Blaylock, Russel L., *Excitotoxins the Taste that Kills*, p. 39.

[366] Blaylock, Russel L., *Excitotoxins the Taste that Kills*, p. 110.

[367] Blaylock, Russel L., *Excitotoxins the Taste that Kills*, p. 255; For more information: *In Bad Taste: The MSG Syndrome* by George R. Schwartz, MD(1988) or contacting NOMSG Consumer Group, Santa Fe, NM.

[368] Blaylock, Russel L., *Excitotoxins the Taste that Kills*, p. 254, This partial list obtained from Jack and Adrienne Samuels, compiled from their extensive research into this field.

[369] Blaylock, Russel L., *Excitotoxins the Taste that Kills*, p. 255; For more information: *In Bad Taste: The MSG Syndrome* by George R. Schwartz, MD(1988) or contacting NOMSG Consumer Group, Santa Fe, NM.

[370] Sonsalla, P.K., Kicklas, W.J. and Heikkila, R.E. "Role for Exitatory Amino Acids in Methamphetamine-Induced Nigrostriatal opaminergic Toxicity." *Sci* 243(1989): 394-400.

[371] Sonsalla, P.K., Kicklas, W.J. and Heikkila, R.E. "Role for Exitatory Amino Acids in Methamphetamine-Induced Nigrostriatal opaminergic Toxicity." *Sci* 243(1989): 394-400.

[372] Olney, J.W., Zorumski, C.F. and Stewart, G.R. "Excitoxicity of L-Dopa and 6-OH-DOPA: Implications for Parkinson's and Huntington's Diseases." *Exp. Neuro.* 108(1990): 269-272.

[373] Blaylock, Russel L., *Excitotoxins the Taste that Kills*, (Health Press, Santa Fe, New Mexico, 1997), p. 106.

[374] Lipton SA (2006). "Paradigm shift in neuroprotection by NMDA receptor blockade: memantine and beyond". *Nature Reviews Drug Discovery* 5(2):160-170.

[375] Cook, *The Brain Wash*, citing: "Epilepsy drug helps fight Parkinson's," Neurology, April 24, 2000. Also citing Fitzgerald, p. 73.

[376] Cook, *The Brain Wash*, p. 42.

[377] Danscher et al. 1990; Hahn et al., 1989, 1990; Lorscheider it al., 1995; Lorscheider and Vimy, 1991; Vimy et al. 1990.

[378] Becker et al., 2002; Gottwald et al., 2001; Kingmann et al., 1998; Pizzichini et al., 2003; Zimmer et al., 2002.

[379] Becker et al., 2003; Gottwald et al., 2001; Kingmann et al., 1998; Zimmer et al., 2002.

[380] Drasch et al. 1992, 1994; Egglestone and Nylander, 1987; Lorscheider et al., 1995; Nylander, 1986; Nylander et al., 1987.

[381] Mercola, MD and Klinghardt, MD, "Mercury Toxicity and Systemic

Elimination Agents," *Journal of Nutritional and Environmental Medicine*, March 2001. Cited by: Cook, *The Brain Wash*, p. 39.

[382] Cook, *The Brain Wash*, p. 39.

[383] Perlmutter, and Colman, *The Better Brain Book*, p. 148. Cited by, Cook, *The Brain Wash*, p. 41.

[384] Mercola, MD and Klinghardt, MD, "Mercury Toxicity and Systemic Elimination Agents," *Journal of Nutritional and Environmental Medicine*, March 2001. Cited by: Cook, *The Brain Wash*, p. 40.

[385] Cook, *The Brain Wash*, p. 41.

[386] Huggins and Levy, *Alt Med Rev.* (August 1998.vol3(4);295-300). Cerebral fluid protein changes in multiple sclerosis after dental amalgam removal.

[387] Godfrey, Mike, Multiple Sclerosis and dental amalgams, *Townsend Letter* Letter to the Editor, (Feb.-March, 2004), Mike Godfrey MD, Tauranga, New Zealand.

[388] Godfrey, Wojcik and Krone. *J. Alzheimer's Disease* 5(2003);185-195; Apolipoprotein E genotyping as a potential biomarker for mercury neurotoxicity.

[389] Godfrey, Wojcik and Krone. *J. Alzheimer's Disease* 5(2003);185-195; Apolipoprotein E genotyping as a potential biomarker for mercury neurotoxicity.

[390] Godfrey, Wojcik and Krone. *J. Alzheimer's Disease* 5(2003);185-195; Apolipoprotein E genotyping as a potential biomarker for mercury neurotoxicity.

[391] Godfrey, Mike, Multiple Sclerosis and dental amalgams, *Townsend Letter* Letter to the Editor, (Feb.-March, 2004), Mike Godfrey MD, Tauranga, New Zealand.

[392] Jones L. J.*NZ Psych Soc.* 1999;97:29-33; Biting the 'silver bullet.'

[393] Godfrey, Mike, Multiple Sclerosis and dental amalgams, *Townsend Letter* Letter to the Editor, (Feb.-March, 2004), Mike Godfrey MD, Tauranga, New Zealand.

[394] Godfrey, Mike, *Townsend Letter* (Feb.-March, 2004).

[395] Klinghardt, Dietrich, MD, PhD, on heavy metals, on website: www.klinghardtacademy.com

[396] Klinghardt, Dietrich, MD, PhD, website on heavy metals.

[397] Martins, Antonio, S.J., *Fatima Way of Peace*, (Still River, MA., The Ravengate Press, 1989), p. 23-24.

[398] Martins, Antonio, S.J., *Fatima Way of Peace*, (Still River, MA., The Ravengate Press, 1989), p. 23-24.

[399] Parry, Ken, *Vegetarianism in Late Antiquity*..., p. 180, citing: Basile de Cesaree. *Su l'origine de l'homme (Hom. X et XI de l'Hexaemeron)*, A. Smets and M. van Esbroeck (eds) (Sources Chretiennes 160, Paris 1970), 2.6-7. Also Novatian, *On Jewish Foods*, 2.6, in *Novatian: The Trinity*, trans. R.J. DeSimone (Fathers of the Church 67, Washington, DC 1972).

[400] Parry, Ken, *Vegetarianism in Late Antiquity*..., p. 174, citing: Basil, *De ieiunio homiliae* 1.3-4, PG 31, 168 A-B. *Sur l'orgine de*

l'homme 2.6-7.

[401] Parry, Ken, *Vegetarianism in Late Antiquity*..., p. 181, citing: Ephrem, *Commentary on Genesis 2, 33, St. Ephrem the Syrian: Selected prose works*, trans. E.G. Matthews and J.P. Amar (Fathers of the Church 91, Washington, DC 1994); Jerome, *Adversus Jovinianum*, PL 23, 221-352.

[402] Parry, Ken, *Vegetarianism in Late Antiquity*..., p. 182, citing: T.M. Shaw, *The Burden of the Flesh: Fasting and sexuality in the early Christianity* (Minneapolis 1988), 233.

[403] Cousens, Gabriel, *Conscious Eating*, (North Atlantic Books, Berkeley, California, 2000), p. 587-8.

[404] Kulvinskas, *Survival into the 21st Century*, (21st Century Publications, Woodstock Valley, CT 1975), p. 27. Citing: (a) Oliver M.F., *Lancet*, 1:653, 1962. (b) McDonald L., Edgill M. *Lancet*, 1:996; 1958.

[405] Day, Lorraine, MD, *Getting Started*..., p. 161, citing: *Environmental Nutrition*, 1994, 3; *The American Journal of Clinical Nutrition*, 1990;51:656-657.

[406] Timon, Mark, "What are Green Foods?" (December 2009) Vibrant Health website.

[407] Carpenter, E., Clinical experiences with chlorophyll preparations with a particular reference to chronic osteomyelitis and chronic ulcers. *American Journal of Surgery*. Feb. 1949: Cited in, ibid. Handel, Jacob, "Chlorophyll Supporter...", p. 33.

[408] John Gainer, "Now the Villain is Protein," *Science News* (August 21, 1971): 123-24.

[409] Gurskin, B. "Chlorophyll - Its Therapeutic Place in Acute and Supportive Disease," *American Journal of Surgery* 49 (1940): 49-55.

[410] Ann Wigmore, *Be Your Own doctor* (Garden City Park, NY: Avery Publishing Group, 1982).

[411] Walters, Richard, *Options the Alternative Cancer Therapy Book*, Avery Pub. Group, Inc., 1992, p. 147.

[412] *Chlorophyllin Reduces Aflatoxin Indicators Among People At High Risk for Liver Cancer*. Johns Hopkins University Bloomberg School of Public Health, Baltimore, MD. Proceedings of the National Academy of Sciences. November 27, 2001. Cited by Boutenko, Victoria, *Green for Life*, p. 94.

[413] Chernomorsky, S. et al. "Effect of Dietary Chlorophyll Derivatives on Mutagenesis and Tumor Cell Growth." *Teratogenesis Carcinogenesis*, 79:313-322, 1999. Cited by Boutenko, *Green for Life*, p. 95.

[414] Vlad M. et al. *Effect of Cuprofilin on Experimental Atherosclerosis*. Romania: Institute of Public Health and Medical Research, University of Medicine and Pharmacy, Cluj-Napoka, 1995. Cited by Boutenko, Victoria, *Green for Life*, p. 95.

[415] Kulvinskas, *Survival into the 21st Century*, p. 53, citing: Paloscia; Pollotten; "Chlorophyl Therapy" Lotta. *Contra. Tuberc.* 22: 738, 1952.

[416] Kulvinskas, *Survival into the 21st Century*, p. 53, citing: "Results of Chlorophyl Therapy," Bull Assoc. Franc Poletude due *Cancer*,

24: 15, 1935.

[417] Kulvinskas, *Survival into the 21st Century*, p. 53, citing: Plagniel, "Remarkable Tonic Power of Chlorophyll Pigment in Asthenic Toxemia of Cancer," *J. de Med.* De Paris, 53: 664, 1933.

[418] Kulvinskas, *Survival into the 21st Century*, p. 53, citing: "Chlorophyll Therapy for Cancer," *Progress. Med.*, Ap. 6, 1935, p. 583.

[419] Meyerowitz, Steve, *Wheat Grass, Nature's Finest Medicine*, p. 70, citing: Dr. Mahnaz Badamchian of the Dept. of Biochemistry and Molecular Biology, George Washing Univ., Medical Center research: Anti-tumor properties of barley leaf extract (BLE) on human prostrate, breast and melanoma cancer.

[420] Meyerowitz, Steve, *Wheat Grass, Nature's Finest Medicine*, p. 69, citing: Inhibition of In Vitro Metabolic Activation of Carcinogens by Wehat Sprout Extracts, By Chiu-Nan Lai, B Dabney, C. Shaw, Dept of Biology, Unive of Texas System Cancer Center, MDAnderson Hospital and Tumor institute, Houston, TX. *Nutrition and Cancer* . Vol. 1, no. 1. P-27-30. Fall, 1978.

[421] Kulvinskas, *Survival into the 21st Century*, p. 54, citing: Smith, "Remarks Upon the History, Chemistry, Toxicity and Antibacterial Properties of Watersoluble Chlorophyll Derivatives as Therapeutic Agents," *Am. J. Med. Soc.* 207:649, 1944.

[422] Kulvinskas, *Survival into the 21st Century*, p. 54, citing: Bowers W.S., "Chlorophyl in Wound Healing and Suppurative Disease", *Am. J. Surg.* 73, 1947.

[423] Kulvinskas, *Survival into the 21st Century*, p. 54, citing: Rafsky, Krieger, "Treatment of Intestinal Diseases with Solutions of Water Soluble Chlorophyl," *Rev. Gastroentology*, 15: 549, 1948.

[424] Siebold, Ronald, M.S., *Cereal Grass: Nature's Greatest Health Gift* (NTC/Contemporary Pub., 1991).

[425] Siebold, Ronald, M.S., *Cereal Grass: Nature's Greatest Health Gift* (NTC/Contemporary Pub., 1991).

[426] Dubin, Reese, *Miracle Food Cures from the Bible*, (Prentice Hall, Paramus, NJ) 1999, p. 130.

[427] Siebold, in *Cereal Grass: Nature's Greatest Health Gift*.

[428] Siebold, in *Cereal Grass: Nature's Greatest Health Gift*.

[429] Siebold, in *Cereal Grass: Nature's Greatest Health Gift*.

[430] Dubin, Reese, *Miracle Food Cures from the Bible*, p. 129.

[431] Dubin, Reese, *Miracle Food Cures from the Bible*, p. 132.

[432] Dubin, Reese, *Miracle Food Cures from the Bible*, p. 133.

[433] Dubin, Reese, *Miracle Food Cures from the Bible*, p. 133.

[434] Handel, Jacob, "Chlorophyll Supporter of all Human and Animal Life", *Healing Our World*, (Hippocrates Health Institute, 2010, Vol. 30, Issue 3), p. 32, 33, 56.

[435] Carpenter, E. 1949. Clinical experiences with chlorophyll preparations with a particular reference to chronic osteomyelitis and chronic ulcers. *American Journal of Surgery*. Feb. 1949: Cited in, ibid.

Handel, Jacob, "Chlorophyll Supporter...". p. 32.

[436] Saunders, C. 1926. The nutritional value of chlorophyll as related to hemoglobin formation. Proceedings of the Society for Experimental Biology and Medicine (3172), p. 788-789: Cited in, ibid. Handel, Jacob, "Chlorophyll Supporter..." p. 32.

[437] Lai, C., Butler, M., and Matney, T. 1980. Antimutagenic activities of common vegetables and their chlorophyll content. *Mutation Research* 77:245-250. Cited in, ibid. Handel, Jacob, "Chlorophyll Supporter...". p. 32.

[438] Spector, H. and Calloway, D. 1959. Reduction of x-radiation mortality by cabbage and broccoli. Proceedings of the Society for Experimental Biology and Medicine 100:405-407. Cited in, ibid. Handel, Jacob, "Chlorophyll Supporter...", p. 32.

[439] Calloway, D., Newell, G., Calhoun, W. and Munson, A. 1962. Further studies of the influence on diet on radiosensitivity of guinea pigs, with special reference to broccoli and alfalfa. *Journal of Nutrition* 79:340-348. Cited in, ibid. Handel, Jacob, "Chlorophyll Supporter...". p. 32.

[440] Smith, L. 1944. Chlorophyll: an experimental study of its water-soluble derivatives. Remarks on the history, chemistry, toxicity and anti-bacterial properties of water soluble chlorophyll derivatives as therapeutic agents. *American Journal of the Medical Sciences* 207:647-654. Cited in, ibid. Handel, Jacob, "Chlorophyll Supporter...". p. 32.

[441] Offenkrantz, W. 1950. Water-soluble chlorophyll in the treatment of peptic ulcers of long duration. *Review of Gastroenterology* 17:359-367. Cited in, ibid. Handel, Jacob, "Chlorophyll Supporter...". p. 32.

[442] Ohtake, H., Nonaka, S., Sawada, Y., Hagiwara, Y., Hagiwara, H., and Kubota, K. 1985. Studies on the constituents of green juice from young barley leaves. Effect on dietarily induced hypercholesterolemia in rats. *Journal of the Pharmaceutical Society of Japan* 105:1052-71. Calloway, D., Newell, G., Calhoun, W. and Munson, A. 1962. Further studies of the influence on diet on radiosensitivity of guinea pigs, with special reference to broccoli and alfalfa. *Journal of Nutrition* 79:340-348. Cited in, ibid. Handel, Jacob, "Chlorophyll Supporter...". p. 32.

[443] Smith, L. 1944. Chlorophyll: an experimental study of its water-soluble derivatives. Remarks on the history, chemistry, toxicity and anti-bacterial properties of water soluble chlorophyll derivatives as therapeutic agents. *American Journal of the Medical Sciences* 207:647-654. Cited in, ibid. Handel, Jacob, "Chlorophyll Supporter...". p. 32.

[444] Smith, L. 1944. Chlorophyll: an experimental study of its water-soluble derivatives. Remarks on the history, chemistry, toxicity and anti-bacterial properties of water soluble chlorophyll derivatives as therapeutic agents. *American Journal of the Medical Sciences* 207:647-654. Cited in, ibid. Handel, Jacob, "Chlorophyll Supporter...". p. 33.

[445] Rothemund, P., McNary, R., and Inman, O. 1934. Occurrence of decomposition products of chlorophyll.II. Decomposition products of

chlorophyll in the stomach walls of herbivorous animals. *Journal of the American Chemical Society* 56:2400-2403. Cited in, ibid. Handel, Jacob, "Chlorophyll Supporter...". p. 33.

446 Hughes, J. and Latner, A. 1936. Chlorophyll and haemoglobin regeneration after haemorrhage. *Journal of Physiology* 86:388-395. Cited in, ibid. Handel, Jacob, "Chlorophyll Supporter...". p. 33.

447 Patek, A. 1936. Chlorophyll and regeneration of the blood. *Archives of Internal Medicine* 57:73-84. Cited in, ibid. Handel, Jacob, "Chlorophyll Supporter...". p. 33.

448 Scott, E. and Delor, C. 1933. Nutritional anemia. *Ohio State Medical Journal* 29:165-169. Cited in, ibid. Handel, Jacob, "Chlorophyll Supporter...". p. 32.

449 Hammel-Dupont, C. and Bessman, S. 1970. The stimulation of hemoglobin synthesis by porphyrins. *Biochemical Medicine* 4:55-60. Cited in, ibid. Handel, Jacob, "Chlorophyll Supporter...". p. 33.

450 Saunders, C. 1926. The nutritional value of chlorophyll as related to hemoglobin formation. Proceedings of the Society for Experimental Biology and Medicine (3172), p. 788-789: Cited in, ibid. Handel, Jacob, "Chlorophyll Supporter...". p. 33.

451 Kimm, S., Tschai, B., and Park, S. 1982. Antimutagenic activity of chlorophyll to direct and indirect-acting mutagens and its contents in the vegetables. *Korean Journal of Biochemistry* 14:1-7. Saunders, C. 1926. The nutritional value of chlorophyll as related to hemoglobin formation. Proceedings of the Society for Experimental Biology and Medicine (3172), p. 788-789: Cited in, ibid. Handel, Jacob, "Chlorophyll Supporter...", p. 33.

452 Ong, T., Whong, W., Stewart, J. and Brockman, H. 1986. Chlorophyllin: a potent antimutagen against environmental and dietary complex mixtures. *Mutation Research* 173:111-15. Saunders, C. 1926. The nutritional value of chlorophyll as related to hemoglobin formation. Proceedings of the Society for Experimental Biology and Medicine (3172), p. 788-789: Cited in, ibid. Handel, Jacob, "Chlorophyll Supporter...", p. 33.

453 Spector, H. and Calloway, D. 1959. Reduction of x-radiation mortality by cabbage and broccoli. Proceedings of the Society for Experimental Biology and Medicine 100:405-407. Cited in, ibid. Handel, Jacob, "Chlorophyll Supporter...", p. 56.

454 Calloway, D., Newell, G., Calhoun, W. and Munson, A. 1962. Further studies of the influence on diet on radiosensitivity of guinea pigs, with special reference to broccoli and alfalfa. *Journal of Nutrition* 79:340-348. Cited in, ibid. Handel, Jacob, "Chlorophyll Supporter...", p. 56.

455 Handel, Jacob, "Chlorophyll Supporter of all Human and Animal Life", p. 32, 33, 56.

456 Young, Robert, website: phMiracleliving.com 2/09.

457 Young, Robert, website: phMiracleliving.com 2/09.

[458] Selig, M.S. Mechanisms by which antibiotics increase the incidence and severity of candidiasis and alter the immunological defense. *Bacteriological Review*, 1966;30: 442-59.

[459] Cousens, Gabriel, *Rainbow Green Live-Food Cuisine*, (North Atlantic Books, Berkely, CA, 2003), p. 5; Also Essene Vision Books, Patagonia, Arizonia, 2003.

[460] Cousens, Gabriel, *Rainbow Green Live-Food Cuisine*, (North Atlantic Books, Berkely, CA, 2003), p. 5; Also Essene Vision Books, Patagonia, Arizonia, 2003.

[461] Cousens, Gabriel, *Rainbow Green Live-Food Cuisine*, (North Atlantic Books, Berkeley, CA. 2003), p. 2.

[462] Cousens, Gabriel, *Rainbow Green Live-Food Cuisine*, p. 8.

[463] Cousens, Gabriel, *Rainbow Green Live-Food Cuisine*, p. 33.

[464] Cousens, Gabriel, *Rainbow Green Live-Food Cuisine*, p. 33.

[465] Schmidt, Michael A., *Brain Building Nutrition* (2007), ibid.

[466] Schmidt, *Brain Building Nutrition*, p. 9, citing: Rudin, DO. Omega-3 essential fatty Acids in medicine. In Bland, JS. 1984-85 *Yearbook in Nutritional Medicine*, New Canaan, Conn.: Keats Pub., Inc., 1985:41.

[467] Schmidt, *Brain Building Nutrition*, p. 9, citing: Simopoulous, AP. Omega-3 fatty acids. In Spiller, GA, ed. *Handbook of Lipids in Human Nutrition*. Boca Raton, Florida: CRC Press, Inc., 1996; 51-73.

[468] Schmidt, *Brain Building Nutrition*, p. 9.

[469] Schmidt, *Brain Building Nutrition*, p. 13.

[470] Julian Whitaker, MD, in her newsletter *Health & Healing,* October 2009; website www.coconutketones.com

[471] *Adv Neurol.* 1993;60:681-4

[472] *Neurology.* 1996 Sep;47(3):636-43

[473] Kalechofsky, *Judaism and Animal Rights*, p. 150-51, citing: Louis A. Berman, *The Dietary Laws as Atonements for Flesh-eating*.

[474] Cousens, Gabriel, *Conscious Eating*, p. 393.

[475] *Encyclopedia of the Early Church*, Institutum Patristicum Augustinianum, Oxford University Press, Inc., New York, N.Y., 1992.

[476] Ibid., *Encyclopedia of the Early Church*, citing: Iren., *Haer.* I 2,1 ; Tertull., *Ieiun.* 15, 1; Epiph., *Haer.* 30,18ff. and 47,1; Aug., *Haer.* 25.46.70.

[477] Ewing, *The Prophet of the Dead Sea Scrolls*, p. 145, citing: *Hastings Encyclopedia on Religion and Ethics* (V.5, p. 143), Charles Scribner=s, Sons, N.Y.

[478] Ewing, *The Prophet of the Dead Sea Scrolls,* p. 145, citing: Teicher, J.L., *Journal of Jewish Studies*, 1951.

[479] As explained in *A Critical Investigation of Epiphanius' Knowledge of the Ebionites: A Translation and Critical Discussion of "Panarion,"* by Glen Alan Kochit.

[480] Cousens, Gabriel, *Conscious Eating*, p. 381.

[481] *Encyclopedia of the Dead Sea Scrolls*, Editors Schiffman, VanderKam, p. 248, citing: *Adversus omnes Haereses* 1.28.

[482] *Encyclopedia of the Dead Sea Scrolls*, Editors Schiffman, VanderKam, p. 248, citing: *Adversus omnes Haereses* 1.28.
[483] St. Francis of Assisi, *Omnibus of Sources*, Celano Second Life, chapter 15.
[484] Hatherhill, J. Robert, PhD, *The BrainGate:...*, p. 32, Cited: Cook, *The 4-Week...*, p. 31.
[485] Cook, *The 4-Week Ultimate Body Detox Plan,* p. 30.
[486] Cohen, Robert, *Milk A-Z*, p. 35, citing: Sandra Steingraber, PhD in *Living Downstream*.
[487] Cohen, Robert, *Milk A-Z*, p. 34, citing: *Food and Water Journal,* Summer 1998; United Press International, March 11, 1983.
[488] According to research that was presented at the American Academy of Neurology 58th Annual Meeting in San Diego, CA, April 1 – 8, 2006.
[489] According to research that was presented at the American Academy of Neurology 58th Annual Meeting in San Diego, CA, April 1 – 8, 2006.
[490] Ellis, F., et. Al, "Incidence of Osteoporosis in Vegetarians and Omnivores," *American Journal of Clinical Nutrition*, 25:555, 1972.
[491] Cohen, Robert, *Milk A-Z*, p. 32, citing: *Science*, 1986;233.
[492] Cohen, Robert, *Milk A-Z*, p. 32, citing: *American Journal of Clinical Nutrition*, 1979;32(4).
[493] Cohen, Robert, *Milk A-Z*, p. 32, citing: *Nutrition Action Healthletter*, June 1993.
[494] Cohen, Robert, *Milk A-Z* (Argus Publishing, Englewood Cliffs, New Jersey, 2001), p. 33, citing: *American Journal of Public Health*, 1997;87.
[495] Day, Lorraine, MD, *Getting Started on Getting Well*, Rockford Press, Thousand Palms, CA, 2003: citing: *American Journal of Clinical Nutrition*, 1991; 53: 132-142; 1987, 46:685-687; *Journal of Nutrition*, 1981, 111:545, 553; 1974;104(6):695-700; *Journal of the American Dietetic Association*, 1980; 76:148-151; *Hospital Practice*, 1994, Nov 15;68.
[496] Wachman, Amnon, et al, "Diet and Osteoporosis," *Lancet*, May 4, 1968, p. 958.
[497] Barnard, Neal, MD, *Breaking the Food Seduction*, p. 68. Citing: Breslau NA, Brinkley L, Hill KD, Pak CYC. Relationship of animal-protein-rich diets to kidney stone formation and calcium metabolism. *J Clini Endocrinol* 1988;66:140-6.
[498] Barnard, Neal, MD, *Breaking the Food Seduction*, p. 68. Citing: Abelow, BJ, Holford, TR, Insogna KI., Cross-cultural association between dietary animal protein and hip fracture: a hypothesis. *Calcif Tissue Int* 1992;50:14-18.
[499] Barnard, Neal, MD, *Breaking the Food Seduction*, p. 68. Citing: Frekanich D, Willett WC, Stampfer MJ, Colditz GA. Protein consumption and bone fractures in women. *Am J Epidemiol* 1996:143:472-9.
[500] Barnard, Neal, MD, *Breaking the Food Seduction*, p. 68.
[501] Chen, Honglei, et al., "Dairy products and the risk of Parkinson's

disease" *American Journal of Epidemiology*, 2007, May 1:165(9):998-1006 (National Institute of Environmental Health Sciences, Research Triangle Park, North Carolina).

502 Chen, Honglei, et al., "Dairy products and the risk of Parkinson's disease" *American Journal of Epidemiology*, 2007, May 1:165(9):998-1006 (National Institute of Environmental Health Sciences, Research Triangle Park, North Carolina).

503 Wendt, L., Wendt, T., and Wendt, A. "Protein Transport and Protein Storage in Etiology and Pathogenesis of Arteriosclerosis, *Ernahrungswiss*. Dietrich Steinkopff Verlag, 1975, pp. 1-38.

504 Wendt, L., Wendt, T., and Wendt, A. "Protein Transport and Protein Storage in Etiology and Pathogenesis of Arteriosclerosis, *Ernahrungswiss*. Dietrich Steinkopff Verlag, 1975, pp. 1-38.

505 Neurology. 2005 Mar 22;64(6):1047-51.

506 Chen H, Zhang SM, Hernan MA, Willett WC, Ascherio A. Diet and Parkinson's disease: a potential role of dairy products in men. *Ann Neurol*. 2002;52:793–801.

507 Holden, Kathrynne, MS, RD, *Parkinson's Disease: Nutrition Matters*, (National Parkinson's Foundation, Inc., Bob Hope Parkinson's Research Center, Miami, Florida, 2003).

508 Hatherill, Robert J., *The Brain Gate*, (Life Line Press, Washington, D.C., 2003).

509 Young, Robert, e-Newsletter, 2007, citing: *American Journal of Epidemiology*, May 1, 2007.

510 Young, Robert, PhD, website (miracle pH) newsletter 2009.

511 Young, Robert, O., *Sick and Tired*, p. 90-91.

512 Frank A. Oski, M.D., Physician-in-Chief, at the John Hopkins Children's Center, *Don't Drink Your Milk! New Frightening Medical Facts About the World's Most Overrated Nutrient*, p. 17, 18, citing: Gryboski JD: Gastrointestinal milk allergy in infants. *Pediatrics* 40:354, 1967.

513 Oski, Frank, *Don't Drink Your Milk*, p. 61, 62, citing: Aagranoff BW and Goldberg D: Diet and the geographical distribution of multiple sclerosis. *Lancet* 2:1061, 1974.

514 Cohen, Robert, *Milk A-Z*, (Argus Publishing, 2001), p. 53, citing: *British Medical Journal*, 1996:313.

515 Saukkonen T, Virtanen SM, Karppinen M, et al. Significance of cow's milk protein and antibodies as risk factor for childhood IDDM: *Dibetologia*. 1998;72-8.

516 CDC U.S. Obesity Trends 1985-2009.

517 Cohen, Robert, *Milk A-Z*, p. 3.

518 Oski, Frank, *Don't Drink Your Milk*, p. 61, 62, citing: Aagranoff BW and Goldberg D: Diet and the geographical distribution of multiple sclerosis. *Lancet* 2:1061, 1974.

519 Simi and Segreti, *Saint Francis of Paola God's Miracle Worker Supreme*, (Tan Book Publishers, Rockford, Illinois), 1977.

[520] Simi, Gino J.; Sergreti, Mario, M., *Saint Francis of Paola God's Miracle Worker Supreme*.

[521] Airola, Paavo, *Are You Confused?* Phoenix, AZ: Health Plus, Publishers, 1974.

[522] Airola, Paavo, *Are You Confused?* Health Plus, Publishers, 1974.

[523] Kulvinskas, Viktoras. *Survival into the 21st Century*. Woodstock Valley. CT/Fairfield, IA: 21st Century Publications, 1975.

[524] Airola, Paavo. *How to Get Well*. Health Plus, Publishers, 1974.

[525] Cousens, Gabriel, *Spiritual Nutrition*, p. 270.

[526] Briskey, E.J., et al, *The Physiology and...*, p. 341.

[527] Wendt, L., Wendt, T., and Wendt, A. "Protein Transport and Protein Storage in Etiology and Pathogenesis of Arteriosclerosis, *Ernahrungswiss*. Dietrich Steinkopff Verlag, 1975, pp. 1-38.

[528] Cousens, Gabriel, *Spiritual Nutrition*, p. 270-71.

[529] Levine, Steve and Kidd, Paris. *Antioxidant Adaption: Its Role in Free Radical Pathology*. San Francisco: Biocurrents Press. 1985.

[530] Cousens, Gabriel, *Spiritual Nutrition*, p. 270-71.

[531] Airola, Paavo. *How to Get Well*. Phoenix, AZ: Health Plus, 1974.

[532] Cousens, Gabriel, *Spiritual Nutrition Six Foundations for Spiritual Life and the Awakening of Kundalini*, (North Atlantic Books, Berkeley, California, 2005), p. 269-270.

[533] Young, Robert, and Young, Shelly, *Back to the House of Health*, and *Back to the House of Health II* (Woodland Publishing, 1999, 2003).

[534] Young, Robert, and Young, Shelly, *Back to the House of Health*, I & II, appendix. (Woodland Publishing, 1999, 2003).

[535] Cousens, Gabriel, *Rainbow Green Live-Food Cuisine*, p. 25, citing: *The Fungal/Mycotoxin Etiology of Human Disease*, Vol. 2, 1994.

[536] Hatherill, Robert J., *The Brain Gate*, (Life Line Press, Washington, D.C., 2003), p. 134.

[537] Hatherill, Robert J., *The Brain Gate*, p. 53.

[538] Barnard, Neal, *Breaking the Food Seduction*, (St. Martins Press, New York, 2003), p. 68.

[539] Clement, Brian, "Killer Fish" article in Healing Our World, (Hippocrates Health Institute, Vol. 32, issue 3, 2012), p. 17, based on Brian Clement's book, *Killer Fish* (2012).

[540] Clement, Brian, "Killer Fish" article in Healing Our World, (Hippocrates Health Institute, Vol. 32, issue 3, 2012), p. 17, based on Brian Clement's book, *Killer Fish* (2012).

[541] Clement, Brian, "Killer Fish", p. 54, 55.

[542] Clement, Brian, "Killer Fish", p. 17.

[543] Clement, Brian, *Killer Fish*, (Hippocrates Publications, 2012), p. 11.

[544] Clement, Brian, *Killer Fish*, p. 7, citing: US Food and Drug Administration, "Mercury levels in commercial fish and shellfish 1990-2010, fda.gove/Food/FoodSafety/Product-SpecificInformation.

[545] Woolsey, Ramond, *Meat on the Menu: Who Needs It?*, 1974, p. 40-41. "The Fish have Cancer. Is the Water Drinkable?" Medical World

News, June 23, 1972, p. 41, 80.

[546] Miller, Bruce, D.D.S., C.N.S., *Protein A Consumer's Concern*, (Bruce Miller Enterprises, Inc., Dallas, TX, 1977), p. 11.

[547] Miller, Bruce, *Protein A Consumer's Concern*, p. 11.

[548] Ballentine, Ro. *Transition to Vegetarianism*, p. 82, citing: Bryan FT: Miscellaneous pathogenic bacteria, in Pearson and Dutson, *Advances in Meat Research*, pp. 250-51.

[549] Ballentine, Rudolph, M.D., *Transition to Vegetarianism, An Evolutionary Step*, (The Himalayan Institute Press, PA, 1999), p. 82, citing: Skirrow MB, Fidoe RG, Jones DM: An outbreak of presumptive food-borne Campylobacter entities. *J Infect Dis* 3:234, 1981. Also, Svedhem A. Kaijser B, Sjogren E: The occurrence of Campylobacter jejuni in fresh food and survival under different conditions. *J Hygiene* 87:421, 1981.

[550] Robbins, J., *Diet for a New America*, HJ Kramer Books, Tiburon, CA, 1987, p. 65, citing: Mason, J., and Singer, P., *Animal Factories*, (Cown Publishers, 1980), pg 5.

[551] Collective-Evolution.com website: "FDA Finally Admits Chicken Meat Contains Cancer-Causing Arsenic." (8/16/13)

[552] Cousens, Gabriel, *Conscious Eating*, p. 389-390.

[553] *The Fathers of the Church a New Translation*, Volume 16, St. Augustine, *Treatises on Various Subjects: The Usefulness of Fasting*; p. 89-92.

[554] Kidd, Parris, PhD, Parkinson's Disease as Multifactorial Oxidative Neurodegeneration,... p.518, citing: Carter JH, Nutt JG, Woodward WR, et al. Amount and distribution of dietary protein affects clinical response to levodopa in Parkinson's disease. *Neurology* 1989; 39:552-556.

[555] Yapa SC 1992; Golbe LI et al 1988.

[556] Powers KM et al 2003; Logroscino G et al 1996.

[557] Kidd, Parris, PhD, Parkinson's Disease as Multifactorial Oxidative Neurodegeneration: Implications for Integrative Management, (*Altern Med Rev* 2000;5(6):502-545), citing: Tsui JK, Ross S, Poulin K, et al. The effect of dietary protein on the efficacy of L-dopa: a double-blind study. *Neurology* 1989; 39;549-522.

[558] Kidd, Parris, PhD, Parkinson's Disease as Multifactorial Oxidative Neurodegeneration,... p.518, citing: Carter JH, Nutt JG, Woodward WR, et al. Amount and distribution of dietary protein affects clinical response to levodopa in Parkinson's disease. *Neurology* 1989; 39:552-556.

[559] *Med Hypotheses*. 2001 Sep;57(3):318-23.

[560] *Eur J Clin Nutr*. 1991 May;45(5):263-6.

[561] *Arch Neurol*. 1987 Mar;44(3):270-2

[562] Barichella M, Marczewska A, De Notaris R, et al. Special low–protein foods ameliorate postprandial off in patients with advanced Parkinson's disease. *Mov Disord*. 2006 Jun 13; DOI 10.1002/mds.21003.

9. Pincus JH, Barry K. Protein redistribution diet restores motor function in patients with dopa–resistant "off" periods. *Neurology*. 1988;38:481–

483. 10. Mena I, Cotzias GC. Protein intake and treatment of Parkinson's disease with levodopa. *N Engl J Med.* 1975;292:181–184. 11. Gillespie NG, Mena L, Cotzias GC, Bell MA. Diets affecting treatment of parkinsonism with levodopa. *J Am Diet Assoc.* 1973;62:525–528.

[563] Pincus JH, Barry K. Protein redistribution diet restores motor function in patients with dopa–resistant "off" periods. *Neurology.* 1988;38:481–483; Mena I, Cotzias GC. Protein intake and treatment of Parkinson's disease with levodopa. *N Engl J Med.* 1975;292:181–184.

[564] *Eur J Clin Nutr.* 1991 May;45(5):263-6.

[565] *Neurology.* 1996 Sep;47(3):636-43.

[566] *Mov Disord.* 1999 Jan;14(1):21-7.

[567] Rogers, Sherry, *The Cholesterol Hoax*, (Prestige Publishing Inc., Albany, N.Y., 2008).

[568] Rogers, Sherry, *The Cholesterol Hoax*, p. 4-12.

[569] Rogers, Sherry, *The Cholesterol Hoax*, p. 91, citing: Hulley S, et al, Childhood cholesterol screening: Contraindicated, *J Am Med Assoc*, 267:100-02, 1992.

[570] Rogers, Sherry, *The Cholesterol Hoax*, p. 101-102, Behar S, et al, Low total cholesterol is associated with high total mortality in patients with coronary heart disease. The Bezafobrate Infarction Prevention (BIP) Study Group, *Heart J*, 1:52-9, Jan. 18, 1997.

[571] Rogers, Sherry, *The Cholesterol Hoax*, p. 102, citing: Cassidy AT, Carroll BJ, Hypocholesterolemina during mixed manic episodes, *Europ Arch Psych Clin Neurosci*, 252, 3:110-14, June 2002. And Engleberg H, Low serum cholesterol and suicide, *Lancet*, 339; 8795:727-79, Mar 21, 1992.

[572] Moynihan and Cassels, *Selling Sickness,* p. 5, citing: N. Choudhry, H. Stelfox, and A. Detsky, "Relationships between authors of clinical practice guidelines and the pharmaceutical industry," *JAMA*, vol. 287, no. 5, 2002, pp. 612-17.

[573] Abramson, John, *Overdosed America,* p. 135.

[574] *Med Hypotheses.* 2001 Sep;57(3):318-23.

[575] *Mov Disord.* 1999 Jan;14(1):21-7.

[576] Yaffe K, Barrett-Connor E, Lin F, Grady D. Serum lipoprotein levels, statin use, and cognitive function in older women. *Arch Neurol* 2002;59:378-84.

[577] *Int J Epidemiol.* 1999 Dec;28(6):1102-9

[578] *Neurology.* 2005 Jun 28;64(12):2040-5.

[579] *Adv Neurol.* 1993;60:681-4.

[580] *Arch Neurol.* 1987 Mar;44(3):270-2.

[581] *Parkinsonism Relat Disord.* 2004 Mar;10(3):137-42

[582] *Mov Disord.* 2006 Oct;21(10):1682-7.

[583] *Mov Disord.* 2006 Aug;21(8):1229-31.

[584] *Int J Mol Med.* 2004 Mar;13(3):343-53.

[585] Pahwa, Lyons, Koller, *Handbook of Parkinson's Disease Third Edition*, p. 231-232.

[586] Smith, Jeffrey M., *Genetic Roulette,* (Yes! Books, Fairfield, Iowa, 2007).

[587] Smith, Jeffrey M., *Genetic Roulette,* p. 111, citing: M. Cretenet, et al, "Submission on the DAR for Application A549 Food Derived from High-Lysine Corn LYO38" citing, for example, M.Bucciantini, et al, "Inherent toxicity of aggregates implies a common mechanism for protein misfolding diseases," *Nature* 416 (2002):507-511.

[588] Russell, Rex, M.D., *What the Bible Says About Healthy Living,* p. 150. Citing: David Macht, M.D., AAn Experimental Pharmacological Appreciation of Leviticus XI and Deuteronomy XIV,@ *Bulletin of Historical Medicine,* Johns Hopkins University, 47:1 (April 1953): pp. 444-450.

[589] Russell, Rex, M.D., *What the Bible Says About Healthy Living,* p. 150. Citing: David Macht, M.D., "An Experimental Pharmacological Appreciation of Leviticus XI and Deuteronomy XIV," *Bulletin of Historical Medicine,* Johns Hopkins University, 47:1 (April 1953): pp. 444-450.

[590] Russell, Rex, M.D., *What the Bible Says About Healthy Living,* p. 150. Citing: David Macht, M.D., AAn Experimental Pharmacological Appreciation of Leviticus XI and Deuteronomy XIV,@ *Bulletin of Historical Medicine,* Johns Hopkins University, 47:1 (April 1953): 444-450.

[591] Grimm, Veronika, E., *From Feasting to Fasting, the Evolution of Sin, Attitudes to food in late Antiquity,* New York, NY: Routledge, 1996, p. 97-98.

[592] Ibid. Grimm, p. 105, 106, citing: Stromateis 2:20.

[593] Cousens, Gabriel, MD, *Rainbow Green Live-Food Cuisine,* North Atlantic Books, Berkeley, CA, 2003, pp. 19-23.

[594] Graham, Doug, *Grain Damage* (Storrington, W. Sussex, 1998, Rozalind Gruben).

[595] Wolfe, David, *The Sunfood Diet Success System, Eating for Beauty,* (Maul Bros. Pub., 2002).

[596] Boutenko, Victoria, *12 Steps to Raw Foods How to End Your Addiction to Cooked Foods,* Raw Family Publishing, Ashland, OR, 2002.

[597] Rhio, *Hooked on Raw, Rejuvenate your Body and Soul with Nature's Living Foods,* (Beso Entertainment, 2000).

[598] Sarno, Chad, *Vital Creations, An Organic Life Experience,* (www.rawchef.org, 2002).

[599] Juliano, *Raw the Uncook Book New Vegetarian Food for Life,* (Harper Collins Publishers, New York, N.Y., 1999).

[600] Shannon, Nomi, *The Raw Gourmet,* (Alive Books, Burnaby, BC, Canada, 1990).

[601] Baker, Elizabeth, The UnCook Book Raw Food Adventures to a New Health High, (ProMotion Publishing, San Diego, CA, 1996).

[602] Patenaude, Frederic, *The Sunfood Cuisine a Practical Guide to Raw Vegetarian Cuisine,* (San Diego, CA, 2001).

603 Cobb, Brenda, *The Living Foods Lifestyle*, (Living Soul Publishing, Atlanta, GA, 2003).

604 Trotter, Charlie; Klein, Roxanne, *RAW*, (Ten Speed Press, Berkley, CA., 2003).

605 Shazzie, *Shazzie's Detox Delights*, (Rawcreation limited, 2001).

606 Ferrara, Alex, *The Raw Food Primer*, (Council Oak Books, San Francisco, Tulsa, OK, 2003).

607 Love, Elaine, *Elaine's Pure Joy Kitchen, Raw, Organic, Vegan, Recipes,* (www.purejoylivingfoods.com) 1998.

608 Kenney Matthew, *Everyday Raw*, (Gibbs Smith Publisher, Utah, 2008).

609 Boutenko, Igor, *Igor's Live Flat Bread*, (Raw Family Publishing, 2005).

610 Boutenko, Sergei; Boutenko, Valya, *Eating without Heating*, (Raw Family Publishing, 2004).

611 Wandling, Julie, *Thank God for Raw*, (Healthy 4 Him Publishing, Akron, OH, 2002).

612 Nison, Paul, *The Raw Life*, (343 Publishing Company, New York, N.Y., 2000).

613 Bisci, Fred, *Your Healthy Journey*, (Bisci Lifestyle Books, NJ, 2008).

614 Arlin, Stephen, *Raw Power*, (Maul Brothers Publishing, San Diego, CA., 1998).

615 Young, Robert, Shelly, *Sick and Tired?*

616 Clement, Brian, PhD., *Living Foods for Optimum Health*, (Prima Pub, Hippocrates Inst. FL, 1996).

617 Clement, Anna Maria, PhD., *Healthful Cuisine*, (Healthful Communications, Juno Beach, FL, 2006).

618 Soria, Cherie, *Angel Foods*, (Heartstar Productions, Santa Barbara, CA., 1996).

619 Tibbetts, James, *Superior Health with a Living Foods Lifestyle*, (2003; www.jimtibbetts.com).

620 Mars, Brigitte, *Rawsome! Maximizing Health, Energy and Culinary Delight with the Raw Foods Diet*, (Basic Health Publications, NJ, 2004).

621 Levin, James, MD; Cederquist Natalie, *Vibrant Living*, (GLO, Inc., La Jolla, CA, 1993; 2001).

622 Safron, Jeremy, A.; Underkoffler, Renee, *The Raw Truth the Art of Loving Foods*, (Loving Foods, Inc., Paia, HI, 1997).

623 Romano, Rita, *Dining in the Raw Groundbreaking Natural Cuisine that Combines the Techniques of Macrobiotic, Vegan, Allergy-free, and Raw Food Disciplines*, (Kensigton Pub., 1992).

624 Jubb, David & Annie Padden, *Life Food Recipe Book, Living on Life Force*, (North Atlantic Books, CA, 2003).

625 Safron, Jeremy, *The Raw Truth, the Art of Preparing Living Foods*, (Celestial Arts, Berkeley, 2003).

626 Calabro, Rose Lee, Living in the Raw Desserts, (Book Publishing Co., TN, 2007).

[627] Markowitz, Elysa, *Warming Up to Living Foods*, (Book Publishing Company, 1998).

[628] Schnitzer, Johann, *Schnitzer-Intensive Nutrition, Schnitzer-Normal Nutrition*, (Schnitzer Publishers, Black Forest, W. Germany, 2002, tenth revised edition).

[629] Gerson, Charlotte, Walker, Morton, DPM, *The Gerson Therapy*, (Kensington Publishing Corp., New York, N.Y., 2001), p. 94, 98.

[630] Sheraton (Dina), Jameth, ND, Sheraton (Sproul), Kim, ND, *Uncooking with Jameth and Kim*, (Healthforce Publishing, 1991-2001).

[631] Malkmus, George H., *God's Way to Ultimate Health*, (Hallelujah Acres Pub, Shelby, NC, 1995).

[632] Malkmus, Rhonda, J., *Recipes for Life*, (Hallelujah Acres Pub., Shelby, NC, 2001).

[633] Dorit, *Celebrating our Raw Nature*, (Book Publishing Co., TN, 2007).

[634] Maerin, Jordan, *Raw Foods for Busy People*, (www.rawfood.com, CA, 2005).

[635] Diamond, Harvey & Marilyn, *Fit for Life II: Living Health*, (Warner Books, New York, NY, 1987).

[636] Smith, Melissa, D., *Going Against the Grain*, (Contemporary Books, New York), 2002.

[637] Horne, Ross, *Improving on Pritikin - You can do Better!*, (Happy Landings Pty Ltd, Australia, 1988), p. 10. citing, Dr. Emmet Densmore and Dr. Charles De Lacy Evenas of England.

[638] Graham, Douglas, *Grain Damage*, (Marathon, FL; Rozalind Gruben, Storrington, W. Sussex, 1998), p. 11, 12.

[639] Graham, Douglas, *Grain Damage*, p. 13, 14.

[640] Graham, Douglas, *Grain Damage*, p. 13, 14.

[641] Graham, Douglas, *Grain Damage*, p. 16.

[642] Graham, Douglas, *Grain Damage*, p. 16.

[643] Graham, Douglas, *Grain Damage*, p. 19, 22, 23.

[644] Graham, Douglas, *Grain Damage*, p. 19, 22, 23.

[645] Graham, Douglas, *Grain Damage*, p. 24.

[646] Graham, Douglas, *Grain Damage*, p. 24.

[647] Graham, Douglas, *Grain Damage*, p. 24.

[648] Cousens, Gabriel, MD. *Rainbow Green Live-Food Cuisine*, p. 21.

[649] Cousens, Gabriel, MD. *Rainbow Green Live-Food Cuisine*, p. 20.

[650] Nison, Paul, *Raw Knowledge II*, p. 223, citing a Dr. Vivian Ventrano interview with Paul Nison.

[651] Smith, Melissa Diane, *Going Against the Grain*, (Contemporary Books/McGraw-Hill, 2002), p. 47; citing: J. Saleron et al, "Dietary fiber, glycemic load, and the risk of non-insulin-dependent diabetes mellitus in women," *Journal of the American Medical Association* 277 (1997): 472-77.

[652] Smith, *Going Against the Grain*, citing: D.R. Jacobs, Jr. et al., "Whole-grain intake may reduce the risk of ischemic heart disease death

in postmenopausal women: The Iowa Women's Health Study," *American Journal of Clinical Nutrition* 68 (1998): 248-57.

[653] Smith, *Going Against the Grain*, p 47.

[654] Walker, Norman, *Raw Vegetable Juices*, (Norwalk Press, Prescott, AZ, 1978), p. 99.

[655] Boroch, Ann, *Healing Multiple Sclerosis* (2007), p. 33, citing: Christina M. Hull, and M. Ryan, "Evidence for Mating of the 'Asexual' Yeast *Candida albicans* in a Mammalian Host," *Science* 289 (5477)(2000): 256-57.

[656] Boroch, Ann, *Healing Multiple Sclerosis*, p. 36, citing: C. Orian Truss, *The Missing Diagnosis* (Birmingham, AL: The Missing Diagnosis, Inc., 1985).

[657] Boroch, Ann, *Healing Multiple Sclerosis*, p. 36, citing: C. Orian Truss, *The Missing Diagnosis* (Birmingham, AL: The Missing Diagnosis, Inc., 1985).

[658] Boroch, Ann, *Healing Multiple Sclerosis*, p. 36, citing: C. Orian Truss, *The Missing Diagnosis* (Birmingham, AL: The Missing Diagnosis, Inc., 1985).

[659] David Perlmutter, *Brain Recovery.com: The Powerful Therapy for Challenging Brain Disorders* (Naples, Fl: Perlmutter Health Center, 2000).

[660] David Perlmutter, *Brain Recovery.com: The Powerful Therapy for Challenging Brain Disorders* (2000).

[661] David Perlmutter, "Fatigue in Multiple Sclerosis," *Townsend Letter for Doctors and Patients* (1995): 6-11.

[662] David Perlmutter, MD, Speaking at the Institute for Functional Medicine's 20th International Symposium, cites, Yao SY, et al. *Neurology*. 2001. 8;56(9):1168-76.

[663] David Perlmutter, MD, Speaking at the Institute for Functional Medicine's 20th International Symposium, cites, Fainardi E, et al. *J Neurovirol*. 2009; 15(5-6); 425-33.

[664] Jim Tibbetts discussion with Dana Flavin cira. 2008.

[665] Meyerowitz, Steve, Sprouts the Miracle Food, the Complete Guide to Sprouting, (Sproutman Publications, P.O. Box 1100, Great Barrington, MA., 01230, www.sproutman.com; 2010).

[666] Cousens, Gabriel, *Spiritual Nutrition*, p. 304.

[667] Cousens, Gabriel, *Conscious Eating*, p. 763.

[668] Cousens, Gabriel, *Conscious Eating*, p. 763.

[669] Cousens, Gabriel, MD. *Rainbow Green Live-Food Cuisine*, p. 19.

[670] Cousens, Gabriel, MD. *Rainbow Green Live-Food Cuisine*, p. 21.

[671] Cousens, Gabriel, *Spiritual Nutrition*, p. 302, citing Szekely, Edmond Bordeaux, *The Essenes, by Josephus and His Contemporaries*. (San Diego, CA: International Biogenic Society, 1981).

[672] Cousens, Gabriel, *Spiritual Nutrition*, p. 303, citing Szekely, Edmond Bordeaux, *The Essenes, by Josephus*.

[673] Cousens, Gabriel, *Spiritual Nutrition*, p. 303, citing Szekely, Edmond

Bordeaux, *The Essenes, by Josephus.*

[674] Parry, Ken, *Vegetarianism in Late Antiquity...*, p. 183, citing: *Pachomian Chronicles and Rules. Pachomian Koinonia,* vol. 2, trans. With an intro by A. Veilleux (Cisterian Studies Series 46, Kalamazoo 1981), 143. Basil of Caesarea suggests one meal a day, vegetables, and fruits (*The Letters* 2).

[675] Parry, Ken, *Vegetarianism in Late Antiquity...*, p. 183, citing: Palladius, *Te Lausiac History,* trans. R.T. Meyer (Ancient Christian Writers, London 1965), 94-95. The fifth-century historian Sozomen mentions a group of Syrian ascetics called 'grazers' who lived on grass cut with a sickle (*Eccesiastical History* 6.33). Te 'grazers' are also mentioned in the Vita of Symeon the Fool; see D. Kruger, *Symeon the Holy Fool: Leontius' life and the late antique city* (Berkeley 1996), 141, 166.

[676] Parry, Ken, *Vegetarianism in Late Antiquity...*, p. 183, citing: P. Rousseau, Pachomius: *The making of a community in fourth-century Egypt* (Berkeley 1999), 102.

[677] Parry, Ken, *Vegetarianism in Late Antiquity...*, p. 186, citing: *Depicting the Word: Byzantine iconophile thought of the eighth and ninth centuries* (Leiden 1996), ch. 17.

[678] Virtue, Doreen, *The Art of Raw Living,* (Hay House, New York, NY, 2009), p. xiv, citing: *Medical News Today* 2004.

[679] Cobb, Brenda, *The Living Foods Lifestyle*, Living Soul Publishing, Atlanta, GA, 2003, p. 88.

[680] *Geriatric Nutrition*, Chernoff, Ronni, p. 137, citing: Doty RL. Odor perception in neurodegenerative disease. In: Doty R, ed. *Handbook of Olfaction and Gustation.* New York, NY: Marcell Dekker Inc.; 2003: 475-501.

[681] *Geriatric Nutrition*, Chernoff, Ronni, citing: Mesholam R, Moberg P, Mar R, Doty R. Olfaction in neurodegenerative disease: a meta-analysis of olfactory functioning in Alzheimer's and Parkinson's disease. *Arch Neurol* 1998;55:84-90.

[682] *Geriatric Nutrition*, Chernoff, Ronni, citing: Bacon Moore , Paulsen J, Murphy C. A test of odor fluency in patients with Alzheimer's and Huntington's disease. *J Clin Exp Neurophychol* 1999;21:341-351.

[683] *Geriatric Nutrition*, Chernoff, Ronni, citing: Nordin S, Monsch A, Murphy C. Unawareness of smell loss in normal aging and Alzheimer's disease: discrepancy between self-reported and diagnosed smell sensitivity. J Gerontol B Psychol Sci Soc Sci 1995;50: P187-192.

[684] *Geriatric Nutrition*, Chernoff, Ronni, p. 138, citing: Doty RL, Deems D, Setella S. Olfactory dysfunction in parkinsonism: a general deficit unrelated to neurologic signs, disease stage, or disease duration. *Neurology* 1988;38:1237-1244.

[685] *Geriatric Nutrition*, citing: Doty RL. Odor perception in neurodegenerative disease. In: Doty R, ed. *Handbook of Olfaction and Gustation.* New York, NY: Marcell Dekker Inc.; 2003: 475-501.

[686] *Geriatric Nutrition*, Chernoff, Ronni, citing: Tews J, Repa J, Nguyen H, Harper A. Protein selection by olfactory bulbectomized rats. *Nutr Rep Int*el 1985:31:797-803.

[687] *Geriatric Nutrition*, Chernoff, Ronni, citing: May K. Association between anosmia and anorexia in cats. Presented at: Ninth International Symposium on Olfaction and Taste. *NY Acad Sci* 1986; 510:480-82.

[688] *Geriatric Nutrition*, Chernoff, Ronni, citing: Mattes R, Cowart B. Dietary assessment of patients with chemosensory disorders. *J Am Diet Assoc* 1994; 94(1):50-56.

[689] Rev. Malkmus, *God's Way to Ultimate Health*, (Shelby, North Carolina, 1990's), p. 132-133.

[690] Baker, Elizabeth, *The Gourmet Uncook Book, The Elegance of Raw Foods*, Promotion Publishing, San Diego, CA, 1996, p. 23-24.

[691] Smith, Jeffrey, M., *Genetic Roulette*, (Yes! Books, Fairfield, Iowa, 2007), p. 105, citing: J.W. J. Heijst, H.W.M. Niessen, K. Hoekman, and C.G. Schalkwijk, "Advanced Glycation End Products in Human Cancer Tissues: Detection of N-(Carboxymethyl) lysine and Argpyrimidine," *Ann. NY Acad. Sci.* 1043(2005); 725-733.

[692] Smith, *Genetic Roulette*, p. 105, citing: T. Goldberg, W. Cai, M. Peppa, V. Dardaine, B.S. Baliga, J. Uribarri, and H. Vlassara, "Advanced glycoxidation and end products in commonly consumed foods," *J. Am Diet. Assoc.* 104(2004):1287-1291.

[693] Smith, *Genetic Roulette*, p. 105, citing: R.B. Elliott, "Diabetes – A man made disease," *Med. Hypotheses*, 67 (March 9, 2006): 388-91.

[694] Smith, *Genetic Roulette*, p. 105, citing: M. Peppa, H. Brem, P. Ehrlich, J.G. Zhang, W. Cai, Z. Li, A. Croitoru, S. Thung, and H. Vlassara, "Adverse Effects of Dietary Glycotoxins on Wound Healing in Genetically Diabetic Mice," *Diabetes* 52(2003):2805-2813.

[695] Smith, *Genetic Roulette*, p. 105, citing: Elliott, "Diabetes – A man made disease," 388-91.

[696] Smith, *Genetic Roulette*, p. 105, citing: T. Henle, "Protein-bound advanced glycation endproducts (AGEs) as bioactive amino acid derivatives in foods," *Am. Acid* 29(2005): 313-322.

[697] Smith, *Genetic Roulette*, p. 105, citing: M. Freixes, A. Rodriguez, E. Dalfo, and I. Ferrer, "Oxidation, glycoxidation, lipoxidation, nitration, and responses to oxidative stress in the cerebral cortex in Creutzfeldt-Jakob disease," *Neurobiol. Aging*, Nov 23 2005.

[698] Farrell, Walter and Healy, Martin, *My Way of Life, Pocket edition of St. Thomas*, Part II, chapter 5, Happiness and Habit, (Confraternity of the Precious Blood, Brooklyn, N.Y., 1952), p. 217-219.

[699] Farrell, Walter and Healy, Martin, *My Way of Life, Pocket edition of St. Thomas*, Part II, chapter 5, Happiness and Habit, (Confraternity of the Precious Blood, Brooklyn, N.Y., 1952), p. 217-219.

[700] Farrell, Walter, O.P., *My Way of Life Pocket Edition of St. Thomas the Summa Simplified for Everyone*, (Confraternity of the Precious Blood,

Brooklyn, NY, 1952), p. 280, 281.

[701] Walker WA. Isselbacher KJ. "Uptake and transport of macromolecules by the intestine. Possible role in clinical disorders." *Gastroenterology*: 67:531-50, 1974. Cited in Boutenko, Victoria, *Green for Life*, p. 47.

[702] Minocha Anil M.D., Carrol David. *Natural Stomach Care: Treating and Preventing Digestive Disorders with the Best of Eastern and Western Healing Therapies*. New York: Penguin Group, 2003. Cited in Boutenko, Victoria, *Green for Life*, p. 62.

[703] Boutenko, Victoria, *Green for Life*, p. 62, citing: Elson M. Haas MD*Staying Healthy with Nutrition*. (California: Celestial Arts, 1992).

[704] Boutenko, Victoria, *Green for Life*, p. 63, citing: Minocha Anil M.D., Carrol David. *Natural Stomach Care: Treating and Preventing Digestive Disorders with the Best of Eastern and Western Healing Therapies*, (New York: Penguin Group, 2003).

[705] Joseph, James, Ph.D.; Nadeau, Daniel, M.D.; Underwood, Anne, *The Color Code a Revolutionary Eating Plan for Optimum Health*, (Hyperion, New York, NY), 2002, p. 3.

[706] Joseph, Nadeau, Underwood, *The Color Code*, p. 8.

[707] Joseph, Nadeau, Underwood, *The Color Code*, p. 9.

[708] Joseph, James, Ph.D.; Nadeau, Daniel, M.D.; Underwood, Anne, *The Color Code a Revolutionary Eating Plan for Optimum Health*, (Hyperion, New York, NY), 2002, p. 11.

[709] Joseph, Nadeau, Underwood, *The Color Code*, p. 14.

[710] *Writings from the Philokalia on Prayer of the Heart*, translated by E. Kadloubovsky and G.E.H. Palmer (Faber and Faber Limited, London, 1977), p. 79-80.

[711] Clement, Brian, *Killer Fish*, (Hippocrates Publications, 2012), p. 61.

[712] Clement, Brian, *Killer Fish*, p. 62.

[713] Dana Flavin, MD communication with J. Tibbetts, 2009.

[714] Logan, Alan C., *The Brain Diet*, (Cumberland House, Nashville, TN, 2006, 2007), p. 129-130.

[715] Eriksson PS, Perfileva E, Bjork-Eriksson T, Aborn AM, Nordbord C, Peterson DA, Gage FH. Neurogenesis in the adult human hippocampus. *Nat Med* 4(11):1313-1317, 1998. Cited in Phosphatidyserine (PS): Mental Clarity at Any Age by Parris M. Kidd, PhD (Natraceutical Publishing, Bohemia, NY, 2007).

[716] Kidd Parris, *Phosphatidyserine (PS)*: citing: McDaniel MA, Maier SF, and Einstein GO. "Brain-specific" nutrients: a memory cure? *Nutrition* 19(11-12):957-975, 2003.

[717] Kidd Parris, *Phosphatidyserine (PS)*: citing: Witkam L, Ramzan I. Ginkgo biloba in the treatment of Alzheimer's disease: A miracle cure? *From Cell to Society*, 2004.

[718] Kidd Parris, *Phosphatidyserine (PS)*: citing: Huskisson E, Maggini S, Ruf M. The influence of micronutrients on cognitive function and performance. *J INt Med Res* 35(1):1-19, 2007.

[719] Kidd Parris, *Phosphatidyserine (PS)*: citing: Crook TH, Tinklenberg J, Yesavage J, Petrie W, Nunzi MG, Massari DC. Effects of phosphatidylserine in age-associated memory impairment. *Neurology* 41(5):644-649, 1991.

[720] Boroch, Ann, *Healing Multiple Sclerosis*, p. 94, citing: John Parks Trowbridge, and Morton Walker, *The Yeast Syndrome* (New York: Bantam Books, 1986).

[721] Boroch, Ann, *Healing Multiple Sclerosis*, p. 96, 98-99.

[722] Hauser, Robert, A., MD, Lyons, Kelly E., PhD, McClain, Terry, ARNP, Perlmutter, David, MD, *Randomized, double-blind, pilot evaluation of intravenous glutathione in Parkinson's disease*, (Glutathione Therapy for Parkinson's Study), email: Robert A. Hauser (rhauser@health.usf.edu); 2009 Movement Disorder Society. Listed on David Perlmutter, blog.

[723] Young, Robert, e-Newsletter, 2007, citing: *American Journal of Epidemiology*, May 1, 2007.

[724] *The Lancet* 344: 796-798, 1994.

[725] Di Monte DA, Cahn P, Sandy MS. Glutathione in Parkinson's disease: A Link Between Oxidative Stress and Mitochondrial Damage? *An Neurol*. 32 Suppl; S111-115, 1992.

[726] Julian Whitaker, MD, in her newsletter *Health & Healing*, October 2009; website www.coconutketones.com.

[727] T.B. VanItallie, MD et al., Treatment of Parkinson disease with diet-induced hyperketonemia: A feasibility study *Neurology* 2005;64:728–730

[728] RL Veech, B Chance, Y Kashiwaya, HA Lardy, GC Cahill, Jr., "Ketone bodies, potential therapeutic uses," IUBMB Life, 2001, Vol. 51 No.4, 241-247

[729] George F. Cahill, Jr., Richard L. Veech, "Ketoacids? Good Medicine?" *Transactions of the American Clinical and Climatological Association*, Vol. 114, 2003.

[730] Richard L. Veech, "The therapaeutic implications of ketone bodies: the effects of ketone bodies in pathological conditions: ketosis, ketogenic diet, redox states, insulin resistance, and mitochondrial metabolism," *Prostaglandins, Leukotrienes and Essential Fatty Acids*, 70 (2004) 309-319.

[731] M Piert, et. al., "Diminished glucose transport and phosphorylation in Alzheimer's Disease determined by dynamic FDG-PET," *The Journal of Nuclear Medicine*, Vol.37 No.2, February 1996, 201-208.

[732] EJ Kim, et. al., "Glucose metabolism in early onset versus late onset Alzheimer's Disease: an SPM analysis of 120 patients," *Brain*, 2005, Vol. 128, 1790-1801.

[733] RF Peppard, et. al., "Cerebral glucose metabolism in Parkinson's disease with and without dementia," *Archives of Neurology*, Vol. 49 No.12, December 1992.

[734] "Cortical and subcortical glucose consumption measured by PET in patients with Huntington's disease," *Brain*, October 1990, Vol 113, part

5, 1405-23.

[735] U Roelcke, et. al., "Reduced glucose metabolism in the frontal cortex and basal ganglia of multiple sclerosis patients with fatigue: a 18F-fluorodeoxyglucose positron emission tomography study," *Neurology*, 1997, Vol. 48, Issue 6, 1566-1571.

[736] Z Guo, et. al., "ALS-linked Cu/Zn-SOD mutation impairs cerebral synaptic glucose and glutamate transport and exacerbates ischemic brain injury," *Journal of Cerebral Blood Flow Metabolism*, March 2000, Vol. 20 No. 3, 463-8.

[737] *The Fathers of the Church a New Translation*, Volume 16, St. Augustine, *Treatises on Various Subjects: The Usefulness of Fasting*: citing St. Jerome, p. 261. Citing: Ps 125.5; cf. Letter 122.1, PL 22.1040(892).

[738] *Handbook of Parkinson's Disease Third Edition*, citing: Cummings JL. Depression and Parkinson's disease: a review. *Am J Psychiatry* 1992; 149(4):443-454.

[739] *Handbook of Parkinson's Disease Third Edition*, citing: Allain H, Schuck S., Mauuit N. Depression in Parkinson's disease. *BMJ 2000*; 320(7245):1287-1288.

[740] *Handbook of Parkinson's Disease Third Edition*, citing: Tandberg E, Larsen JP, Aarsland D, et al. Risk factors for depression in Parkinson's disease. *Arch Neurol* 1997; 54(5):625-630.

[741] *Handbook of Parkinson's Disease Third Edition*, citing: Kuopio AM, Marttila RJ, Helenius H, et al. The quality of life in Parkinson's disease. *Mov Disord* 2000; 15(2):305-308.

[742] *Handbook of Parkinson's Disease Third Edition*, citing: Committee TGPsDSS. Factors impacting on quality of life in Parkinson's disease: results from an international survey. *Mov Disord* 2002; 17:60-67.

[743] *Handbook of Parkinson's Disease Third Edition*, citing: M Hietanen, H Teravainen. The effect of age of disease onset on neuropsychological performance in Parkinson's disease. *J Neurol Neurosurg Psychiatry* 1988; 51:244-249.

[744] *Handbook of Parkinson's Disease Third Edition*, citing: WE Martin, RB Loewenson, JA Raesch, AB Baker. Parkinson's disease: clinical analysis of 100 patients. *Neurology* 1973; 23:783-790.

[745] *Handbook of Parkinson's Disease Third Edition*, citing: BE Levin, MM Llabre, WJ Weiner. Cognitive impairments associated with early Parkinson's disease. *Neurology* 1989; 39:557-561.

[746] *Handbook of Parkinson's Disease Third Edition*, citing: WP Goldman, JD baty, VD Buckles, S Sahrmann, JC Morris. Cognitive and motor functioning in Parkinson disease – subjects with and without questionable dementia. *Arch Neurol* 1988; 55:675-680.

[747] *Handbook of Parkinson's Disease Third Edition*, citing: SE Starkstein,PL Bolduc, HS Mayberg, TJ Preziosi, RG Robinson. Cognitive impairments and depression in Parkinson's disease: a follow up study. *J Neurol Neurosurg Psychiatry* 1990; 53:597-602.

[748] *Handbook of Parkinson's Disease Third Edition*, citing: Pahwa, Lyons, Koller, *Handbook of Parkinson's Disease Third Edition*, p. 31.
[749] *Handbook of Parkinson's Disease Third Edition*, citing: Stein MB, Heuser IJ. Juncos JL, Uhde TW. Anxiety disorders in patients with Parkinson's disease. *Am J Psychiatry* 147:217-220, 1990.
[750] *Handbook of Parkinson's Disease Third Edition*, citing: Pahwa, Lyons, Koller, *Handbook of Parkinson's Disease Third Edition*, p. 116.
[751] Healy, David, *Let Them Eat Prozac the Unhealthy Relationship between the Pharmaceutical Industry and Depression*, (New York University Press, New York, 2004), p. 65.
[752] Young, Robert, web (October 2007): www.phmiracleliving.com
[753] Young, Robert, web (October 2007): www.phmiracleliving.com
[754] Mayer, John; Tibbetts, James, "Emotion Over Time Within a Religious Culture: A Lexical Analysis of the Old Testament." *Journal of Psychohistory*, fall, 1994, p. 244.
[755] Lipton, Bruce, *The Biology of Belief*, p. 121, citing: Segerstrom, S.C., and G.E. Miller (2004). "Psychological Stress and the Human Immune System: A Meta-Analytic Study of 30 Years of Inquiry." *Psychological Bulletin* 130(4): 601-630.
[756] Lipton, Bruce, *The Biology of Belief*, p. 121, citing: Kopp and Rethelyi (2004). "Where psychology meets physiology: chronic stress and premature mortality – the Central-Eastern European health paradox." *Brain Research Bulletin* 62:351-367.
[757] Lipton, Bruce, *The Biology of Belief*, p. 121, citing: McEwen, B. and with Elizabeth N. Lasley (2002). *The End of Stress As We Know It.* Washington, National Academies Press.
[758] Lipton, Bruce, *The Biology of Belief*, p. 121, citing: McEwen, B.S. and T. Seeman (1999). "Protective and Damaging Effects of Mediators of Stress: Elaborating and Testing the Concepts of Allostasis and Allostatic Load." *Annals of the NY Academy of Sciences* 896:30-47.
[759] Lipton, Bruce, *The Biology of Belief*, p. 121, citing: Atkinson, William (2000). "Strategies for Workplace Stress." Risk and Insurance Online (www.riskandinsurance.com).
[760] Lipton, Bruce, *The Biology of Belief*, p. 121, Hay House, Inc. New York City (2005), Mountain Love Productions (2008, 2011).
[761] Lipton, Bruce, *The Biology of Belief*, p. 114.
[762] *The Art of Prayer an Orthodox Anthology*, compiled by Igumen Chariton of Valamo, (Faber and Faber Limited, London and Boston, 1978), p. 233.
[763] Paradise M, Cooper C, Livingston G., Systematic Review of the Effect of Education on Survival in Alzheimer's Disease. *Int Psychogeriatr*. 2009;21(1):25-32.
[764] National Institute on Aging. 2006-08-29. Retrieved 2008-02-29.
[765] *Frontiers in Neuroscience*, Aug 2010. Enhancing brain activity such as with *Nrf2*.
[766] citing: summary at Dr. Perlmutter's site

www.vanguardneurologist.com
[767] citing: article at Dr. Perlmutter's site; vanguardneurologist.com
[768] citing: article at Dr. Perlmutter's web site
[769] Verghese, Joe, MD, and et., Leisure Activities and the Risk of Dementia in the Elderly, New England Journal of Medicine, June 19, 2003, vol 348:2508-2516, no. 25.
[770] Katz, Lawrence, Rubin, Manning, *Keep Your Brain Alive*, (Workman Publishing Company, NY, New York, 1999), p. 140.
[771] Hamler, Brad, *Exercises for Multiple Sclerosis*, (Healthy Living Books, New York, 2006), p. 42.
[772] Hamler, Brad, *Exercises for Multiple Sclerosis*, (Healthy Living Books, New York, 2006), p. 42.
[773] For more information, apply to the Secretariat of the Medical Society for Ozone Therapy (Arztliche Gesellschaft für Ozontherapie), Nordring 8-10, D-7557 Iffezheim, Fed. Rep. of Germany.
[774] Ed McCabe is a best-selling oxygen author in the 1980's and 1990's *Oxygen Therapies;* and *Flood Your Body with Oxygen, Therapy for Our Polluted World.*
[775] Wolfe, David; *Eating for Beauty*, p. 206.
[776] Wolfe, David; *Eating for Beauty*, p. 206.
[777] Adams JS, Clemens TL, Parrish JA, Holick MF. Vitamin D Synthesis and metabolism after ultraviolet irradiation of normal and vitamin D deficient subjects. *N Engl J Med* 1982, Mar 25;306(12):722-5.
[778] Adams JS, Clemens TL, Parrish JA, Holick MF. Vitamin D Synthesis and metabolism after ultraviolet irradiation of normal and vitamin D deficient subjects. *N Engl J Med* 1982, Mar 25;306(12):722-5.
[779] Adams JS, Clemens TL, Parrish JA, Holick MF. Vitamin D Synthesis and metabolism after ultraviolet irradiation of normal and vitamin D deficient subjects. *N Engl J Med* 1982, Mar 25;306(12):722-5.
[780] Adams JS, Clemens TL, Parrish JA, Holick MF. Vitamin D Synthesis and metabolism after ultraviolet irradiation of normal and vitamin D deficient subjects. *N Engl J Med* 1982, Mar 25;306(12):722-5.
[781] *The Fathers of the Church a New Translation*, Volume 58, (The Catholic University of America Press, Washington, D.C., 1966), St. Gregory of Nyssa, *Ascetical Works*, p. 153.
[782] Sister Marie Simon-Pierre on her cure from Parkinson's. 2/11/04 translated on *Zenit, the World Seen from Rome*, paper online (Zenit.org) Rome April 30, 2011.
[783] Flavin, Dana, communication with Jim Tibbetts (2009).
[784] Cousens, Gabriel, *Spiritual Nutrition*, p. 135, citing: Airola, Paavo, *Worldwide Secrets for Staying Young*, Phoenix, AZ: Health Plus, 1982.
[785] Bronshtein, Shai D., *The Harvard Crimson* (University Daily, December 16, 2005).
[786] Bronshtein, Shai D., *The Harvard Crimson* (University Daily, December 16, 2005).

[787] Verghese, Joe, MD, and et., Leisure Activities and the Risk of Dementia in the Elderly, New England Journal of Medicine, June 19, 2003, vol 348:2508-2516, no. 25.

[788] Shmerling, Robert, M.D., 'Can Prayer Heal the Sick?' Harvard Health Publications, Harvard College, 2009.

[789] Shmerling, Robert, M.D., 'Can Prayer Heal the Sick?' Harvard Health Publications, Harvard College, 2009.

[790] Shmerling, Robert, M.D., 'Can Prayer Heal the Sick?' 2009.

[791] Tibbetts, James, *Christian Meditation, the Jesus Prayer and Praise*, (LF Tech Inc., Schenectady, NY, 2008), www.jimtibbetts.com

[792] Cousens, Gabriel, *Conscious Eating*, (North Atlantic Books, Berkeley, CA, 2000), p. 367-68.

[793] Cousens, Gabriel, *Conscious Eating*, p. 370.